Preparing for International Health Experiences

At some point in their careers, many health professionals engage in elective overseas exchange work. The benefits of practicing in different environments and learning healthcare methods from other global perspectives is invaluable.

This book is a unique resource that offers necessary insights into making the most of the experience, from pre-departure training through to return orientation. It provides information on navigating the legalities and bureaucracies of international medical training and gives insights into cultural and language competencies, including how to be ethical and deferential in the exchange of situational knowledge.

Preparing for International Health Experiences is a must-read for any healthcare student considering volunteering abroad as it covers specific professions from pediatrics to psychiatry to dentistry. Its balance of case studies that cover a broad spectrum of medical professions and practical tips will be valued by readers.

Akshaya Neil Arya is an Adjunct Professor in Environment and Resource Studies at the University of Waterloo and Assistant Clinical Professor in Family Medicine at McMaster University (part-time). He is currently president of the Canadian Physicians for Research and Education in Peace (CPREP).

Preparing for International Health Experiences

A Practical Guide

Edited by
AKSHAYA NEIL ARYA

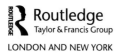
Routledge
Taylor & Francis Group

LONDON AND NEW YORK

First published 2017
by Routledge
2 Park Square, Milton Park, Abingdon, Oxon OX14 4RN

and by Routledge
711 Third Avenue, New York, NY 10017

Routledge is an imprint of the Taylor & Francis Group, an informa business

British Library Cataloguing-in-Publication Data

A catalogue record for this book is available from the British Library

Library of Congress Cataloging-in-Publication Data
Names: Arya, Akshaya Neil, author.
Title: Preparing for international health experiences : a practical guide / Akshaya Neil Arya.
Description: Milton Park, Abingdon, Oxon ; New York, NY : Routledge, 2017.	Includes bibliographical references and index.
Identifiers: LCCN 2016056492| ISBN 9781498780803 (hbk)	ISBN 9781138627277 (pbk)	ISBN 9781498780810 (ebk)
Subjects: LCSH: World health.	Medical personnel--Employment--Foreign countries.	Public health--International cooperation.
Classification: LCC RA441 .A78 2017	DDC 362.1--dc23
LC record available at https://lccn.loc.gov/2016056492

ISBN: 978-1-4987-8080-3 (hbk)
ISBN: 978-1-138-62727-7 (pbk)
ISBN: 978-1-4987-8081-0 (ebk)

Typeset in Garamond
by diacriTech

Contents

Acknowledgements

I would like to thank Melissa Whaling and Rebekah Baumann for editorial assistance. In addition, I would like to thank the following internal and external reviewers.

Chapter	Reviewers
Section I: Putting Global Health Electives in Context	
Chapter 1. Introduction	Rob Chase and Jill Allison
Chapter 2. Should I Stay or Should I Go? And What Can I Do When I Get There?	Carolyn Beukeboom and Alyssa Smaldino
Chapter 3. Maximizing Benefits and Minimizing Harm of IHEs on Trainees, Programs and Hosts	Jill Allison and Rob Chase
Chapter 4. Doing Your Homework: Choosing an Organization, Project or Opportunity in Global Health	Kevin Chan, Lorena Bonilla and Caity Jackson
Chapter 5. Mentorship	Bill Cherniak and Shweta Dhawan
Chapter 6. Technology and Social Media	
Chapter 7. Preparation to Go Abroad	Jill Allison and Carolyn Beukeboom
Section II: Aspects of Pre-Departure Preparation	
Chapter 8. Staying Safe While Abroad	Jill Allison and Kevin Chan
Chapter 9. Travel Health Considerations	Jill Allison
Chapter 10. Seeking Cultural Competence	Carolyn Beukeboom and Matt DeCamp
Chapter 11. Communicating Effectively	
Chapter 12. Ethics: Four Key Questions You Need to Ask	Mary White, Barry Pakes and Melissa Whaling
Section III: Specific Professions	
Chapter 13. Emergency Medicinee	Kevin Chan and Brian Bell
Chapter 14. Pediatrics and Child Health	
Chapter 15. Obstetrics and Gynecology	Heather Thompson
Chapter 16. Midwifery: 'With Women' across the Globe	Manavi Handa

Chapter	Reviewers
Chapter 17. Nursing during Global Health Experiences	Olive Wahoush
Chapter 18. Disability and Rehabilitative Experiences	Mona Negoita
Chapter 19. Developing and Preparing Appropriate Social Work Placements	
Chapter 20. Surgical Team Experiences	Bill Cherniak
Chapter 21. Dentistry and Oral Health	Rahim Valani, Kerr Banduk and Tim Lee
Chapter 22. Eyecare	Carol Cressman
Chapter 23. Global Public Health: Preparation and Training	Donald Cole
Chapter 24. Global Health Research: Practical Guidelines	
Section IV: Moving On	
Chapter 25. Returning Home: Debriefing and Managing Reverse Culture Shock	Melissa Whaling and Matt DeCamp
Chapter 26. Moving Forward	Don Sutherland

Contributors

Jill Allison's, PhD, 25-year career as a nurse in numerous cultural contexts, both in Canada and internationally, became the backdrop for doctoral studies in medical anthropology. She has published in a variety of social science and healthcare journals and currently works as a global health coordinator in the Faculty of Medicine at Memorial University of Newfoundland, Canada. She teaches in the undergraduate and postgraduate programs as well in community health and humanities.

Michelle M. Amri, BHSc, MPA, is a public health and public policy specialist. Her initial introduction to global health was at the World Health Organization's (WHO) Western Pacific Regional Office (WPRO), primarily working on smoke-free cities and health promotion leadership and financing. Amri later returned as a health promotion consultant working on urban health for the region and returned to WHO subsequently to develop the draft national action plan on antimicrobial resistance for the Lao People's Democratic Republic to guide the nation's work for 2 years. She holds the degrees of honors bachelor's of health sciences (specialization in health promotion) from the University of Western Ontario and a master's of public administration from Queen's University. She is currently a PhD student in public health at the University of Toronto, Ontario, Canada.

Kelly Anderson, MD, CCFP(EM), is a family physician with a special focus in human immuno-deficiency virus (HIV) primary care at St. Michael's Hospital in Toronto, Ontario, Canada. Prior to medicine she worked in Rwanda and Canada in HIV-related non-governmental organizations, where she developed a strong interest in examining the ethics of global health work.

Jane Barrow, MS, is an assistant dean for the Office of Global and Community Health at the Harvard School of Dental Medicine (HSDM), Boston, Massachusetts. She directs school-wide efforts in education, research and clinical services that further the school's strategic goals for oral public health and the integration of oral health and medicine. Barrow has a master's degree in health policy and management from Harvard (1987). She has an extensive background in healthcare systems planning at the community and national levels, as well as experience in institutional strategic planning, finance and operations.

Carolyn Beukeboom, MSc, BScN, RN(EC), is a primary healthcare nurse practitioner working in a Community Health Centre in rural Ontario, Canada. She has worked overseas in various capacities, including with Médecins Sans Frontiéres as an inpatient supervisor and overseeing the malnutrition clinic in a rural surgical hospital in South Sudan; in an HIV/AIDS clinic in Lesotho; in Pakistan, post-earthquake in 2005; as a health promoter and educator in primary healthcare in Ecuador; in children's homes in India; on an evaluation of a maternal child health program in Liberia; as well as many other short-term missions. Beukeboom's main areas of interest include healthcare for people living in poverty as well as new immigrants and refugees to Canada. Recently, she completed a master's of science in public health from the London School of Hygiene and Tropical Medicine.

Jason T. Blackard, PhD, earned a PhD in biological sciences in public health at Harvard University, and in January 2014, he was appointed as the director of the newly formed Office of Global Health at the University of Cincinnati, Ohio, advising students about research and education as well as facilitating clinical electives for international medical students. His current work focuses on several viral hepatitides as well as HIV with collaborations in South Africa, Botswana, India and Ghana.

Lorena Bonilla, RN, BA, BSN, MN, EdD(c), is a professor in the School of Nursing at Fanshawe College, and an adjunct assistant professor in the School of Nursing at Western University in London, Ontario, Canada. She has volunteered as a nurse and clinical educator in medical missions to the Dominican Republic, Peru, Ecuador and Nepal. Bonilla has lectured at the Universidad Catolica de Santa Maria and Honorio Delgado Hospital in Arequipa, Peru, as well as the Kathmandu University School of Medical Sciences, Nursing School, Nepal. Bonilla's research interests include international nursing practice, global health as well as ethical and legal issues in interprofessional healthcare practice. Her doctorate work examined the process of nursing clinical decision making and a nurse's ability to provide safe, ethical and competent care during medical missions in developing countries.

Debra Cameron, PhD, MEd, BSc(OT), is an assistant professor and international fieldwork coordinator in the Department of Occupational Science and Occupational Therapy at the University of Toronto, Ontario, Canada. With 30 years of experience working with children and families as an occupational therapist, in the last few years she has been passionately interested in international health and is education lead for the International Centre for Disability and Rehabilitation (ICDR). As part of her work within the Department of Occupational Science and Occupational Therapy, she facilitates students who wish to pursue placements in international settings, and in the past few years her students have been in Cameroon, Kenya, Tanzania, Trinidad, the Philippines, Hong Kong, Sweden and Holland. Cameron has also taught in an interprofessional preparatory education program for nursing and occupational therapy (OT), physical therapy (PT) and speech-language pathology (SLP) students going on international placements.

Kevin Chan, BSc(Hon), MD, FRCPC, MPH, is the chair of pediatrics at Memorial University, Newfoundland, Canada; the clinical chief of Children's Health at Eastern Health; and the division head of Pediatric Emergency Medicine at St. John's, Newfoundland, Canada. After a pediatric residency at BC Children's Hospital, and his pediatric emergency fellowship at Children's Hospital of Eastern Ontario and Boston Children's Hospital, he has held the Frank Knox Fellowship at Harvard University where he did his MPH, the Pierre Elliott Trudeau Scholarship, and has been a Yale/Johnson & Johnson Physician Scholar in International Health. Chan has worked for over 25 years in sub-Saharan Africa, mostly in Somalia, Tanzania, Uganda and Malawi, including disasters in Rwanda, Kosovo, El Salvador and India and has been an advisor to UNICEF, the World Health Organization, World Bank, CIDA and the Canadian government. He served as the chair of the Canadian Society for International Health, president of the International Child Health Section of the Canadian Paediatric Society, chair of the Canadian International Health

Education Network and currently is an executive member of the Section on International Child Health of the American Academy of Pediatrics.

Maija Cheung, MD, is a general surgery resident at Yale New Haven Hospital, New Haven, Connecticut. She received her MD in 2014 from Dartmouth Medical School after receiving her BA in 2005 from Middlebury College. She has a special interest in global surgery and has spent time on medical trips to South America and Africa. Her major research interests are in surgical education and clinical outcomes and capacity building in developing countries.

Lesley Cooper, BSW, PhD, has extensive professional and academic experience as a social worker, community worker and educator in Australia, New Zealand and Canada. These positions have taken her to work with rural and remote communities in Queensland, the Northern Territory and Western Australia. She has worked closely with Aboriginal communities in Australia, in the areas of housing, sustainable tenancy, family violence and diabetes education. She worked as the dean of the Faculty of Social Work and vice president of the Brantford Campus at Wilfrid Laurier University and is now the foundation professor of social work at the University of Wollongong, New South Wales, Australia.

Matthew DeCamp, MD, PhD, is an assistant professor at the Johns Hopkins Berman Institute of Bioethics and in the Johns Hopkins Division of General Internal Medicine, Baltimore, Maryland. A practicing internist, his current research interests include global health (with a special emphasis on short-term global health training), social media and medical professionalism and ethical issues in health reform (focusing on accountable care organizations). His PhD (philosophy) thesis examined the intersection of human rights, distributive justice and global access to essential medicines. His teaching and mentorship has been recognized with an Excellence in Global Health Advising Award from Johns Hopkins, and he regularly teaches on topics in global health and human rights at the graduate and undergraduate levels.

Hawazin Elani, BDS, MS, PhD, DMsC, is a dentist who completed her master of science and PhD degrees at McGill University, Quebec, Canada, and received a master of medical sciences and a clinical certificate in prosthodontics from HSDM. Elani is currently working at HSDM as an instructor at the Department of Restorative Dentistry and Biomaterial Science Global and Community Health. Her research interests include disparities in oral health, access to oral healthcare and topics related to integrating research into dental curriculums.

Jessica Evert, MD, is the executive director of Child Family Health International (CFHI), a UN-recognized leader in Global Health Education Programs for health and social science students with over 25 programs in 7 countries. She is on faculty at the Department of Family and Community Medicine at the University of California, San Francisco, where she previously graduated from residency and helped create and complete the Global Health Scholars Program. Evert is a graduate of the Ohio State University College of Medicine and a long-time advocate for global health education quality and ethical standards. She has completed international work in Kenya, Guatemala, Australia and Cuba and served as an officer and board member of IFMSA-USA. She is an author and editor of multiple chapters, articles and books in global health with a focus on education, ethics and asset-based engagement. Evert is a recipient of the Global Health Education

Consortium's prestigious Christopher Krogh Award for her dedication to underserved populations at home and abroad.

Alison Eyre, MDCM, CCFP, FCFP, is an assistant professor at the University of Ottawa, Department of Family Medicine. There she is the director of Postgraduate Medical Education. Her clinical practice is at an inner city Community Health Centre. She has worked and lived abroad in Haiti and Sri Lanka with the Red Cross and other agencies. In her roles as physician and educator, she has supported the safe journeys of many travels and students.

Michael R. Hall, MD, graduated from Tufts University School of Medicine and from Yale New Haven Hospital for general surgery residency where he was part of the Global Health Division of the Section of Surgical Education, and he is now pursuing a career in vascular surgery. His global health experiences include medical mission trips to Costa Rica and a surgical mission trip to Haiti.

Dan Hayhoe, OD, FAAO, is an optometrist engaged in private practice, teaching as adjunct clinical faculty at the Health Sciences Optometry Clinic (University of Waterloo/McMaster University Michael G. DeGroote School of Medicine joint campus), Hamilton, Ontario, Canada, and coordinating primary care clinical rotations for optometry interns in Malawi, Central Africa. Hayhoe has been involved in collaborating with African leaders in healthcare and education, beginning with the establishment of the School of Optometry at the University of Benin in Nigeria in 1976. Currently, his international focus is on encouraging North–South dialogue and collaboration in Malawi. In Canada, he works extensively with new Canadians while mentoring interns on cultural sensitivity.

Karen Hays, DNP, CNM, ARNP, is a certified nurse midwife and advanced registered nurse practitioner in Seattle, Washington. She is adjunct faculty in the Bastyr University Department of Midwifery, Kenmore, Washington, in both the clinical midwifery program and the new master's degree in Maternal–Child Health Systems, and she is a research nurse practitioner with the Obstetric–Fetal Pharmacology Research Unit in the Department of Pharmacy at the University of Washington, Seattle. For the past 30 years, Hays has also had a global health focus, working with several non-governmental organizations, promoting maternal–newborn clinical care and education in low-resource settings, with Jhpiego (Asia), Health Leadership International (Lao PDR); Global Health Media Project (Africa and Asia); PRONTO (East Africa); Adara (Uganda) and Medical Teams International (Africa, Central America, and Asia). She has been exploring the ethics and challenges of placing American midwifery students in maternity care clinical sites.

Andrea Hunter, MD, FRCPC, DTM&H, is an associate professor of pediatrics and a consultant general pediatrician at McMaster University, Hamilton, Ontario, Canada. She has been involved in community settings such as the Shelter Health Network and coordinating community-based pediatric refugee/immigrant health clinics in Hamilton, Ontario, since 2004, and is an editor and task force member for *Caring for Kids New to Canada*, a Canadian Pediatric Society peer-reviewed guide for health professionals working with immigrant and refugee children and youth. Internationally, she is the co-external program director for a pediatric residency program at the University of Guyana and has been involved in ongoing pediatric education programs with Uganda. She has extensive involvement in preparing medical students and residents for global health electives as well as curriculum design experience in newcomer child health and social pediatrics.

Caity Jackson, MSc, is a global health consultant, specializing in education and training and communications. As a young professional, she co-founded and ran the MentorNet global health mentorship program and is the co-founder and director of communications for the Women in Global Health movement. She is the director of European Engagement for CFHI and the international program coordinator for Swedish healthcare in Stockholm, where she resides. Jackson holds an HBHSc from the University of Ottawa, Ontario, Canada; an MScMed in global health from Karolinska Institute and was recently named one of the top 300 women leaders in global health by the Graduate Institute, Geneva.

Anne McCarthy, MD, FRCPC, DTM&H, is a professor of medicine at the University of Ottawa, Ontario, Canada and a member of the Division of Infectious Diseases at the Ottawa Hospital, Ontario, Canada. She is the lead for undergraduate medical education, global health and a previous director of the Office of Global Health for the Faculty of Medicine, University of Ottawa. Over the past two decades, she has been involved with preparing, particularly, medical trainees for safe and ethical electives in resource-poor settings. Her clinical work includes many new Canadians, including a number of refugees.

Stephanie A. Nixon, PhD, MSc, BHSc(PT), is a physiotherapist and an associate professor in the Department of Physical Therapy and Dalla Lana School of Public Health at the University of Toronto, Ontario, Canada. She is also the director of the ICDR. She conducts critical social science research on HIV and disabilities in Canada and sub-Saharan Africa.

Doruk Ozgediz, MD, MSc, FACS, is a faculty pediatric surgeon at Yale University, New Haven, Connecticut. He trained in medicine and general surgery at the University of California, San Francisco and pediatric surgery at the University of Toronto. He has also completed a master's in public health in developing countries from the London School of Hygiene and Tropical Medicine. Ozgediz is a co-founder of the group Global Partners in Anesthesia and Surgery, a long-term collaboration to support surgery and anaesthesia capacity in Uganda.

David Ponka, MDCM, CCFP(EM), FCFP, MSc, is a family doctor and an associate professor at the Faculty of Medicine at the University of Ottawa, Ontario, Canada. He is also a medical advisor (acting) at the Migration Health Policy and Partnership Division within the Migration Health Branch of Immigration, Refugees and Citizenship Canada. Although he pursues various clinical, teaching and scholarly interests, the common thread is working with vulnerable populations. Ponka has worked in many parts of the world, including in Chad with Médecins Sans Frontières, in Haiti with Médecins du Monde and currently with a project to build capacity in family medicine in Guyana. He is supported by Academics without Borders in delivering this work. He advises the newly created Besrour Centre of the College of Family Physicians of Canada with disseminating evidence for task shifting towards primary care in emerging health systems.

Caley A. Satterfield, EdD, is the assistant director for the University of Texas Medical Branch (UTMB) Center for Global Health Education, Galveston, Texas. In this role, she manages the Global Health Education Training program at UTMB. Her research interests are in global health pre-departure preparation and research skills training in global health.

Brittany Seymour, DDS, MPH, is an assistant professor at the Harvard School of Dental Medicine, where she holds a full-time appointment in the Department of Oral Health Policy and Epidemiology and the Office of Global and Community Health. She earned her DDS from the University of Colorado and completed her MPH at Harvard. Her overall research focus is on interdisciplinary approaches for oral health improvement at the global level through prevention, policy and health promotion and she conducts funded research on how misinformation online impacts important public health programs such as community water fluoridation and childhood vaccinations. She is the director of the Consortium of Universities for Global Health's Global Oral Health Interest Group and has contributed to the FDI World Dental Federation's *Oral Health Atlas*, Second Edition. Seymour has won numerous honours and awards, including the Award for Community Dentistry and Dental Public Health, the Herschel St. Horowitz scholarship presented by the American Association of Public Health Dentistry, an Outstanding Achievement in Teaching Award from HSDM and an Excellence in Mentoring Award from the Harvard Medical School.

Alyssa Smaldino, BSc, is the executive director of GlobeMed. She studied public health at George Washington University, where she acted as a co-president of GlobeMed. With GlobeMed she conducted in-person capacity assessments with 50 grassroots organizations across 18 countries, provided leadership training to over 500 students and started a program for grassroots changemakers to co-develop new strategies for effective cross-cultural collaboration. Prior to joining the GlobeMed staff, she worked at the GlobalGiving Foundation and volunteered at the National Institute for Mental Health and the Rwanda Village Concept Project.

Rachel F. Spitzer, BSc, MD, FRCPS, MPH, is an associate professor in the Department of Obstetrics and Gynecology and cross appointed to the Dalla Lana School of Public Health at the University of Toronto, Ontario, Canada. She obtained a BSc at McGill University, MD at McMaster University, residency training in Obstetrics and Gynecology, fellowship training in Pediatric and Adolescent Gynecology at the University of Toronto and MPH at Harvard University. She is faculty lead for Global Health in the undergraduate Medical Program and vice chair of Global Health in the Department of OB–GYN, University of Toronto, Ontario, Canada. Spitzer combines clinical practice of general, pediatric and adolescent with the practice and teaching of global women's health and has been involved as an investigator and collaborator in numerous projects related, in particular to the evaluation of programs to reduce maternal morbidity and mortality and conditions leading to obstetric fistula, for which she has received numerous prestigious grants, including those from Grand Challenges Canada and Saving Lives at Birth.

Paul Thistle, BSc(Hon), MD, FRCSC, LLD, has 20 years of full-time medical missionary experience in Zimbabwe, first as the chief medical officer at the Salvation Army Howard Hospital (1995–2012), and most recently at Karanda (since 2012). He received his medical degree and fellowship in Obstetrics and Gynaecology from the University of Toronto. He is an honorary lecturer at the University of Zimbabwe, and an associate professor at the University of Toronto, Ontario, Canada. Thistle has mentored hundreds of Zimbabwean and international medical students, residents and graduates in his rural practice. In 2008, he received an Honorary Doctor of Laws from the University of Windsor, a Paul Harris Fellowship from Rotary International and the inaugural Teasdale-Corti Humanitarian Award from the Royal College of Physicians and Surgeons of Canada.

Rahim Valani, CCFP-EM, FRCP, M. Med. Ed, MBA, is an associate professor of medicine and pediatrics at McMaster University, Hamilton, Ontario, Canada. He is an emergency medicine consultant and completed additional training in pediatric emergency medicine at the Hospital for Sick Children. He also undertook additional training in the United Kingdom and Australia, building on his international experience. Rahim is a co-director of the International Pediatric Emergency Medicine Elective, bringing together medical students from the Middle East and Canada with the goal of increasing cross-border cooperation. After completing his master's in medical education from the University of Dundee, his interest in medical education focused on curriculum development. More recently, Rahim's focus has shifted towards quality metrics and value-based care using medical informatics as a vehicle. He recently completed his MBA from the Wharton School of Business.

Melissa Whaling, MA, has a master's degree in health geography as well as a variety of experience within the global health and community health fields. She currently works as the fund development coordinator for Regional HIV/AIDS Connection, London, Ontario, Canada. She formerly worked for the Office of Global Health at the Schulich School of Medicine & Dentistry. Whaling has extensive international experience, working in East Africa (mainly Tanzania, Kenya and Rwanda) for over 7 years as a program officer for the Kivulini Women's Rights Organization and as the executive director for the African Probiotic Yoghurt Network Organization.

Mary T. White, PhD, is a professor of ethics and medical humanities at the Boonshoft School of Medicine in Dayton, Ohio, where her teaching includes public health ethics and a pre-departure course in global health for medical students. Her global health experience includes teaching and partnership development in Uganda and Ethiopia, and involvement with immigrant and refugee assimilation in Dayton, Ohio. Her interests include global health education, ethical issues in short-term educational experiences and research ethics.

PUTTING GLOBAL HEALTH ELECTIVES IN CONTEXT

Chapter 1

Introduction

Neil Arya

Contents

So you're considering going abroad for an international health experience (IHE)? You may have friends who have returned, or perhaps your educational program has an overseas partnership. No doubt you wish to make new friends, to learn about the world and other cultures. Perhaps you have the laudable desire to make a difference in the world, to become a change leader or be changed yourself in the process. All these are certainly possible. But well before that, you need to ensure you are safe and not harming yourself or others, and for this, preparation is paramount.

This guidebook is designed to help you, whether you are a health professional or trainee embarking on a placement abroad towards a medical, allied health or research career. It is also intended to be a handbook for faculty and administrators involved in international health who facilitate pre-departure and return orientation sessions for medical students, residents, nursing, rehabilitative and health sciences students. Near-retirees and retirees being engaged in clinical service and education, those working with non-governmental organizations (NGOs) or consultants to global health projects may also benefit as they prepare for international engagement.

There are general texts on global health, guides to finding jobs or organizations, books devoted to medical issues, especially directed to professionals in a specific discipline (e.g. gynecology, pediatrics, surgery), but this work is meant to fill a gap: it includes foundational aspects, looking at experiences in a larger context with their attendant benefits and harms, and reflective elements such as whether you should go at all. This guide covers the breadth of practical dimensions for preparation with specific aspects of pre-departure training (PDT) including ethical and cultural considerations. By introducing relevant aspects of particular health disciplines, this guide addresses issues of interest to a general audience, and in passing, offers an introduction to global burden of disease and health, and health systems in low- and middle-income countries (LMICs). It discusses what to do when you return home, as well as possible directions for your education or career.

A student's IHE, be it an alternative spring break, a public health practicum, research project or medical electives, has life- and career-changing potential and has been the start for many now working at the forefront of North–South partnerships. Having a positive experience and creating positive relationships can be the start of positive impact that you hope to make, creating a positive culture and environment for others, as administrators, supervisors, researchers or program directors.

Interest in international opportunities across professions, public health and health sciences is rising, although less studied in non-medical health professional training. The proportion of U.S. students going overseas on electives during medical school has risen steadily from 6.4% in 1984 (Heck and Pust, 1993) to 16.7% in 1990 (Heck and Wedemeyer, 1991), to over 31% in 2011 (Nelson et al., 2012). While research on the importance of global health opportunities on students' selection of medical schools is limited, in 2013, the Association of American Medical Colleges (AAMC) found that 65% of incoming medical students expressed interest in participating in global health learning experiences (Krisberg, 2015). But can such interest be reflected in positive impacts on trainees and those with whom they interact and hope to serve? Unfortunately, this does not appear to be a universal phenomenon.

Harms of Inadequate Preparation for both Host and Visitor

Those participating in their first health experience abroad may well experience some culture shock. Pedersen (1994) classifies 'culture shock' in five stages: the exciting honeymoon phase, where all seems fascinating; followed by the second, rejection phase, where there are difficulties accepting differences from the home country; the third, regression phase, where one has an attitude of superiority glorifying one's home country; the fourth, acceptance/negotiation phase, where one achieves perspective and the fifth, 'new-self' phase, returning to the home culture and old life (where reverse culture shock is also possible). Culture shock can lead to inappropriate judgment, misunderstandings, culturally insensitive behaviours and interpersonal conflicts that affect relationships, both personal and institutional. Social media may be a support, but hurtful posts or disrespectful pictures can have damaging consequences. Students may also themselves be scarred. Based on interviews conducted with medical students returning from an IHE, Elit et al. (2011) identified issues of discomfort related to (1) *uncertainty about how best to help;* (2) *perceptions of Western medical students as different;* (3) *moving beyond one's scope of practice;* (4) *navigating different cultures of medicine* and (5) *unilateral capacity building.*

The harms to host personnel, students and communities should not exceed the benefits of hosting. Trainees often assume that they are better than nothing and would be surprised to have heard Monsignor Ivan Ilich imploring not to impose themselves as 'volunteers', in a speech now entitled 'To Hell with Good Intentions' (Illich, 1968). Reflecting on unconscious neocolonial attitudes of students and premises of programs, Illich pointed out harms of volunteering, and unfortunately these persist a half century later. Madsen-Camacho (2004) found a student depicting a person with whom s/he worked in a service learning opportunity as *proud, sincere and noble,* which she summarizes as *the quintessential noble savage* (Madsen-Camacho, 2004, 38). Another illustrated *a tension between multiple roles she experienced,* describing herself as *hero, observer and intruder* (Madsen-Camacho, 2004, 37).

Kraeker et al. (2014) found Ugandan medical students working alongside students from the North were concerned with objectification of their compatriots, with their continent perceived as a *museum of disease*. 'I think here because of the lax in our laws, that's why they come here because they get the opportunity to touch the patient, to do the procedures and everything' and lack of real communication and reciprocity of opportunity. 'Sometimes we work on projects with them while they are here, but the tendency is when they go, they never really get back to us with what happened'. Even hosts can internalize such issues. Radstone cited Solomon Islands medical personnel's belief that students be allowed to diagnose, do procedures and prescribe without supervision, well beyond what was allowed in England, enabling them to *practise on the poor* (Radstone, 2005).

My Journey

Unfortunately in my international interactions, I have not been immune to potentially causing harm and being harmed; reflecting on my story may help you avoid some of the mistakes I have made over the years.

> My immigrant parents had previously been refugees as children with the partition of their native land. I inherited my father's keen interest in other cultures, languages, religions and ways of life. Dad fought a lifelong battle for justice for those marginalized which motivated me as we settled into this new culture in small town Canada. His optimism, despite losing everything as a child, inspired me, and our Hindu faith, focused on process rather than outcome, guided me. My mother taught me not to judge people that there are no 'bad people', just people who do bad things. After an engineering degree, I chose to study medicine because I wanted to make a difference.
>
> My first clinical international experience in third year medical school was in East Africa. I appreciated the difference in terms of case mix, facilities, treatment and consideration of patients and their choices between a semi-private hospital where I spent the first half of my time and a teaching hospital where I spent the second. During the latter half of my elective time, which I largely spent in internal medicine and nutrition, one weekend, at the recommendation of other medical students, I 'hung around' the high-risk maternity ward, the only one in the country as most women gave birth at home with traditional birth attendants. There was 'no one' around the labour and delivery area that weekend day, save more experienced nurses, with the overworked and sleepless intern assisting in a C-section. Encouraged by the nurses and lightly overseen by one, I did my first delivery. All turned out fine (I believe the mother's 'high-risk' condition was pregnancy-induced hypertension). I took a photograph of this child, but strangely rather than feeling proud, I sheepishly and anxiously skulked out of the ward.
>
> The next year, I returned to the Indian city where I was born, for an elective, going to a well-known Christian institution headed by nuns. Although I had written confirmation of acceptance, on arrival, the nuns had no idea what I would do and

who could supervise me. Eventually, I hooked up with a mentor, an Indian physician volunteer who came to their various facilities several times a week. The experience with him, and the nuns, was outstanding. On outreach missions, I accompanied the nuns who despite a lack of formal education offered symptomatic treatment and supplies – a cough indicative of tuberculosis (TB) might be treated with a cough suppressant; a fever related to hepatitis with paracetamol. In a facility for children with severe disabilities, incontinent children paralyzed by polio or with contractures related to cerebral palsy lay on hot vinyl mattresses to avoid soiling sheets and did not even receive simple mobilization for contractures. In a third facility, the destitute might be mixed with those dying of TB-related 'consumption'. I saw all this suffering and neglect, with attendant consequences, ignored by those with a dogmatic lack of faith in technology, but . . . when I chose to hold judgment, to look deeper, I was able to appreciate care inspired by God, the stubborn belief that He would provide, that God's time was not as finite as I thought. I was then able to enter into a dialogue with these nuns and the supervising physician, to appreciate the realities of functioning with limited resources and to seek solutions. The remarkable physician mentor I was with more than a quarter-century ago volunteers to this day.

Three and a half years later, having finished my residency, I worked in small town Canada in a few provinces, doing emergency work and deliveries, I felt more prepared when invited to accompany this same physician to a medical camp in the mountains a year after an earthquake, this time as a colleague. I now felt that having these skills and knowing the national language, I could make a difference. To my surprise, the most useful thing I did in one week was syringe out a few ears. I did not understand the context, would not prescribe injections of antibiotics or saline for what appeared to be viral infections and could neither address the psychological pain of loss in the local dialect nor the various determinants of health that people were lacking.

After this, I chose to avoid any clinical setting abroad for many years, favouring instead more local work on environmental issues and peace. Having finished a family medicine residency based at a francophone multicultural centre, I chose to develop a multicultural and multilingual practice. Later, I helped develop a program for mental health of people experiencing, or at risk of, homelessness and founded a refugee health clinic.

When a friend asked me to assist him in supervising an interprofessional team, primarily of medical and nursing students from two different parts of Canada in a Central American country, I hesitated. However, I was impressed with the level of planning and training of my co-facilitator, who developed a curricula with no pre-existing model that would largely mirror pre-departure guidelines developed a couple of years later. The five domains of Section II on pre-departure were reflected in preparation. In addition there were social justice readings applicable to the country, and our students for the most part had great attitudes and had learned basic Spanish. We worked with a local NGO well known to my friend who had assisted them on several prior trips; the NGO integrated with the local healthcare team. So off we went, ready to make a small difference with a small bag of simple sustainable medicines. We found women appreciating their first respectful interactions with a health professional as they agreed to a first Papanicolaou cervico-vaginal (Pap) smear, and children undergoing useful screens for nutritional status.

Communication with patients translating from English to Spanish to the indigenous language could be compromised or distorted in a major way. At the behest of our social worker we occasionally did a test, playing a type of 'telephone' game: student–translator–patient–translator–student, getting the patient to repeat the message we thought we were relating back to us. We thus found that simple messages could be 'lost in translation'. Given that people were relating issues of trauma from a recent earthquake and mudslides, family violence and alcoholism, this was not insignificant. One medical student proclaimed after consulting his pocketbook that Paxil must be given to the post-traumatic stress disorder (PTSD) patients he saw. After discussion about sustainability, cost and cultural acceptance, he agreed that the social worker who recommended chamomile tea may not have been so wrong.

However, what proved critical, and led to the ultimate demise of the program, were communication issues without language barriers – between the NGO and the university, the university and us and among the medical and nursing staff and students from different institutions each of which lived within different 'microcultures', experiencing particular constraints, expectations and understanding of ownership and responsibility.

Through this and a research project in Palestine, I gained new perspectives on biomedicine, the centrality of justice, the power of language, the limits of good intentions. In Palestine, I not only developed a new perspective on historical and epidemiological 'truth', but also an appreciation of how human beings could dehumanize and objectify 'the other', rendering their discourse null. I also discovered that the benevolent NGO and mental health industries that meant to 'help' had their own interests and agenda.

A few years later, I was invited to found a Global Health Office at a Canadian university, providing me the opportunity to understand university administrative constraints, to develop overseas partnerships and to appreciate linkages between local and global activities. Further, I was introduced to many authors of this text and was mentored by many. Foremost among these mentors were several of my students.

Through such experiences, I gained perspective on the importance of humility and respect, interprofessionalism, mentorship, the potential for harm, the impact of accident of birth on self-determination and access to resources and conditions for health. These experiences convinced me that a book of this nature was essential and guided its development and organization.

Book Organization

This book focuses on the health sciences student and is meant to give depth and detail to concepts only touched on in online training resources. With a stellar list of contributors, who are not merely academics, but people just like you, who learned in training and in the field, through the school of hard knocks. We hope not just to inform you, but support you, and to cultivate in you, an appropriate understanding, attitude and the skills to cope with challenges such as those we faced. Though providing assistance, our book cannot act as an alternative to PDT.

Section I

Chapter 1 sets the stage, putting IHEs in context. It provides advice on finding opportunities, mentors and organizations that might best fit you in terms of your interests, experiences and values. Chapter 2 addresses pros and cons of going abroad and the alternatives to a global health experience, at home, helping you assess your motivations, attitudes, skills and talents, as well as developing the learning objectives of an international experience. Chapter 3 is meant to get you to consider the impact of your experience, not just on you, but those hosting you. With the rise of social media, it behooves us to address its opportunities and dangers, and suggest its respectful, ethical use. Chapter 4 goes through how to find and evaluate various opportunities. Chapter 5 addresses the types of mentors and mentorship models at home and in the country you are visiting, and how to be a good mentee so you can get the most out of the experience. We finish Section I by exploring planning and pitfalls, practical aspects of preparation, protocols, packing lists, orientation, how to contact your host and providing a last minute checklist.

Section II

Next, we address PDT. Some have drawn attention to the need to develop attitudes, beyond knowledge and skills, mitigating potential for harm to students and host communities. Wallace considered such training as part of the social accountability agenda (Wallace and Webb, 2014). A decade ago, Brewer found no road map for global health in North American medical schools (Brewer et al., 2006) and proceeded to facilitate a national movement to create and mandate PDT at Canadian medical schools. With the guidance of Tim Brewer and leadership of one of our authors, Kelly Anderson, engaged medical students, concerned about impacts of past international experiences, by and on themselves, spearheaded these efforts. They developed PDT guidelines beyond personal safety and health to include issues around culture, language and ethics (Anderson and Bocking, 2008); they then developed curricula (Anderson and Bocking, 2008), helped organize and implement and deliver content nationally, evaluated, generated evidence and lobbied for incorporation of these as standards between 2008 and 2012. PDT training exploded in Canada in this time frame, was universalized by 2012 and became an accreditation standard for Canadian medical students doing clinical placements in developing world settings by the 2013 (Anderson et al., 2012; AFMC, 2016). Such preparation, while most developed in medical schools, is equally relevant to other clinical professions, as well as research and public health.

Personal health prior to departure and during travel, particularly in a healthcare context is highlighted in Chapter 8 with sources of information and information on diseases, vaccines and medications. Personal safety, understanding risk, preparing for the unforeseen and getting proper advice, is addressed in Chapter 9 by using case examples/scenarios. Beginning with theoretical-defining culture and addressing concepts such as competence, awareness, receptiveness, respect and reflection, examining how culture shapes values, perceptions and expectations, Chapter 10 moves to concrete advice on appropriate dress and behaviour, and provides activities to guide learning. Together with Chapter 11 and its focus on language – with advice on effective verbal and non-verbal communication skills – can help facilitate more meaningful relationships but also assist in safety and immunize against culture shock. Chapter 12 moves from principles of bioethics to critical reflection and to practical steps that might help avoid trauma and guilt years later.

Section III

Particularities related to experiences in specific disciplines in the Global South are addressed in Section III. Each chapter addresses safety, health, language, culture and ethics as well as preparation more specific to the discipline. However, we go beyond looking at the discipline in terms of general safety, burden of illness, pathology and its management, to addressing learning opportunities and objectives, principles related to training and practice of these professions in settings in the Global South. We must remember that local professionals may be different in terms of education, skill level and relationships within the hierarchy.

While in current interprofessional environments, knowing more about disciplines with which you are interacting is valuable, a major purpose of these chapters is to give you a chance to integrate lessons from the introductory chapters. Even if you never interact with professionals of the chapter, on reading you will learn about placements and team function, medical missions and health systems, approaches to cultural differences and ethical issues, be able to reflect on who benefits and how, who bears which costs, and how best to develop authentic partnerships. Thus, we have devoted more than a third of the volume to this section and recommend reading each chapter.

Chapter 13, opens the section, addressing burden of disease, common presentations and pathologies in outpatient care, allocation of healthcare resources in an environment of scarcity, the challenges of late presentation as well as emergency preparation. Chapter 14 also highlights common causes of mortality and morbidity in children, management of these problems and the specific skills required to work with them. Learning about the complexities of obstetrics and gynecology as a medical/surgical speciality in a context of varied international laws and cultural norms and the reality of neonatal and maternal deaths is fascinating in itself, but the authors in Chapter 15 relate three traits of a health practitioner relevant to global health in any setting – ability, availability and affability.

After the medical professions, we examine other health professions including midwifery, nursing, rehabilitation and social work. Each carries its own unique considerations, standards and expectations in a particular cultural context. Chapter 16 concentrates on how to accompany women in an environment that is not your own and also gives advice on seeking appropriate programs, placement and mentorship. Since the nursing profession may work more intimately with patients and families, Chapter 17 discusses the value of open communication and also examines the 'hows' of organizing missions and interprofessional collaboration. With increasing recognition of rights of those disabled, perceptions of ability and disability, the role of rehabilitative specialties in improving ability and inclusion, the subject of Chapter 18, are especially worthy of examination. Chapter 19 not only looks at the range of placements, differences in practice and developing practicums from administrative point of view, but also questions international experiences.

Chapters 20 through 22 cover surgical, dental and eye care professions, which often go on short-term medical missions (STMM) with teams 'parachuted in' to perform interventions. Only recently has any attention been paid to community development, capacity building and cross-cultural sensitivity, but these chapters include these elements. Chapter 20 includes consideration of personnel and equipment needs and the importance of case selection providing clear guidelines to those organizing any mission. Chapter 21 describes how to choose missions and gives examples of interesting partnerships. Chapter 22 is a real window not only onto individual barriers to care, indigenous systems of belief and the role of complementary practices but also onto health systems and the importance of integration with the host country's local healthcare personnel.

Foundational and practical aspects of global public health and research are addressed in turn in Chapters 23 and 24. Chapter 23 not only looks at dilemma in particular situations, but also at preparation for a career, comparing training with a master's in public health or global health. Chapter 24 guides you step by step in terms of considerations, as you move ahead at any level of research.

Thus, we hope to reiterate the principles and concretize the lessons of Sections I and II, as well as give more of an understanding of the types of settings, assist those planning missions and projects, allow appreciation of common medical issues, pathologies and burdens of illness, and lead to reflection of common issues among the professions.

Section IV

Section IV guides 'what next' post return, beginning with a piece on the value of debriefing and management of reverse culture shock. For those interested in continuing an engagement with global health, we conclude with a discussion on how to continue being active in global health at different levels and provide links to guide your search whether you just want to read more, further your education or develop a career.

Without further ado, let's get on with the show. We trust that you will enjoy reading this cover to cover, as much as I have and will be going back years later to reflect, with different eyes each time.

References

Anderson K and Bocking N. 2008. *Preparing Medical Students for Low-Resource Setting Electives: A Template for National Pre-Departure Training.* AFMC Global Health Resource Group and CFMS Global Health Program. Ottawa, Canada: Association of Medical Faculties of Canada. http://www.old.cfms.org/downloads/Pre-Departure%20Guidelines%20Final.pdf; http://caep.ca/sites/caep.ca/files/pre-departure_guidelines_final_0.pdf

Anderson KC, Slatnik MA, Pereira I, Cheung E, Xu K, and Brewer TF. 2012. Are we there yet? Preparing Canadian medical students for global health electives. *Acad Med*, 87(2):206–9.

Association of Faculties of Medicine of Canada (AFMC). 2016. Accreditation Standards. AFMC. https://www.afmc.ca/accreditation/committee-accreditation-continuing-medical-education-cacme/accreditation-standards; https://www.ualberta.ca/medicine/-/media/medicine/ume/policy/qualityreviewelectives.pdf

Brewer, T. et al. 2006. *Towards a Medical Education Relevant to All: The Case for Global Health in Medical Education.* A Report of the Global Health Resource Group of the Association of Faculties of Medicine of Canada. Ottawa, Canada: Association of Medical Faculties of Canada. http://www.old.cfms.org/downloads/The%20Case%20for%20Global%20Health%20in%20Medical%20Education-%20AFMC.pdf

Elit L, Hunt M, Redwood-Campbell L, Ranford J, Adelson N, and Schwartz L. 2011. Ethical issues encountered by medical students during international health electives. *Med Educ*, 45(7):704–11. doi:10.1111/j.1365-2923.2011.03936.x.

Heck JE and Pust R. 1993. A national consensus on the essential international health curriculum for medical schools. *Acad Med*, 68(8):596–8. doi:10.1097/00001888-199308000-00004.

Heck JE and Wedemeyer D. 1991. A survey of American medical schools to assess their preparation of students for overseas practice. *Acad Med*, 66(2); 78–81.

Illich I. 1968. To Hell with Good Intentions. Speech presented at the Conference on InterAmerican Student Projects (CIASP), Cuernavaca, Mexico, April 20. http://www.swaraj.org/illich_hell.htm

Kraeker C, Khalifa A, Delahunty-Pike A, Waiswa M, O'Shea T, and Damani A. 2014. Host perspectives of visiting medical trainees: A Qualitative analysis of global health electives. *J Global Health Perspect.* http://jglobalhealth.org/wp-content/uploads/2014/11/Kraeker_Christian.pdf

Krisberg K. 2015. Global community: Medical schools meet student desire for international learning experiences. *AAMC Reporter.* https://www.aamc.org/newsroom/reporter/september2015/442220/global-community.html

Madsen-Camacho M. 2004. Power and privilege: Community service learning in Tijuana. *Michigan J Community Service Learning*, 10(3):31–42. http://hdl.handle.net/2027/spo.3239521.0010.303

Nelson BD, Kasper J, Hibberd PL, Thea DM, and Herlihy JM. 2012. Developing a career in global health: Considerations for physicians-in-training and academic mentors. *J Grad Med Educ*, 4(3)3: 301–6. http://www.jgme.org/doi/full/10.4300/JGME-D-11-00299.1

Pedersen P. 1994. *Five Stages of Culture Shock: Critical Incidents Around the World*. ABC-CLIO. Contributions in Psychology, No. 25. Westport, CT: Greenwood Press, 1995.

Radstone SJJ. 2005. Practising on the poor? Healthcare workers' beliefs about the role of medical students during their elective. *J Med Ethics*, 31(2):109–10. doi:10.1136/jme.2004.007799.

Wallace LJ and Webb A. 2014. Pre-departure training and the social accountability of International Medical Electives. *Educ Health*, 27:143–7. https://www.researchgate.net/publication/261180403 _Pre-Departure_Training_and_the_Social_Accountability_of_International_Medical_Electives

Chapter 2

Should I Stay or Should I Go? And What Can I Do When I Get There?

Neil Arya and Kevin Chan

Contents

So you wish to embark on a global health experience? In this chapter, we explore the motivations, objectives and skills that you can bring abroad. But let us begin with the first question to consider prior to considering an international elective: 'Should you go abroad in the first place?'

Why Go Abroad? The Pros for Going International

Global health experiences (GHEs) provide opportunities for personal and professional growth, exchange of information and development of lifelong relationships and friendships. Trainees often develop fresh insights and attitudes with exposure to a broad spectrum of health and wellness, illness and disease, healthcare systems and social conditions unique to regions with different ethnic groups in resource-poor settings.

Cons

Electives abroad are not for everyone as they can be challenging – physically, mentally, ethically, emotionally, spiritually and financially – so it is best to ask yourself some hard questions before you consider an elective.

Remember, going abroad presents a whole set of logistical and ethical issues including systems not working, people denied access to appropriate care because of resource constraints, cultural differences, religious attitudes, lack of education, lack of informed consent, social class, family hierarchy and perceived variance in work values.

Global Health Is Not Only 'Abroad'

One of the persistent myths is that global health is only abroad. Sometimes, individuals who work in the international health arena think we *own* global health. But experiences with local indigenous populations, refugee and undocumented populations and those experiencing poverty in our inner cities may be equally or even more rewarding and provide valuable learning experiences – from treating psychosocial or physical needs of immigrants and refugees to focusing on research and advocating for health equity to developing more system-based approaches to addressing societal health needs. And the benefits of going abroad including sharpening clinical and language skills, facilitating population health perspectives, and developing a stronger sense of social inequities and injustices are equally applicable to resource-constrained settings in North America.

In fact, one of the best ways to prepare for going abroad is working with disadvantaged populations at home, as this provides a framework, emphasizing the social determinants of health (food insecurity, housing insecurity, poverty, etc.) and rights for health through a social justice lens.

Going abroad has the reverse benefit of providing a greater appreciation of social challenges at home. Many leading global health experts (e.g. Paul Farmer and James Orbinski) have utilized their considerable expertise while working abroad to address issues at home, in domestic under-resourced areas. The challenges and the lessons learnt from working in resource-poor settings in an international setting are similar to those in resource-poor settings at home.

Why Do I Want to Go Abroad?

Trainees who go to developing world settings often have mixed motivations, some of which may not always be in the interests of the facilities and communities in which they are placed. It is important to identify and recognize these motivations before going abroad.

Jane Philpott, in a brainstorming session with a group of postgraduate medical trainees at the University of Toronto, asked about the motivation of trainees wanting to work abroad (Philpott, 2010). She separated them into three broad categories. You might ask yourself if you have some of these motivations cited by the residents:

1. Motivations to which I aspire:
    a. Do I want to be part of a global community?
    b. Do I want to experience and learn from other cultures?
    c. Do I want to help disadvantaged populations (including those in my own country of origin/ancestry) with fewer resources and access to healthcare?
    d. Do I want to learn about health, how it's interpreted and the healthcare system of an international location?

2. Motivations I can tolerate:
   a. Do I want to travel around the world?
   b. Do I want to broaden my life experience?
   c. Will I see new diseases or face new medical problems?
   d. Will I develop new skills or languages?
   e. Do I wish to discover if global health should be part of my career?
3. Motivations I'd rather suppress:
   a. Do I want to go abroad because of the sensation, glamour and mystique of global health?
   b. Do I want to go abroad because I know better (self-aggrandizement and/or superiority)? Philpott identifies this latter set of motivations as problematic, perhaps leading to condescending, domineering and exploitative behaviour. Another thing to reflect on is
   c. Do I want to go abroad so I can get away from problems at home?

This should not be an absolute contraindication to going, but problems may sometimes be exacerbated and fewer supports may be present in an overseas context in a foreign culture.

Do I Have What It Takes?

Do I Have the Proper Attitude?

Pinto and Upshur cite attitudes and values such as humility, introspection, social justice and solidarity to help guide students as they approach a decision to go abroad (Pinto and Upshur, 2007).

For any GHE, you need to be understanding, flexible and adaptable. A major challenge is to manage your own expectations. There *will* be elements beyond your control. Have a more open sense of *success*. Accept your own boundaries and remember that it is natural for you to be less *able* in a context that is not yours. Be inquisitive before and appreciate that others' sense of right or wrong may be different than yours and equally valid. When you are feeling frustrated, remember how this will look in a decade. It might even be a story to tell.

For your own mental health and for the sake of relationships, learn to suspend judgment. From a Yale colleague,

> My internal medicine residents chose Uganda to improve their physical diagnosis skills and clinical reasoning in the context of lower resources, but the harsh daily reality of death is difficult to contemplate. With a 25% mortality on the ward, seeing a patient dying in the middle of rounds is not a rare occurrence. As rounds continue without pause, the slightest attempt at CPR and with no code being called, my residents ask incredulously, 'Don't the doctors here care?' I try to get them to reframe the question and their point of reference. For our system to work, providers need to be trained in ACLS, you need drugs readily available, you need an ICU bed and you need monitors. Can such critical care be practised in this context?

Try not to be procedure-oriented as there is so much more to learn. Medical students may be even less active clinically then at home, especially with limited knowledge of the language and cultural context. Learn to arrange for, and enjoy, downtime. Take a book. Learn more about the context, language and culture. Open-ended questions about things you don't understand can be an opportunity for meaningful dialogue.

Respect local customs that are a part of your host country's heritage. Be the kind of guest that you would welcome to Canada. Remember that overworked doctors, nurses, midwives, public health nurses and other staff of the host institution are contributing to supervisory time out of a sense of hospitality and friendship.

Even if there is a small charge for local accommodation, food or transport, or a token tuition or host organization fee, you are getting much more than you are paying for.

Be careful how you travel and try to bring a friend. If you wouldn't do it at home, don't do it there (sex, drugs, etc.)!

Websites such as https://www.instagram.com/barbiesavior/ and http://humanitariansoftinder .com/?og=1 attempt to name and shame. If the attitudes of people depicted are yours international experiences may not be the best for you. Others look at ways to end worst practices. http:// endhumanitariandouchery.co.nf/.

What Skills/Talents Do I Have?

Another part of self-reflection is to identify your personal skills or talents. Everyone has a skill or talent that can be imparted, but it's important to be sure what you can and cannot do. As a medical student or nursing student, you may have limited clinical knowledge, but perhaps you can teach basic sciences or provide basic cardiopulmonary resuscitation (CPR) skills. As a physician, nurse or healthcare professional, you may have some very specific skills that you can teach and impart. One of the most useful members of many global health teams has been a mechanic/ handyman, who has helped set up oxygen tanks, fixed electrical wiring and provided alternateive energy generation.

Of course, the more skills and talents you have, the more likely you will be useful abroad. Often, it helps to prepare well in advance and to go through an orientation course prior to going abroad.

Many medical and nursing students have tried to perform procedures and skills without appropriate training. It's important to remember that going abroad doesn't mean that those abroad don't deserve the same level of care and respect as back home. If anything, they require more protection.

How Can I Afford to Go Abroad?

One of the most challenging questions is funding for a GHE abroad. The good news is that over the past 25 years, there has been increasing amounts of money set aside for global health travel.

The most common means for most people is still self-funding. For some students, it may mean borrowing from a student loan, asking parents/friends, and/or doing fundraisers or applying through academic institutions. In the United States, the government has helped those who are receiving federal student aid (under the Free Application for Federal Student Aid [FAFSA]) by having their loans and interest deferred. Many student groups do things like bake sales, car washes, raffles, concessions sales, auctions of items from local vendors and art objects from abroad, selling T-shirts, concerts, raffles/lotteries and dinners.

For some professionals, it may mean using one's salary or income to finance a trip. Many nongovernmental organizations with charitable status provide tax receipts. Many student offices have various grants/stipends for travel abroad.

For those with specific skills or a more established global health career, some projects/research have funding for travel abroad. Many religious groups and diaspora populations have funding available for global health work. Increasingly, professional organizations have grants/stipends for travel abroad, and alumni associations have grants and travel funds. Local newspapers and magazines and local clubs (such as the Lions Club, Rotary Clubs and Jaycees) have travel funds. Some national chapters or sororities and fraternities also have funds. Also, various corporations, drug companies and private foundations are increasingly supporting global health work.

What Are My Specific Goals?

There are some fundamental guiding principles that should be part of any GHE that ensures the safety and well-being of the communities that we work with.

Some basic principles include the following:

- Responsibility and accountability
- Equity and the just distribution of, and access to, resources
- Respect for the history, context of individuals and communities
- Humility in recognizing our own values and culture as well as those of communities with whom we engage
- Honesty and openness in planning and implementation of all collaborations
- Multidirectional sharing of knowledge of experience among collaborating partners

Your program may provide some learning objectives. These objectives may include the following:

- Increased knowledge and sensitivity towards different cultures and contexts
- Expose yourself to a variety of global ethical issues in healthcare to promote transformative learning processes
- Allow an understanding of transdisciplinary and interprofessional care and a range of activities and organizations that can promote the well-being of their patients (e.g. community agencies, self-help groups, advocacy)

As a trainee, you should develop specific goals related to your GHE that can help you in your future practice, career trajectory and values as a global citizen. Some sample goals include the following:

- Gain a broader understanding of global health concepts and develop awareness of social, economic and political factors in health and disease
- Enhance understanding of illness and wellness and examine the root causes or determinants of health issues and outcomes
- Identify what health promotion and disease prevention activities are most appropriate for these populations
- Develop diverse skills or learning techniques specific to your profession
- Reflect critically on community service, and social responsibility in a clinical practice setting
- Reflect on differences in cultural practice, values, interests, standards of care, resource availability, politics and patient rights

While difficult to plan, a GHE might lead to (1) development of an ethical framework and more culturally appropriate care methods or (2) build abilities and skills and methodologies in decision making, problem-solving, reasoning and modelling.

Educational value is important but remember that the GHE is not all about the value to the trainee and there are potential harms to many with whom you interact. So clearly define and articulate your goals to yourself and also to those overseas helping you on the journey.

Specific Considerations When Choosing to Go Abroad

After you explore your own personal motivations and goals, there are four fundamental topics that should be addressed. These have been reiterated in a number of different books (Chan et al., 1997; Chan and Brodie, 1999; Evert et al., 2008; Drain et al., 2009):

1. Identify what broad scope of global health opportunities you are interested in (see below):
   a. Clinical, research, education and/or public health/advocacy
   b. Rural versus an urban setting
   c. Individual elective versus a group project
   d. New versus established project/program
   e. Funded versus self-financed project/program
   f. Paid versus unpaid position
   g. Are you looking to establish a career in global health?
   h. Are you looking to build sustainability in a project?
   i. How much supervision is required?

   The various scopes of global health opportunities can be indicated by four major categories: clinical, education, research and public health/advocacy (Chan et al., 1997; Chan, 2000). You may have one or more areas of expertise in these arenas. When going abroad, it's important to know which role you're playing because it requires different preparation and expectations going abroad.

   For many people, going into an established project/program often has the advantage of reducing the time and effort required to develop logistics, and often if the project is funded, reduces the time and effort needed to raise funds to establish your program. The other important consideration is how much will this program be a long-term goal and career for the individual. For some, it's a sidebar to their major career activities. For others, global health is the career that they want to have.

2. Identify how long you would like the experience to be and when you should go:
   a. Undergraduate/graduate student – summer time, as part of a course, after graduating/internships
   b. Medical, nursing and health professional students – summer vacation, elective time
   c. Medical resident/Fellows – part of a rotation, vacation
   d. Junior faculty and healthcare staff – before starting a career, vacation
   e. Mid-career faculty and healthcare staff – part of career/projects, vacation, sabbatical
   f. Retirees – full-time, part-time

   The duration may be different dependent on the stage of the career or personal stage in life that the individual is in. Despite general concerns about follow-up, sustainability and long-lasting impact of a project, for some surgical specialties, a short duration trip (2 weeks) may be sufficient. For recent graduate and junior faculty/healthcare staff trying to establish a career, it may be difficult to be away from a new job or from a young family or to have the financial resources to be able to do the job, so consideration of these impacts need to be factored in. Remember, it will take you time to orient yourself at the beginning of the trip – for personal reasons (finding markets, health centres as well as professional or project) – knowing key people, understanding relationships, institutions, influences and at the end to develop longer term goals and perhaps ensuring sustainability.

3. Is there a country or locale you would like to be in? Are there special language requirements (e.g. French Africa, or Spanish/Portuguese in South America)?

   There may be special considerations to locale to work in. For example, Paul Farmer, one of the co-founders of Partners in Health chose Haiti, because of geographic accessibility to his school and work at Harvard Medical School. Some groups prefer working in certain areas because of their specific language skills or some infectious disease doctors need to work in sub-Saharan Africa because certain tropical diseases exist only in a narrow range of areas/countries. Consideration should also be made to how stable and safe a location is, and the risks that may be important.

4. Are there any special needs or requirements? For example, laboratory facilities with bench-top research? Do you need to consider a spouse or children?

   For example, as a critical care doctor, you may feel comfortable working in areas with critical care equipment, which may require electricity. Or you may have specific health needs, such as insulin-dependent diabetes, which may require refrigeration for insulin. For those with families, it's important to consider how your partner/spouse and/or children will adapt to conditions abroad. An honest discussion within the family may be able to address some concerns prior to going abroad.

Conclusion

In this chapter, we've explored the question – should you go abroad in the first place? If you decide to go, explore your personal motivations and your objectives when going abroad. Make these explorations explicit and specific, and consider whether you should be going abroad in the first place. In the end, the challenge is should you be going abroad in the first place, and this chapter will hopefully help you decide if you think you're ready to go abroad or not.

References

Chan K. (2000). How do I do International Health? Presented at the *Canadian Conference on International Health*, Hull, Quebec. Nov. 2, 2000.

Chan K, Brodie J. (1999). Orientation and Debriefing. In: *International Health Medical Education Consortium (IHMEC) Handbook for Preparing International Health Rotations*. Heck J, Wedemeyer D, eds. Chapel Hill, NC: International Health Medical Education Consortium.

Chan K, Hillman D, Hillman E. (1997). *An International Workbook Guide for Students and Residents*. Ottawa, Canada: Centre for International Health and Development.

Drain P, Huffman S, Pirtle S, Chan K. (2009). *Caring for the World*. Toronto, Canada: University of Toronto Press.

Evert J, Stewart, K, Chan K, Rosenberg M, Hall T eds. (2008). *Developing Residency Training in Global Health: A Guidebook*. San Francisco, CA: Global Health Education Consortium.

Philpott J. (2010). Training for a global state of mind. *Virtual Mentor,* 12(3):231–236. http://journalofethics.ama-assn.org/2010/03/mnar1-1003.html\

Pinto AD, Upshur REG. (2007). Global health ethics for students. *World Bioethics*, 9(1):1–10. jointcentreforbioethics.ca/people/publications/dwb2007.pdf

Chapter 3

Maximizing Benefits and Minimizing Harm of IHEs on Trainees, Programs and Hosts

Neil Arya

Contents

Trainees (and sending institutions) have a great desire for more international health experiences (IHEs) in medical school (Drain et al., 2007). IHEs are viewed as a major plus to those seeking admittance into professional schools and appear to be beneficial to medical, health professional and health sciences students. However, while programs in the Global North celebrate the positive outcomes of international engagements, they historically have ignored potentially negative impacts of their students and on their students. It is therefore important to examine potential benefits and harms and look at ways of maximizing the positives not only for the individual but also for sending programs and hosts.

Benefits to Students and to Global North Society

Participation in global health tracks in medical training (including electives and sometimes didactic teaching involving global health topics, local experiences, pre-departure training including language, culture and ethics) helps develop knowledge, skills and values in a number of areas including greater awareness of social and public health issues, increased understanding of the challenges of working in areas with scarce resources, improved clinical skills, better understanding of appropriate resource utilization, improved communication and cultural sensitivity and higher levels of compassion and respect towards patients (Haq et al., 2000; Godkin and Savageau, 2001). A 2003 meta-analysis of 8 studies involving 522 medical students and 166 residents found that IHEs improved knowledge of topics such as tropical medicine and public health, and clinical skills such as managing with limited resources and cross-cultural communication (Thompson et al., 2003). Dowell and Merrylees found benefits in four key learning domains: (1) clinical knowledge and skills, (2) attitudes, (3) global perspectives and (4) personal and professional development (Dowell and Merrylees, 2009).

Students who participated in the global health track demonstrated a stronger preference for working with underserved communities and engaging in community service activities (Ramsey et al., 2004). In addition, a review by Jeffrey et al. of 11 seminal articles that suggested IHEs influenced medical students to choose careers in areas of priority in the Global North, such as a primary care and/or a public service (Jeffrey et al., 2011) and another by Thompson et al found that this was true particularly with underserved communities (Thompson et al., 2003). Bazemore and Dey found that the presence of IHEs was important to those students ranking family medicine and emergency residency programs (Bazemore et al., 2007; Dey et al., 2002). At the University of Toronto, a qualitative assessment of psychiatry residents determined that participation in an international rotation influenced their inclination to work with immigrants and vulnerable populations, and to get involved in health advocacy 1–2 years after the field experience. Participating residents also reported awareness of global health and ethical issues as well as skills which included teaching, clinical skills for practising with few resources, transcultural collaboration, advocating for patients and disadvantaged populations (Brook et al., 2010). Family residents who participated in an international health track at the University of Cincinnati were more likely to practice with underserved communities in the United States or internationally when compared to their peers who did not take part in the IHE (Bazemore et al., 2011).

Harms to Students

Dell et al. (2014) interviewed 23 students who personally faced or witnessed ethical or safety-related challenges during their undergraduate medical global health experience (GHE).

> We were surprised when every participant we approached met this criterion. . . . participants repeatedly and emotionally recounted incidents of ethical and safety-related dilemmas, including risks of needle sticks, doing clinical work that exceeded skill levels, and being publically(sic) ridiculed by host-country physician mentors
>
> **Dell et al. (2014)**

Safety Issues

In Dell's study, 83% of participants described witnessing or being involved in scenarios where a GHE-participant's physical safety was jeopardized, occupational safety concerns cited by 61% including 21% needle-stick injuries, while 52% described life-threatening scenarios outside the clinical setting including nearby murder of Western tourists.

I was less prepared for some of the cultural [and] social differences and how to protect myself. . . . So I was kind of stuck in this car with a drunk man who was trying to do things that he shouldn't have been doing and I didn't know how to get out. I didn't know what to do.

Dell et al. (2014)

Two studies spoke about reasonable concerns of administrators of IHEs over liability related to physical safety, travel and emotional well-being and harm to students travelling to areas with higher prevalence of communicable diseases, such as HIV, hepatitis and tuberculosis (TB). Sharafeldin et al. (2010) surveyed Dutch medical students from the University of Leiden doing IHEs in tropical locations over 2.5 years and found that two-thirds engaged in procedures that constituted a risk of exposure to blood-borne viral infection, often in countries with high HIV prevalence rates, but none of the students exposed to potentially infectious body fluids reported the exposure at the time it occurred nor used post-exposure prophylaxis. A further 20% of students who were in malaria-endemic areas reported that they stopped using mefloquine to prevent malaria infection due to the adverse effects from taking the drug (Sharafeldin et al., 2010). Tyagi et al., reviewing data from nine medical schools in the United Kingdom, found that accidents posed a greater threat for UK students participating in IHEs (five serious injuries from motor vehicle accidents – two post-elective on holiday from an estimated population between 2400 and 3000) than infections (no deaths or serious health problems except mild cases of malaria and a couple of parasites). Personal violence and events related to the political situation of the elected country were also reported and there were a few psychiatric issues, including one suicide. The literature does not identify student behaviour that might put students at risk or strategies for prevention to provide appropriate advice for personal safety (Tyagi et al., 2006).

Addressing Safety Issues

Pre-departure and in-country training can prepare students to avoid and manage dangerous situations. Jeffrey noted that the quality and availability of IHEs vary considerably by institution, at least in the United States (Jeffrey et al., 2011). Steiner et al. described three crises in 1 year that affected groups at one institution. These included an H1N1 flu epidemic that impacted one group bound for Mexico, a political upheaval that affected one headed to Honduras and a hurricane that threatened a group in Nicaragua. These groups found the barriers to address safety concerns included the lack of consistent, categorical funding, and limited faculty experience and resources to support and guide students during their rotations abroad (Jeffrey et al., 2011; Steiner et al., 2010). As a result of this post crisis analysis, Steiner determined that institutions could better respond to unpredictable events by developing well-defined institutional travel policies, clear communication plans in the event of an emergency, a responsible administative entity for global experiences and formal pre-departure training for students and faculty.

Ethical Dilemmas

While international health elective programs have increasingly focused on ensuring health, security and learning needs, standards and requirements around licensing and visas for higher-income country trainees in the last few years, ethical considerations may lag behind. Some promising efforts evolving are promotion of individual ethics around privacy, consent, and scope of patient care, but these neglect systemic issues. Dell et al. found 57% involved in, and/or witnessing, an ethical dilemma including resource disparity, for example limited affordable medical supplies, impacting on patient care.

> Patient care was very compromised. A lot of patients really needed tests or blood transfusions and could not afford them and therefore they were just left to just bleed to death. . . . Whereas over there, they use no anesthetic because they just don't have the resources or the money to pay for anesthetic unless the patient pays, which no one can.
>
> **Dell et al. (2014)**

Experiencing poverty was especially frustrating, especially when they realized limited impact of their own clinical skills.

> The main ethical issue I had was my own feelings of [being] a medical tourist.... I had a lot of trouble with that.... Although I took money and donated it to the hospitals and I did try and contribute, I basically told myself I would never go back to a developing country until I had something to offer, I felt like it was very one-sided, that all I did was take, take, take.
>
> **Dell et al. (2014)**

Elit et al. conducted semi-structured interviews with 12 medical students returning from IHEs and found similar issues such as uncertainty on how to be of best use in low-resource communities where healthcare needs were high.

Additional challenges for students arose as they navigated unfamiliar medical and social cultures, where they were easily identified as a Westerner and considered to be 'different' by colleagues and patients (Elit et al., 2011). Students may experience culture shock (Furnham and Bochner, 1986) (see also Chapter 10) or come back with reverse culture shock, a *process of readjusting, reacculturating and reassimilating into one's own home culture after living in a different culture for a significant period of time* (Gaw, 2000) (also see Chapter 25).

As one of Dell's students articulated,

> Honestly it was probably one of the most traumatic things to have happened to me and it took a very long time [pause] after we came back [to Canada] to be able to even go through the motions. . . . When it happened, I crashed. I got home in the afternoon and stayed in bed until the morning and I didn't speak to anyone. It was ridiculously hard on me.
>
> **Dell et al. (2014)**

Some students questioned the underlying premise of most of these international electives, mainly whether these are 'doing good' or at the very least, 'do no harm'. Dell and Elit both cited pressures to go beyond level of training, scope of practice or appropriate supervision, a sense of being a burden rather than an aid to local communities, working with limited clinical resources or providing unsupervised care beyond scope of training partly because of medical resource shortages.

A lot of times I was put in situations where there was somebody bleeding in front of me, and I really didn't know what to do. So I would just do what I could, and hope [I was] doing the right thing. A lot of times there was just nobody to help you and so you are all by yourself

Dell noted, 'However, limited skills were not always viewed by local supervisors as a reason to avoid performing procedures, requiring trainees to persist in declining such opportunities' (Dell et al., 2014) with a classic example of a student suggesting fluid restriction for a patient with polyuria realizing only many months later that it could have been a symptom of uncontrolled diabetes. Several papers cite concerns about trainees who do not adequately understand the local culture or context when they embark on IHEs (Shah and Wu, 2008; Hanson et al., 2010).

Addressing Ethical Gaps

Banatvala and Doyal (1998) asserted that well-structured, supervised electives might better enable students to say no in unfamiliar environments where they had insufficient experience to perform the task at hand (Banatvala and Doyal, 1998). Elit recommended formal pre-departure training including exploration of ethical and professionalism issues; careful selection of the IHE, including evaluation of expectations and motivations; and learning about the local context, communication with an invested on-site colleague or supervisor and maintaining an ongoing connection with the home institution, along with formal debriefing (Elit et al., 2011). Dowell agreed that greater planning and structure could be beneficial educationally, with the opportunity to contribute and to minimize risk (Dowell and Merrylees, 2009). Dell recommended that discussions go beyond competence to prior communication of trainee skill level with host supervisor. However, even with the best of preparation, such discussions with local residents and staff, sometimes led to ridiculing or shaming. This together with a trainee's desire to learn, may contribute to trainees going beyond their level of competence. Crabtree stressed the importance of preparation, reading to understanding contemporary and historical context, layered reflection dialogue with the host partner and community, and debriefing and integrating experience once home (Crabtree, 2013).

Responding to Host Societal Needs

Individual trainees, sponsoring institutions and host community each may have different perspectives on (1) cultural challenges, for example work ethic, (2) expectations and perceptions of skills and what trainees might do, (3) relationships – with trust affected by power dynamics and access to resources and (4) learning objectives. McCarthy et al. (2013) reflected that communication among the three about this discordance, and in particular seeking to find common ground or an intersection of interests was desirable. Emanuel et al. (2004) went beyond controversies around standard of care to develop benchmarks on the ethical conduct of research. These include being responsive to the community's health problems, true collaborative research with shared responsibility for assessing problems and the value of research, for planning and conducting the study and disseminating the results. For sustainable partnerships, there should be minimizing exploitation (unfair level of benefits or unfair burden of risks), fair distribution of the tangible and intangible rewards of research among the partners and the community and minimizing disparities between researchers and sponsors from developed countries and the host community (Emanuel et al., 2004). Such considerations might apply to any international experience, whether research, short-term medical missions or medical electives.

Social accountability is considered increasingly important in medical schools in Canada and around the world (Health Canada, 2001). In a landmark paper, Crump and Sugarman cite ethical issues, such as foreign students getting preferential treatment over local trainees, and clashing with local personnel due to a lack of cultural sensitivity (Crump and Sugarman, 2008). Kraeker's example of Ugandan medical students in Chapter 1 (Kraeker et al., 2014) pointed to resentment about patients being perceived as part of a zoo or museum and a concern about reciprocity. It is therefore certainly possible that negative impacts on hosts could outweigh the positive educational outcomes for trainees. John Crump, site director for the Kilimanjaro Christian Medical Centre-Duke collaboration in Moshi, Tanzania states: 'The worst-case scenario is that a host institution in a poor country carries the cost and bears unintended negative consequences of training people who do not contribute to improvements in global health now or in the future' (Zamora, 2010).

To respond to this concern, Crump et al. (2010) including team members from Global North and South, devised the WEIGHT guidelines. They claimed that to achieve the goal of reciprocal benefits and to mitigate adverse consequences of IHEs, well structured long-term, programs required that partners derive mutual and equitable benefit and would begin with open discussion of expectations, responsibilities and terms for implementation, a comprehensive accounting of costs and benefits to institutions, personnel, trainees, patients and the community in host countries. Furthermore, after careful selection of motivated, adaptable trainees, ensuring adequate trainee preparation, mentorship, supervision was essential.

While this book is meant to address such issues from an individual perspective, those wishing to explore these issues further may be interested in a companion volume *From Theory to Practice*, meant more to reflect on the programmatic level and provide examples of best practices dealing with ethical and pedagogical issues.

References

Banatvala N, and Doyal L. (1998). Knowing when to say "no" on the student elective: Students going on electives abroad need clinical guidelines. *BMJ*, 316(7142):1404–5. http://www.bmj.com/content/316/7142/1404.fullEditorial

Bazemore A, Henein M, Goldenhar LM, Szaflarski M, Lindsell CJ, and Diller P. (2007). The effect of offering international health training opportunities on family medicine residency recruiting. *Fam Med*, 39(4):255–60. http://www.ncbi.nlm.nih.gov/pubmed/17401769

Bazemore A, Goldenhar L, Lindsell CJ, Diller PM, and Huntington MK. (2011). An international health track is associated with care for underserved U.S. populations in subsequent clinical practice. *J Grad Med Educ*, 3(2):130–37. doi:10.4300/JGME-D-10-00066.1.

Brook S, Robertson D, Makuwaza T, and Hodges BD. (2010). Canadian residents teaching and learning psychiatry in Ethiopia: A grounded theory analysis focusing on their experiences. *Acad Psychiatry*, 34(6):433–7. doi:10.1176/appi.ap.34.6.433.

Crabtree R. (2013). The intended and unintended consequences of international service-learning. *J High Educ Outreach*, 17(2):43–66.

Crump JA and Sugarman J. (2008). Ethical considerations for short-term experiences by trainees in global health. *JAMA*, 300(12):1456–1458. doi: 10.1001/jama.300.12.1456.

Crump JA, Sugarman J, and Working Group on Ethics Guidelines for Global Health Training (WEIGHT). (2010). Ethics and best practice guidelines for training experiences in global health. *Am J Trop Med Hyg*, 83(6), 1178–182.

Dey CC, Grabowski JG, Gebreyes K, Hsu E, and VanRooyen MJ. (2002). Influence of international emergency medicine opportunities on residency program selection. *Acad Emerg Med*, 9(7):679–83. http://onlinelibrary.wiley.com/doi/10.1197/aemj.9.7.679/pdf

Dell EM, Varpio L, Petrosoniak A, Gajaria A, and McCarthy AE. (2014). The ethics and safety of medical student global health electives. *Int J Med Educ*, 5:63–72. doi: 10.5116/ijme.5334.8051.

Dowell J and Merrylees N. (2009). Electives: Isn't it time for a change? *Med Educ,* 43(2):121–6. doi:10.1111 /j.1365-2923.2008.03253.x.

Drain PK, Primack A, Hunt DD, Fawzi WW, Holmes KK, and Gardner P. (2007). Global health in medical education: A call for more training and opportunities. *Acad Med,* 82(3), 226–30. doi:10.1097/ACM.0b013e3180305cf9.

Elit L, Hunt L, Redwood-Campbell L, Ranford J, Adelson N, and Schwartz L. (2011). Ethical issues encountered by medical students during international health electives medical education. *Med Educ,* 45(7):704–11. doi:10.1111/j.1365-2923.2011.03936.x.

Emanuel EJ, Wendler D, Killen J, and Grady C. (2004). What makes clinical research in developing countries ethical? The benchmarks of ethical research. *J Infect Dis,* 189(5): 930–37. doi:10.1086/381709.

Furnham A and Bochner S. (1986). *Culture Shock: Psychological Reactions to Unfamiliar Environments.* London: Methuen.

Gaw, K. (2000). Reverse culture shock in students returning from overseas. *Int J Intercult Rel,* 24(11):83–104. doi:10.1016/S0147-1767(99)00024-3.

Godkin MA and Savageau JA. (2001). The effect of a global multiculturalism track on cultural competence of preclinical medical students. *Fam Med,* 33(3) 178–86.

Hanson L, Harms S, and Plamondon K. (2010). Undergraduate international medical electives: Some ethical and pedagogical considerations. *J Stud Int Educ,* 15(2):171–85. doi:10.1177/1028315310365542.

Haq C., Rothenberg D, Gjerde C, Bobula J, Wilson C, Bickley L, Cardelle A, and Joseph A. (2000). New world views: Preparing physicians in training for global health work. *Fam Med,* 32(8):566–72.

Health Canada. (2001). *Social Accountability: A Vision for Canadian Medical Schools.* Ottawa, ON: Publications Health Canada, Online version, http://www.afmc.ca/pdf/pdf_sa_vision_canadian_medical_schools_en.pdf

Jeffrey J, Dumont RA, Kim GY, and Kuo T. (2011). Effects of international health electives on medical student learning and career choice: Results of a systematic literature review. *Fam Med,* 43(1):21–8. https:// www.stfm.org/fmhub/fm2011/January/Jessica21.pdf

Kraeker C, Khalifa A, Delahunty-Pike A, Waiswa A, O'Shea T, and Damani A. (2014). Host perspectives of visiting medical trainees: A qualitative analysis of global health electives. *J Global Health Perspect.* Nov 16. http://jglobalhealth.org/wp-content/uploads/2014/11/Kraeker_Christian.pdf

McCarthy AE, Petrosoniak A, and Varpio L. (2013). The complex relationships involved in global health: A qualitative description. *BMC Med Educ,* 13:136. http://bmcmededuc.biomedcentral .com/articles/10.1186/1472-6920-13-136

Ramsey AH, Haq C, Gjerde CL, and Rothenburg D. (2004). Career influence of an international health experience during medical school. *Fam Med,* 36(6):412–6. http://www.stfm.org/FamilyMedicine/Vol36Issue6 /Ramsey412

Shah S and Wu T. (2008). The medical student global health experience: Professionalism and ethical implications. *J Med Ethics,* 34(5):375–8. doi:10.1136/jme.2006.019265.

Sharafeldin E, Soonawala D, Vandenbroucke JP, Hack E, and Visser LG. (2010). Health risks encountered by Dutch medical students during an elective in the tropics and the quality and comprehensiveness of pre and post-travel care. *BMC Med Educ,* 10:89. doi:10.1186/1472-6920-10-89.

Steiner B, Beat D, Carlough M, Dent G, Peña R, and Morgan DR. (2010). International crises and global health electives: Lessons for faculty and institutions. *Acad Med,* 85(10):1560–3. doi:10.1097 /ACM.0b013e3181f04689.

Thompson MJ, Huntington MK, Hunt DD, Pinsky LE, and Brodie JJ. (2003). Educational effects of international health electives on U.S. and Canadian medical students and residents: A literature review. *Acad Med,* 78(3):342–7. http://journals.lww.com/academicmedicine/Abstract/2003/03000/Educational _Effects_of_International_Health.23.aspx

Tyagi S, Corbett S, and Welfare MR. (2006). Safety on elective: A survey on safety advice and adverse events during electives. *Clin Med (Lond),* 6(2):154–6. http://www.clinmed.rcpjournal.org/content/6/2/154 .short

Zamora A. Guidelines for global health training eliminate pitfalls: Programs should improve public health without adding problems. *Duke Today,* December 1, 2010, accessed July 18, 2016, http://m.today.duke .edu/2010/12/GHethics.html

Chapter 4

Doing Your Homework: Choosing an Organization, Project or Opportunity in Global Health

Alyssa Smaldino and Jessica Evert

Contents

Introduction

Global health encompasses health equity at home and abroad and it is common for students and others to seek experiences internationally, particularly in low- and middle-income countries. Collectively, these are called short-term experiences in global health (STEGH) and can encompass a variety of activities, including service learning, volunteering, educational programs, field research and internships (Loh et al., 2015). While most, if not all, of these programs are grounded in good intentions, they are not all created equally in their philosophy of responsible engagement, impact measurement or mindfulness of unintended harms. How should students, faculty and advisors decide which global health programs to participate in and endorse? What questions should you ask? How can you understand these programs? And, are offering ethical opportunities?

It is important to remember that the selection of a particular program reflects an endorsement of that program's model, and you are 'speaking with your feet' by participating, and thus can perpetuate efforts that may result in unintended harms. With the appropriate level of thoughtfulness and strategy, you can support efforts that are constructive for both you and the host community.

A goal of global health is to provide resources and expertise that can help underserved and under-resourced populations to access greater well-being and productivity. Without recognition of local institutions already working to advance healthier livelihoods, international support can be disruptive and lead to sidelining of local capacity, which disempowers the exact settings outsiders aim to help.

What follows is a case study that suggests questions for you to ask, as well as pre-departure tips to promote fruitful global health engagement. By properly selecting and preparing for an international experience, you can nest your short-term experience in locally led longitudinal efforts that carry forward benefits long after your own international experience ends.

Case Study

A team of U.S. students was volunteering through a national network of university-based chapters to partner with an organization in rural Nicaragua, which we will call Better Health. The students had supported the organization's domestic violence shelter through fundraising for 3 years. The students who volunteered in the summer of 2013 had a goal to identify more services that could be incorporated at the shelter because they were able to raise more money. They planned to do this through interviews with the organization's staff, community members and shelter employees.

Better Health is part of a larger organization whose main office is in London, United Kingdom. The London office coordinates with the Managua office, which then coordinates with the local office. Communication goes from the top down but rarely are the voices of the local staff considered at the highest levels of strategy.

When the students arrived in the community, ready to expand upon their project, they asked the local leader: *What does your community need most in the next phase of the project?* They were prepared with the right question, but the answer they received surprised them: *Well, you are the donors. What do you want to do?*

These conversations quickly became frustrating to the students. *How do they not know what they want?* Through a series of conversations, it became clear that the local staff did, in fact, know what their community wanted and needed, but they knew that anytime they expressed those ideas to their superiors in Managua or London, they were told that they were wrong or that the international donors' and volunteers' priorities come first. As a result, they were not empowered to guide the students from the United States and instead felt that the students could develop their own objectives, potentially leading to damaging or less effective results for the community in the long term.

What Did We Learn from This Case?

Not all grassroots organizations are created equally. While it is important to support work that is being sustained and led by local people, we must ask questions to determine their effectiveness before we arrive in a country. We must understand *What is the organization's long-term goal? Who determined that goal? And, how have volunteers advanced it?* If the staff of Better Health had been accustomed to facilitating volunteer experiences in a way that advances community goals, the students' experience would have been better for their learning process and their ability to make an impact.

Grassroots organizations are embedded in a context and history that is essential to understand. The students went into the internship thinking about Better Health as the voice of their community. To an extent, that was true, but the context and history in which the organization has grown was deeply influential to the students' experience. We must understand *How has the organization come to be in this community? And, what conditions make it necessary for them to exist in the first place?*

For centuries, people of European descent have ventured to African, Asian and American territories. Often, using the delivery of 'tropical medicine' as a means to enter foreign communities, there has been a historical tendency to displace local people, separate them from resources and town centres and create new hierarchies in society (Barron, 2008). This happened all over the world, with colonial governments and arbitrary borders established by Europeans consistently throughout the sixteenth to nineteenth centuries.

By the time countries in Africa, Asia and Latin America gained independence in the mid-twentieth century, many inequitable programs and policies were established by Western and multilateral institutions. The result of this period was that formerly colonized countries were left with massive amounts of debt, locking them in poverty and keeping them dependent on Western governments for aid. Development programs and trade policies, for example, continue to lock these same countries in a cycle of poverty, debt and dependence (Barder, 2015).

In order to be most effective and empathetic in your work with communities that have been affected by poverty and inequitable health outcomes, you must become aware of the history that produced the challenges that you are addressing. You must try to understand and tackle root causes of issues, rather than putting forward more band-aid solutions that may have negative consequences in time.

Finding the Right Opportunity for You

Once you have developed the knowledge and commitment to participate in a short-term global health experience, there are many factors to consider. Within every community, there are many layers that form the systems and social services that either facilitate or hinder progress and well-being. In the context of global health volunteering or scholarly work, it is important to consider the needs and capacity of local organizations, as they often create the connections among international volunteers, local hospitals/clinics, social service organizations or government agencies.

One of the biggest challenges you might face in finding an opportunity is understanding the array of options and narrowing them down. There are two steps to this: finding all of the options that exist and then making your selection from a list that you've narrowed down. Following are some suggested ways to find out about the options for your global health experience.

Where Do You Find Information on What's Available?

One of the biggest challenges that trainees and people new to global health find when going abroad is trying to find out what's available out there. Here are some suggested ways to find your global health experience:

- **Word of mouth:** The best way to find a program is through trusted sources on your campus or in your network. Since thoughtfulness around international programs and engagement varies, speaking to your peers is just a start to doing your homework. Going beyond the 'it was great' is essential. Asking questions to understand if you are 'value-aligned', meaning your values, ethics and belief around global engagement, types of volunteering and related dynamics is essential.
- **Students/alumni/colleagues/university faculty and established programs/ongoing projects/research within the medical, health professional and public health schools:** There are many people connected to your academic institution who may be able to direct you to a trusted program. In addition to asking your medical/health professions or other school faculty, many campuses have an international education (or study abroad) office. These folks are experts in best practices of international programs for trainees, as well as safety and security while abroad.
- **Diaspora living in your country:** If you have a particular country or region in mind for your experience, consider connecting with the diaspora community from that country and gaining insight from their perspective. You may find them through community groups that have been formed, restaurants, religious institutions or community centres. Global health means health at home and abroad, so don't overlook the opportunities in your own backyard. Oftentimes, your ability to have continuity, relevance and impact is greater when you are in your own community.
- **Conferences:** There are many global health events that you could attend to meet key players in global health. A few of them include Consortium of Universities for Global Health (CUGH), Canadian Conference on Global Health (CCGH), Clinton Global Initiative University (CGIU) and the Unite for Sight Global Health and Innovation Conference.
- **Non-governmental organizations (NGOs) involved in global health work:** Many NGOs have programs for students to engage in global health. There are tips at the end of this chapter that can help you to understand the quality and effectiveness of the different options. The Global Health Council (GHC) is a membership organization for a wide variety of global health–oriented NGOs and is a great resource. Also, smaller in-country NGOs often cannot afford to belong to membership organizations that charge a fee, so looking for smaller grassroots organizations can be done directly or through organizations that partner with them. Organizations that subscribe to Fair Trade Learning can be found at www.globasl.org.
- **Government and international governmental organizations:** Agencies such as Global Affairs Canada, U.S. Agency for International Development (USAID) and the United Nations Agencies and World Health Organizations often have internships abroad or notices about various opportunities to engage in their international missions.

Once you've narrowed down your list to a few options, we encourage you to undertake further research about those options. The organizations' websites may only give a simplified, glowing perspective on their approach, so it is important to ask difficult questions and seek perspectives from a variety of sources. Below is a list of questions for you to consider when seeking out opportunities. At the end of this chapter you can find a list of websites and resources to help facilitate this process.

- **Who has volunteered there in the past?** It can be very valuable to speak with previous volunteers, read their blogs and learn about their experience.
- **How does the international community perceive this organization?** You can find out a lot of information about an organization by looking on non-profit transparency and accountability websites such as Guidestar and Charity Navigator. You can also review the non-profit organization's annual report to understand how their money is spent and how they evaluate their impact.

■ **What is the expected role of the student during the experience?** Per the Forum on Education Abroad and Working Group on Ethics Guidelines for Global Health Training (WEIGHT) guidelines, students should be primarily learners. You must not engage in clinical activities beyond your capabilities or violate local licensure and medical professionalism requirements (The Forum on Education Abroad, 2015). In addition, the Forum on Education Abroad Standards specify that it's critical to 'Ensure students receive training that articulates and limits their patient interaction to the same level of patient/community interaction that they would have in a volunteer position in the United States'. Keep in mind that health competencies are much more comprehensive than just clinical practice or service; programs that provide broader learning objectives are important for your professional development.

■ **Who is organizing the opportunity?** It is important for you to understand who exactly is organizing the experience, their past experience and legacy in doing so and their accountability to the student and to the local institutions.

■ **How long have they been involved in the community/location?** Oftentimes, program longevity is a proxy for successful partnership. Continuity is key to providing ongoing program quality improvement, as well as longitudinal development goals for the community.

■ **Is there support going to the community for the time, resources and effort spent on hosting and mentoring the student?** WEIGHT Ethics and Best Practice Guidelines for Training Experiences in Global Health state that programs should 'recognize the true cost to all institutions and ensure they are appropriately reimbursed', for community-based programs, including all costs of hosting students and/or faculty in community-based settings (Crump and Sugarman, 2010).

■ **Is the organization a non-profit or a for-profit? Is there a religious, governmental or other affiliation?** You may be seeking certain types of affiliation or may prefer not to be associated with affiliations. It is important that it is clear if such affiliations exist so that you can make informed choices.

■ **What type of safety procedures, insurance and incident response is in place?** You should be aware of the program's risk management policies and procedures, including the presence of a policy committee, an emergency fund, relationships with local embassies and a clear decision-making process for crisis management.

■ **What type of preparation, in-country support and post-experience debriefing is provided?** There are a variety of best practices for pre-departure training, in-country support and debriefing, and they will vary depending on the objectives of your experience. A program that offers comprehensive support and guidance, from pre-departure through debriefing, is ideal for both your experience and community impact.

■ **If students are paying a fee, is the use of the fees transparent and are there appropriate fiduciary practices by the organization?** Most non-profit organizations are required to have an audit, and if the organization is based in the United States, the IRS Form 990 can be obtained freely online at www.guidestar.com. These can be useful to ascertain financial transparency and diligence.

■ **Does the organization have an ethical code of conduct?** Ethical codes of conduct should be easily accessible to you in the early stages of your experience and should address both cultural and behavioural codes of conduct. At its core, an organization's code of conduct should emphasize the importance of respecting local law and respecting the local community. The code should also ensure that you understand that you are prohibited from practicing medicine beyond your capabilities.

■ **How are student activities linked with long-term reciprocal gains for the host community?** It is important for the local host organization to be involved in the selection and evaluation of volunteers and to be responsible for designing your agenda. You should therefore consider the capacity of the local organization to manage and support you throughout your experience. This can be assessed based on proven experience hosting other volunteers or exhibiting a strategy for providing fruitful volunteer experiences.

How to Make the Most of Your Opportunity

Both your needs and the organization's needs will vary from situation to situation, but data captured through a program evaluation revealed some key activities that grassroots organizations have benefited from (GlobeMed Partner Forum, 2014).

■ **Locally requested and institutional review board (IRB)-approved research studies.** Chapter 25 includes a number of recommendations and processes necessary for conducting research during your STEGH.
■ **Grant writing and fundraising strategy.** Can you leverage your networks and communication skills to help a grassroots organization increase their capacity and better sustain their work?
■ **Documenting and sharing stories.** Do you have high-quality equipment to help the community capture the impact they are experiencing? Who should you talk to in order to ensure your media collection is done in collaboration with the community and with their consent? What are the positive stories of change you can capture to amplify the work of your host organization? How can the community actively participate in capturing and sharing media and stories?
■ **Designing data collection tools and systems.** Have you developed skills in Excel or other data analysis platforms in your education? Can you utilize those skills to capture the real impact that's happening so the organization can be a model for others and continue to develop in a strategic way for their community?

These activities often do not involve clinical work, but they can help advance the local institutions that are fostering sustained, long-term improvements in health and development. If you are a medical student, resident or physician, ensure that you are not acting beyond your level of expertise and that you prioritize capacity building over ad hoc patient care.

Depending on your medical expertise, different factors should be considered in the process of selecting your experience. A number of recommendations exist for medical trainees to help them frame 'success' in terms of understanding and uniting pre-existing resources and building local capacity to sustain a thriving health system in the long term (Evert et al., 2007). As a high-ranking Guatemalan official in the Ministry of Health explained,

> [Short-term medical work] does not, and cannot, address these primary health issues of Guatemala. We already have many surgeons and other physicians who are well trained to take care of all problems common in our country. The lack of healthcare in rural areas is not due to a lack of physicians; it is due to a lack of resources to provide clinics, hospitals, and supplies to these areas.
>
> **Green et al. (2009)**

Table 4.1 Red Flags for Global Health Opportunities That Jeopardize Patient Safety and Development Quality

• Organizations that see high numbers of patients in a very short time
• Organizations that allow unlicensed or non-professional students to do professional activities such as triaging patients, taking history and physicals, doing physical exams and dispensing medications (particularly when there is no redundancy with a licensed/trained health professional repeating all patient care activities done by the students)
• Opportunities that over-promise big impacts in a short time
• Organizations that simplify the challenges of global health disparities to simple causes and/or simple fixes
• Organizations that are not transparent about the use of fees and/or are trying to profit off of volunteering goodwill
• Organizations that focus narrowly on the benefit for volunteers (such as the benefits to your resume), rather than the benefit to the community
• Organizations that do not measure their impacts on communities or evaluate their work (evaluation by independent researchers is ideal as it has less bias)

Conclusion

Many are familiar with the adage 'Speak with your feet'. This saying is especially relevant when you are choosing STEGH. Not only promises that you will be 'saving' people or impacting community health immediately can be very alluring, but can also be red flags for opportunities (Table 4.1) that do not have the necessary continuity, longevity, safety and humility built into them. It is our hope that you will take the time and apply the intention necessary to foster your professional development while preventing any possibility of unintended harm.

References

Barder, O. 2015. A Development Policy for the 21st Century. *The Center for Global Development Blog*, February 2. http://www.cgdev.org/blog/development-policy-21st-century.

Barron, D. 2008. Tropical medicine's contribution to colonial racism, *Crossroads*, 111(1): 86–91.

Crump, JA, Sugarman J and the Working Group on Ethical Guidelines for Global Health Training (WEIGHT). 2010. Ethics and best practice guidelines for training experiences in global health, *American Journal of Tropical Medical Hygiene*, 83(6):1178–1182. doi:10.4269/ajtmh.2010.10-0527.

Evert, J. 2007. Going Global: Considerations for Introducing Global Health Into Family Medicine Training Programs, *Family Medicine*, 39(9):659–65.

Forum on Education Abroad. 2015. Standards of Good Practice for Education Abroad. Last modified 2015. https://forumea.org/wp-content/uploads/2014/08/Standards-2015.pdf. Accessed October 24, 2016.

GlobeMed. 2014. How to Make the Most of Your Organization's Volunteers, data collected at Africa Partner Forum, Entebbe, Uganda, May 1-3.

Green, T, H Green, J Scandlyn, and A Kestler. 2009. Perceptions of short-term medical volunteer work: A qualitative study in Guatemala, *Globalization and Health*, 5:4. doi:10.1186/1744-8603-5-4.

Loh, LC, W Cherniak, BA Dreifuss, MM Dacso, HC Lin, and J Evert. 2015. Short term global health experiences and local partnership models: A framework, *Globalization and Health*, 11:50. doi:10.1186/s12992-015-0135-7.

Chapter 5

Mentorship

Kelly Anderson and Caity Jackson

Contents

All phases of the global health elective cycle – from contemplating, planning, participating and returning – can leave you craving for seasoned mentorship. A skilful mentor can shed light on your pressing questions, clarify problems, provide a sounding board and guide you in further academic and educational pursuits. Even a small act of support or nugget of inspiration from a mentor can renew, inspire and transform your work as a global health student.

Definition of Mentorship

A mentor has been described as an influential and trusted counsellor, guide, teacher, coach or supporter. Through sharing expertise, a mentor contributes to the development of a mentee in personal and professional capacities. According to Berk et al., the academic mentoring relationship: 'may vary along a continuum from informal/short term to formal/long term in which faculty with useful experience, knowledge skills and/or wisdom offers advice, information, guidance, support or opportunity to another faculty member or student for that individual's professional development' (Berk et al., 2005). This chapter focuses on the 'functional mentoring' that can surround a global health elective experience, including how to initiate, foster and evaluate those relationships (Thorndyke et al., 2008).

Mentorship Models

As a trainee, it can be useful to understand the various models of mentorship that exist in different institutions.

One-on-One (Non-Mediated)

In this model, as a trainee you would search out and approach a desired mentor informally. This model tends to be unofficial, casual and personal. Indeed, you may already inadvertently be on this search and have just not articulated it as such. This type of mentoring emerges over time or can often be recognized in retrospect. The mentor may also feel that he or she is mentored by the fresh perspectives brought by you as a learner, and thus the relationship can be reciprocal.

Instead of creating formal mentorship programs, some institutions may facilitate opportunities for this type of informal one-on-one mentorship to arise, such as bringing students and faculty together to meet, through interest groups or activities. Bringing interested students and potential mentors together, both socially and professionally, in a systematic way can facilitate connections between keen, passionate and motivated learners with potential like-minded mentors early on.

In terms of other informal mentorship opportunities, local mentorship through partners in the Global South may arise during your global health electives. Many learners may need to be primed to look for this type of mentorship as it moves them out of their comfort zone. Often, the depth of experience, practical knowledge and expertise can be overlooked by students who prioritize their home institution mentors while on elective. The cross-cultural exchange and on-the-ground viewpoint is something a mentor from your home institution may not be able to offer (Shah et al., 2011).

In addition to providing systematic ways for learners and mentors to meet, learners should be prompted to seek out their own mentorship (Thorndyke et al., 2008; Sambunjak et al., 2009; Straus et al., 2009). Trainees should identify and reach out to thought leaders in a field of interest or faculty members further along in their career path who have similar backgrounds. Finding someone who has the breadth and appropriate resources (time, etc.), including an interest in mentoring, increases the success of a mentoring relationship.

Informal mentorship models may work well for you if you are keen, with the skills to seek out and connect with experienced teachers; however, challenges can lie in continuing the connection between you and an informal mentor when no formal responsibilities are articulated. Challenges also lie in the fact that not all learners may have the enthusiasm, discipline or creativity required to seek out and maintain appropriate mentorship.

One-on-One (Mediated)

In this model, which requires more specific organizational input from an institution, both you and potential mentors would apply to a program, and thereafter a third party would match you together. This is more resource-intensive, requiring a point person as an organizational hub, and there may be a discrepancy in the number of students and mentors applying. The MentorNet program, through the Canadian Society of International Health, is a strong example of a program matching learners with mentors who are experts in the global health field across Canada. Mentors and students connect across various media, including phone, e-mail, text and skype for a period of 8 months. Prepared topic-based modules and a liaison to weather challenging relationships add to this model's success. These programs are formalized further by the use of mentorship agreements and contracts, addressing frequency and modality of meetings and mentorship timelines, expectations and objectives, as well as frequency of revisiting the agreement (Sunley et al., 2014; CSIH MentorNet, 2013).

Group Mentorship (Mediated)

In this model, a point person would establish a group of learners to be guided and to engage in conversation with a single mentor. This model is illustrated by the Canadian Coalition for Global Health Research (CCGHR) mentorship module work, as well as the 'Global Health Me' program (Global Health Me, 2015) run jointly by the Next Generation Network and the Swedish Network for International Health. This model differs from the one-on-one mediated program model by increasing the number of individuals included in the mentorship relationship. Multiple learners to one mentor can increase the quality of the discussion and even lead to some peer mentoring, if the skill and knowledge levels of the learners vary slightly. This model mimics a small classroom, with mentors able to share their wisdom to many individuals at the same time and learners able to teach each other.

What Is the Role of a Mentor in the Context of Global Health Electives?

Ideally, an experienced mentor will be able to guide and reflect with you while you consider and plan an elective. In addition to hard logistics (such as personal health and safety, travel plans, insurance and what to do in case of emergency), your motivations should be addressed – why do you feel a global health elective is important now? Is there a risk of harm to your host community? How will you know whether or not you are a burden? How might this elective contribute to future career goals? These critical ethical discussions may not be easy and are best facilitated by a supportive, open-minded mentor that is also open to considering new perspectives.

During the elective stage, mentorship can become important should you encounter an ethical situation or a logistical impasse. In these situations, along with mentorship, a program must consider what immediate resources might be available for you: is there someone available to coach you through a situation that feels unethical, for example, if asked to perform a medical procedure for which you are not adequately trained? It may be the case that a local mentor can serve in this capacity.

Mentors can play a pivotal role in post-return debriefing, where discussion can highlight successes, regrets and learning areas. Proper facilitation of this stage can increase the likelihood of trainees to pursue elements of a global health career and fostering a global state of mind (Petrosoniak et al., 2010).

Selecting and Supporting Faculty Mentors

There is no algorithm to ensure success in selecting mentors; the experience level of a mentor may vary from recent residency graduates to senior health professionals committed to globally focused research or long-term clinical work. Faculty at different stages in their career may be able to serve in different yet equally valuable mentoring roles (Rose et al., 2005). Early career professionals may be better able to relate to you, and may be more familiar with training program requirements, applications and logistics of global health electives. Having often forged their own path in global health, such early career mentors may be very eager to share their experience with others. Faculty who are in the middle to late career stages may have more expertise to share, more established reputations, more contacts in the field and more institutional influence; however, they may have less time to dedicate to mentorship. The former may be better suited to serve as a mentor for you as you prepare for your global health electives or projects, while the latter may be better suited to serving as career or curriculum advisors. You may value having two or more mentors who are at different stages of their careers, layering your mentors: for example, discussing the details of a global health elective with a mentor who recently finished training, while seeking broader professional guidance from more experienced advisors.

Academic institutions looking to recruit mentors, but with a limited pool of local expertise, may recruit local and international affiliates and extramural advisors for their programs. Global health mentors can come from multiple fields and will not necessarily be found exclusively within the faculty base. Resources include special interest sections and groups of professional societies, young physician networks, public health schools, non-governmental and community-based organizations. Community physicians, allied health professionals and NGO or non-profit workers may welcome the opportunity to share their expertise as global health mentors with students currently in training.

Cultivating effective global health mentors requires that institutions specifically provide support for their mentors. Institutions undertaking a new formal or informal mentorship program should consider how to support mentorship as part of the culture of their organization. In a recent review of the literature, five articles discussed the need for improved institutional support and recognition of mentors. Rammani et al. conducted a series of workshops with medical faculty to identify key elements of training in mentorship programs (Rammani et al., 2006). These workshops identified focus areas of interpersonal boundaries, forums to discuss uncertainties and problems, evaluation strategies, protected time, reward systems and recognition. In their systematic literature review, Sambunjak et al. cited several structural barriers to effective mentorship including lack of time, lack of energy due to overwhelming logistical and tactical problems, lack of recognition and incentive for mentors and a limited pool of available mentors. They proposed incentives of protected time, formal evaluations and awards. Many young mentors would like to receive feedback on their mentorship style and approach and would like their mentorship journey to be complemented by training and workshops. Mentorship teaching should be part of continuous faculty development, helping established faculty members to improve skills in mentorship.

Cultivating Effective Mentees

Many studies emphasize the importance of a learner's active management of the mentoring relationship (Thorndyke et al., 2008; Sambunjak et al., 2009; Zerzan et al., 2009; Straus et al., 2009; Gusic et al., 2010). Effective mentorship truly begins when as a mentee, you possess the right degree of interest, motivation and skills to initiate, and cultivate and facilitate a relationship with a mentor. This mentee-based leadership has been described as sitting in the driver's seat (Straus et al., 2009). In their systematic review, Sambunjak et al. explored and summarized the development, perceptions and experiences of mentoring relationships in academic medicine. They noted that passion to succeed, proactivity and willingness to learn are critical attributes in an effective mentee. They also suggested that mentees should prepare for meetings with their mentors, provide a suggested outline for each discussion and complete assigned tasks. As a mentee, you should also respond honestly to feedback and accept suggestions constructively, regularly self-reflecting and bring these insights to the discussion, so the mentor can provide input.

If institutions prefer that students seek out their own mentors for global health electives, some coaching may be required and as a learner, you may need persistence. In order to further investigate mentoring and to examine effective mentorship alliances, Jackson et al. conducted individual telephone interviews of 16 young faculty members about seeking mentorship (Jackson et al., 2003). One interviewee suggested, 'Advice that I do give . . . is to go set up a half hour appointment with everyone in your department. Just go sit and talk with them and that way you start to find out who would be the natural mentors'. Another participant added, 'I would persevere and if you don't find someone who's suitable in your department or in your institution, then think of people beyond. But I think you have to go get it set up yourself. People aren't just going to fall into your lap and say, "I want to be your mentor"'. The study noted that you may find that several people, rather than one individual, are better at providing comprehensive mentorship.

This is not to diminish the role of a mentor in cultivating the relationship but to encourage programs to train learners on how to be mentored. Indeed, even formalized, facilitated mentorship programs do not guarantee the right chemistry between mentors and mentees, but innovative and initiative-taking learners often find the right fit through an informal mentor search (Jackson et al., 2003).

Evaluation of Mentorship

The personal and fluctuating nature of mentorship makes evaluation difficult and subjective. Buddeberg-Fischer and Herta conducted a Medline review of formal mentoring programs for students and physicians and concluded that the majority of programs lack concrete structure as well as short- and long-term evaluation strategies (Buddeberg-Fischer and Herta, 2006). Similarly, Gusic et al. conducted workshops called 'The Mentorship Toolbox: How to Build Better Mentors and Mentoring Programs' at three annual meetings of the Pediatric Academic Society. With over 100 participants, there was unanimous agreement that measurable outcomes must be used to demonstrate success of mentorship programs. Suggested outcomes and measurement tools include self-evaluation, focus groups, retention data and data on number of scholarly projects and promotions to measure satisfaction, growth, productivity and success within the program.

There are some tools available to guide institutions on how they evaluate their mentorship programs. Three recent peer-reviewed articles discussed specific tools and strategies to evaluate mentorship programs based on tangible, measurable outcomes.

Berk et al. reported the findings of an ad hoc faculty mentoring committee established at the John Hopkins School of Nursing, identified 10 measurable roles and responsibilities for the mentor. These included (1) committing to mentoring; (2) providing resources, experts and source materials in the field; (3) offering guidance and direction regarding professional issues; (4) providing timely, clear and comprehensive feedback to mentee's questions; (5) encouraging the mentee's ideas and work; (6) providing constructive and useful critiques of the mentee's work; (7) respecting a mentee's uniqueness and his or her contributions; (8) challenging the mentee to expand his or her abilities; (9) appropriately acknowledging contributions of a mentee; and finally, (10) sharing success and benefits of the products and activities with the mentee. Based on these responsibilities, the authors developed 'The Mentorship Effectiveness Scale'. It consists of a series of 12 questions, each utilizing a six-point agree-disagree Likert scale. Each question corresponds to one of the roles and responsibilities of the mentor. To complement this scale, the authors also developed the mentorship profile questionnaire to describe the nature of the mentoring relationship. A copy of both tools can be found in their article. The authors also call for more research on the definition, conceptual issues, and tools of mentorship, so that we can measure effectiveness.

Rogers et al. developed a second tool: a quantitative instrument to measure domains of the mentee's experience in a mentorship program (Rogers et al., 2008). They demonstrated statistical evidence in support of the tool, which was tested on 96 faculty members from one medical department. The proposed measurement tool has 27 items which follow a five-point Likert-type scale. A full copy of the instrument can be found in the article. The authors of this chapter developed points of reflection for mentors and trainees to consider prior and during their mentorship experience, to increase effectiveness (Box 5.1).

BOX 5.1

The following list of points may be helpful for mentors and trainees regarding global health training experiences:

- Mentors should consider having the student reflect on where they would like to go and why. Ask the learner to reflect on whether they see themselves immersing in an urban or a rural setting, in an inpatient or an office-based experience or are considering a research experience and how the mentor can best contribute to this reflection and experience and how they can guide the learner.
- Mentors should ask the learner if there are any specific learning objectives they would like to achieve (e.g. a resident interested in human immunodeficiency virus [HIV] care should be guided towards a site where HIV prevalence is high enough to gain significant exposure within a short period of time) and the learner should communicate their learning objectives in relation to both the experience and the mentorship.
- The mentor should encourage the learner to consider the safety and political stability of the site. To consider what level of risk are they comfortable with, what level of accommodation are they prepared for (i.e. different communities have different degrees of resources availability – electricity, running water, access to Internet/communication, etc.).
- Both learner and mentor should consider how much time is available for planning the elective and mentorship component. (Consider beginning this discussion as much as a year in advance, as some elective sites may fill up early or require privileging, VISA clearance, community partner identification, mentor might have other time obligations, etc.).

The mentor must also take into account other important considerations from an institutional point of view:

- Is there availability of an on-site mentor? Do they have time and resources to dedicate to a trainee? What level of supervision will the resident have? What clinical activities will be expected of the resident?
- What are the available funds and estimated budget?
- Can clear communication with the on-site mentor be established prior to the rotation, in order to guide expectations and preparation?
- Are there residents who have rotated at the site before? What resources and needs have been identified regarding the site in consideration?

Conclusion

As a learner seeking mentorship, you are not treading a common or well-worn path. Very little research has been done to look at mentorship in this flourishing field of global health, and many options exist for how to structure these relationships. But no matter which format is chosen or sought out, mentorship increases the richness and diversity in any setting (Allen et al., 2004; Sunley et al., 2014). It provides for cross pollination – encouraging creative exchange across generations, increasing the amount of self-reflection had by both parties. It may allow for new projects and new collaborations to emerge. It offers you the chance to benefit from mistakes made and lessons learned from wise mentors; it offers mentors the chance to see experience through new eyes, to keep their feet on the ground vicariously through trainees and to keep discovering, assimilating new elements of the global health field. It may change your career pathway as a trainee; it may revive and re-inspire the career aspirations of the mentor. Mentorship can be a fruitful two-way street, ideally, everyone involved can benefit remarkably.

References

Allen, TD, Eby, LT, Poteet, ML, Lentz, E, and Lima, L. Career benefits associated with mentoring for protégés: A meta-analysis. *Journal of Applied Psychology*, 89, no. 1 (2004): 127–36. doi:10.1037/0021-9010.89.1.127.

Berk, RA, Berg, J, Mortimer, R, Walton-Moss, B, and Yeo, TP. Measuring the effectiveness of faculty mentoring relationships. *Academic Medicine*, 80, no. 1 (2005): 66–71.

Buddeberg-Fischer, B, and Herta, KD. Formal mentorship programs for medical students and doctors: A review of the medline literature. *Medical Teacher*, 28, no. 3 (2006): 248–56. doi:10.1080/01421590500313043.

Mentorship and Leadership Resources. *Canadian Coalition for Global Health Research*. http://www.ccghr.ca/resources/mentorship-and-leadership/

CSIH MentorNet. *Canadian Society for International Health*. 2013. https://csihmentornet.wordpress.com.

Global Health Me Mentorship Program. 2015. Partnership between Global Health Next Generation Program and Swedish Network for International Health. http://globalhealthmentor.wixsite.com/ghme.

Gusic, ME, Zenni, EA, Ludwig, S, and First, LR. Strategies to design an effective mentorship program. *Journal of Pediatrics*, 156, no. 2 (2010). doi:10.1016/j.jpeds.2009.11.012.

Jackson, VA, Palepu, A, Szalacha, L, Caswell, C, Carr, PL, and Inui, T. Having the "right chemistry": A qualitative study of mentoring in academic medicine. *Academic Medicine*, 28, no. 3 (2003): 328–34.

Petrosoniak, A, McCarthy, A, and Varpio, L. International health electives: Thematic results of student and professional interviews. *Medical Education*, 44, no. 7 (2010): 683–9. doi:10.1111/j.1365-2923.2010.03688.x.

Rammani, S, Gruppen, L, and Kachur, E. Twelve tips for developing effective mentors. *Medical Teacher*, 28, no. 5 (2006): 404–8. doi:10.1080/01421590600825326.

Rogers, J, Monteiro, FM, and Nora, A. Toward measuring the domains of mentoring. *Family Medicine*, 40, no. 4 (2008): 259–63.

Rose, GL, Ruckstalis, MR, and Schuckit, MA. Informal mentoring between faculty and medical students. *Academic Medicine*. 80, no. 4 (2005): 344–8.

Sambunjak, D, Straus, S, and Marusic, A. A systematic review of qualitative research on the meaning and characteristics of mentoring in academic medicine. *Journal of General Internal Medicine*, 25, no. 1 (2009): 72–8. doi:10.1007/s11606-009-1165-8.

Shah, SK, Nodell, B, Montano, S, Behrens, C, and Zunt, J. Clinical research and global health: Mentoring the next generation of health care students. *Global Public Health* 6, no. 3 (2011): 234–46. doi:10.1080/17441692.2010.494248.

Sunley, SLK, Dhawan, S, Wong, K, Jackson, C, Frain, A, Macphail, C, and Padayachee, L. CSIH MentorNet: Impact of an innovative national global health mentorship program on students and young professionals. *Annals of Global Health*, 80, no. 3 (2014): 180. doi:http://dx.doi.org/10.1016/j.aogh.2014.08.062.

Straus, SE, Chatur, F, and Taylor, M. Issues in the mentor–mentee relationship in academic medicine – A qualitative study. *Academic Medicine*, 84, no. 1 (2009): 135–9. doi:10.1097/ACM.0b013e31819301ab.

Thorndyke, L, Gusic, M, and Milner, R. Functional mentoring: A practical approach with multilevel outcomes. *Journal of Continuing Education in the Health Professions*, 28, no. 3 (2008): 157–64. doi:10.1002/chp.178.

Zerzan, JT, Hess, R, Schur, E, Phillips, RS, and Rigotti, N. Making the most of mentors: A guide for mentees. *Academic Medicine*, 84, no. 1 (2009): 140–4. doi:10.1097/ACM.0b013e3181906e8f.

Chapter 6

Technology and Social Media

Michelle M. Amri

Contents

A picture is worth a thousand words.

Background

Images have the power to ignite drastic change. The photos of 9-year-old napalm victim Kim Phuc running naked down a street during the Vietnam War or of young Syrian Alan Kurdî washed up on the shores of the beach are just two examples.

Many individuals functioning in global health are working in contexts and conditions that are unique and quite different than their home countries. By utilizing means such as photography to capture their experiences, global health practitioners are able to use images to portray messages and convey emotions that words alone sometimes cannot. Alternatively, practitioners use other avenues of technology to share their experiences, educate, raise funds and recruit staff (Médecins Sans Frontières [MSF], n.d.), which can include blogging, YouTube videos, Facebook, Instagram, Twitter, LinkedIn, personal and organizational websites, all of which can have varying levels of use. The appropriate use of technology and social media in global health, by students, clinicians and practitioners, is the focus of this chapter.

Current Considerations

Currently, there is no standardized guidance provided to those setting off to utilize technology in global health (Macintosh, 2006). Not only are existing guidelines difficult to enforce or apply universally, but also obstacles such as linguistic and cultural differences, lack of local infrastructure and low literacy rates are faced (Macintosh, 2006). Despite the lack of standardized guidance, institutions and international organizations have developed their own guidelines, such as the American Medical Association (Lagu and Greysen, 2011) and MSF (MSF, n.d.).

While journals such as the *Lancet* and *British Medical Journal* require informed consent forms to be submitted with a submission, others such as *Disasters* and *Tropical Medicine and International Health* require instead a statement of ethical approval (Macintosh, 2006) – demonstrating the lack of consistency even among journals of similar scope.

For practitioners, it is important to consider technology, whether engaging in blogging, writing research articles or merely posting pictures (1) before departure, (2) before and during technology use and (3) after technology use. For the purpose of this chapter, individuals taking photos in global health contexts from here on will be referred to as 'photographers'.

Before Departure

Because images convey meaning and experiences, a photographer has influence over the audience's impression, whether positive or negative (University of Toronto, 2016). The emotions a traveller experiences vary drastically during different stages of culture shock, from honeymoon, rejection, regression and acceptance/negotiation to reverse culture shock (Pedersen, 1995). Therefore, as a photographer or blogger, it is crucial to consider the potential implications of your emotional state when you communicate your feelings and ideas.

It is also important to consider that the standpoint images are captured in. Future viewers may define populations by the photographer's portrayal (Macintosh, 2006). In fact, media-depicted suffering bodies in developing nations would not be on par with ethical standards required in developed countries (Calain, 2013). Before departure, consideration should be given to how the context of an individual can be retained while depicting images of societal problems, such as famine (Young, 2004, as cited in Macintosh, 2006).

Therefore, it is important to consider the subject being photographed in combination with the partner worked with (Estrin, 2012). Because many global health photographers are typically working with non-governmental organizations (NGOs), it is key to reflect on whether the mission of the NGO and how the photos will be used is one that you as a photographer would like to support. For example, the images captured will be used to further the left- or right-leaning goals of the newspaper or publication. As Stephen Mayes, the Director of Magnum Photo Agency states, 'by working with them, you're effectively endorsing that world view' (Estrin, 2012).

Careful reflection, perhaps assisted through readings (e.g. MSF photographer guidelines), on the differing levels of power of individuals in each unique context should be undertaken. If you are a practitioner and are providing clinical care to a local, an imbalance of power may leave the patient feeling treatment may be jeopardized if a photograph is refused. This imbalance of power can have implications on receiving informed consent, which will be discussed below. If you are ever unsure of guidelines or best practices, reach out to your home institution, whether a university or hospital, as they typically host their own social media and communications teams. Home institutions may consider implementing a social media contract that you would be required to sign before departure, highlighting guidelines.

You should obtain approval from the authorities of the premises or host site, such as the Ministry of Health, before any photographs are taken. This is to avoid any potential issues with the military (MSF, n.d.), and try to gain an understanding of local traditions and customs to ensure good relations (AusAID, 2012).

Before and During Technology Use

Due to the disproportionate prevalence of disease and starvation in many low- and middle-income countries, many subjects being photographed are perceived as not 'normal' (Macintosh, 2006). Therefore, it is of utmost importance to strive to protect the identities of the individuals captured or receive consent for the photographs being taken (Macintosh, 2006), all while being transparent about the role you are undertaking (Estrin, 2012): for example, if you are working with an NGO versus writing an editorial publication.

Informed consent is largely understood by Beauchamp and Childress to include certain components; when one is competent to act, receives a thorough disclosure, acts voluntarily and consents to the intervention (Berle, 2002). However, more recently, due to the pervasive nature of the Internet, it is advisable to relay an understanding of the potential for misuse and/or greater spread of the individual's image when receiving consent (Macintosh, 2006). While it cannot be predetermined what product could potentially be used for when made public, it is important you relay a general understanding of the possibility of reproduction beyond initial intent when obtaining consent.

There is a misconception that requesting informed consent may result in higher rates of refusal. However, researchers have found evidence to suggest the contrary, that individuals are willing to provide informed consent and have photographs taken when the intended use of photographs is expressed (Dysmorphology Subcommittee of the Clinical Practice Committee, 2000). Thus, having the possibility to increase participation rates and improve relationships with community members.

However, at times receiving written consent may go against the subject's best interests (MSF, n.d.). When written consent cannot be received due to illiteracy or language barriers, for example, you may employ other methods. For a largely illiterate group of individuals in Paraguay, a group of researchers provided study information and protocol aloud with translators, for which consent was received through audiovisual documentation. This process was determined to be largely successful, as it allowed participants to express refusal, which may not have been possible with traditional written informed consent (Benitez et al., 2002). In these instances, consent should be received in the native tongue, not in the presence of armed guards, and translators should understand subjects are permitted to not provide consent (MSF, n.d.). This works to remove a power imbalance present in many low-income settings, as people being photographed do not feel free to refuse in these scenarios (Devakumar et al., 2013).

In other instances, individuals may not be able to provide consent given their current state (e.g. mentally ill or in distress). In these instances, a family member or caregiver can step in and act as a power of attorney to provide consent to you (MSF, n.d.).

However, while receiving consent is thought to be for the protection of identity, the primary reason is for the right of the individual to choose and to equal dignity (Macintosh, 2006). This fundamental right to informed consent is expressed in Articles 1, 5 and 12 of the *Universal Declaration of Human Rights*. Therefore, receiving informed consent is seen as crucial, as many experts advise to focusing efforts on receiving consent of individuals photographed , rather than on trying to achieve anonymity (Taub, 2001).

Upon completion of photography, you are strongly advised against giving photographed subjects financial or other gifts as compensation (MSF, n.d.; AusAID, 2012). Instead, ensure that the names of photographed subjects are recorded or written with relevant history (Partners in Health, 2013) and if possible, show the photographed image to the person captured (University of Toronto, 2016).

After Technology Use

Because, as discussed above, every effort should have been made to receive informed consent of individuals photographed, photos that may unveil the identity of individuals are omitted if there is no consent (Macintosh, 2006). For instances where consent was not received but the image is essential, you should remove identifiable aspects of the image (Macintosh, 2006). This also applies when photographing individuals at-risk, such as human immunodeficiency virus (HIV)-positive children or children charged with or convicted of a crime, the identity should be protected (United Nations Children's Fund [UNICEF] Guyana, n.d.). While widely used, a black bar to cover the eyes of the individual is not effective, as the individual is still recognizable to friends and family (Slue, 1989) and can connote criminality (UNICEF Guyana, n.d.). Alternatively, digital editing may be utilized to alter identifiable factors from images (Pallen and Loman, 1998) but with caution, as some consider it ineffective (Welsby, 1998).

Because photographs in global health seek to capture images that differ from the 'norm', what is visible in a photograph is only superficial and fails to allow for a deeper understanding of the complexities of the human subject (Macintosh, 2006). Therefore, ensure photographs intended to highlight subjects 'before' treatment are featured alongside those of 'after treatment' (Partners in Health, 2013). Many times, a caption is provided to assist the viewer in understanding the action(s) occurring while the photograph was shot – in fact, images are more compelling when they tell stories (UNICEF Guyana, n.d.). However, by providing a photographer-written caption, the agency is removed from the individual photographed (Powerful Images event, personal communication, June 28, 2016). This can result in gross misunderstandings and negative judgments about people and their societies (Powerful Images event, personal communication, June 28, 2016). An example of this was an image of a breastfeeding mother in South America featured in a magazine. While the image is of a natural occurrence, the description and backstory provided resulted in viewers misconstruing the event (Powerful Images event, personal communication, June 28, 2016). To overcome this, you should fact check written narratives and captions with the individual photographed.

This can also be problematic if you share photographs with a caption or narrative on blogs or social media through platforms such as Facebook, Instagram and LinkedIn. While some may argue social media would bring this content to the masses, which may not otherwise be received, it is advised you receive informed consent to share on any platform, including social media. However, in the instance that informed consent cannot be attained, there may be instances where image sharing on social media is acceptable. For example, sharing an image of an unusual spider bite on a tropical medicine page that is utilized by healthcare clinicians to determine an appropriate treatment. However, even in this instance, there are other preferred options than sharing to social media (Palacios-González, 2014).

Because each social media platform has developed unique terms of use and privacy settings, there is a risk that content initially uploaded intending to be private ends up in a public domain. For example, Facebook's terms of use state the company possesses permission to share a user's content, such as photos or videos, if the privacy settings allow it. Specifically, subject to your Facebook settings, you grant Facebook, '[...] a non-exclusive, transferable, sub-licensable, royalty-free, worldwide license to use any IP content that you post on or in connection with Facebook (IP License)' (Statement of Rights and Responsibilities, 2015).

If content intended to be private becomes public, such as when another individual 'shares' a Facebook post, it risks damaging relationships formed with partners or colleagues. This is particularly problematic for Facebook posts, as they are instantly shared, often as an instant reaction of the author without editing. Therefore, it is advisable to avoid posting to social media (consider taking a 'social media holiday') and ensure appropriate steps are taken to treat photographs like data to protect their storage and use. However, if desired, it is crucial to receive informed consent with the intended use of photos on social media platforms and clearly state possible risks. An alternative to posting on social media is to express your thoughts in a personal journal.

When you return from a global health opportunity abroad, you may be asked to give a presentation at your home institution. Consideration should be given to the images used and whether or not consent was received. Images presented should not be used to exploit poverty and should never be used to evoke shock or pity (Partners in Health, 2013). Additionally, you should ensure the content is not seen as being on behalf of your institution, but rather, yourself. This can be accomplished by adding a disclaimer, such as 'the views expressed are my own and do not represent those of my institution'.

A final review of the medium in which the photos are being presented in, is recommended to ensure the message portrayed is accurate and provides subjects with agency, privacy and dignity. Ensure the best interests of the subject are put before any other considerations, such as advocacy or promotion of rights (UNICEF, 2005). If you have any doubt regarding putting the subject at risk, report on the situation rather than a specific individual (UNICEF, 2005) or reach out to the individual subject(s) of photographs to ask for a review of image and associated commentary. If contact is maintained, provide a copy of the document or a link for the individual subject to access the photograph(s) (University of Toronto, 2016). Exercise judgment when sharing content, for example you should ensure it is accurately depicted, as it will likely be difficult to remove in its entirety once online and respects patient privacy and dignity.

Problems and Pitfalls

As briefly alluded to above, while technology in global health can lead to tremendous positive impacts, for example, to mobilize individuals into action for social change and by increasing professional networking and education, there are also potential pitfalls.

The distribution of inaccurate or poor quality information can pose risks to both patients and providers, which include: damage to professional images, breaches of confidentiality and violation of personal–professional boundaries (Ventola, 2014).

You should pay particular attention to social media, given its widespread use and possible misunderstandings of terms of use. Numerous individuals have faced repercussions for posting images on social media platforms in poor professional taste and without patient consent. Prominent cases include those of a Swedish nurse posting an image of a brain surgery to her Facebook page in 2008 (Salter, 2008) and four nursing students posting an image with a patient's placenta in 2011 (Gibson, 2011). Less drastically, many individuals are engaging in 'voluntourism' and posting images of global humanitarian work online to social media platforms – typically, portraying images such as a white individual hugging an orphaned child from a developing nation. Questions have risen about the impacts these images have, as they can further perpetuate judgments by those developing societies and engrain norms by people in developing nations. Two individuals have sought to raise awareness of this issue by developing a satirical 'Barbie Saviour' Instagram page to poke fun and spark debates, discussions and resolutions (Murphy, 2016).

Recommendations

Many individuals in global health are flocking to Africa, in part, due to the lack of ethical guidelines and regulations on research (Macintosh, 2006). It is recommended to apply the principles and strategies put forth in this chapter to work in not just Africa, but abroad.

While ideally, a standardized framework of global guidelines that could be tailored to each unique setting would be developed, this does not currently exist (Macintosh, 2006). Therefore, it is up to the photographer to strive to achieve a high standard of best practice:

- To fight to collect voluntary informed consent from all photographed individuals
- To work collaboratively to negotiate terms of inclusion with those photographed to guarantee they have a stake in the results (Macintosh, 2006)
- To give agency and human dignity back to those photographed and remove breaches of privacy and exploitation

Summary

Current considerations of technology use in global health are summarized in Table 6.1.

Table 6.1   Current Considerations of Technology: (1) Before Departure, (2) Before and During Technology Use and (3) After Technology Use

Before Departure	*Before and During Technology Use*	*After Technology Use*
• Reflection on organization's worldview • Do you support it? • Considerations of how the individual's voice can be captured in photos depicting societal problems	• Be transparent about your role • Editorial or NGO, etc. • Ensure voluntary informed consent or refusal • Ideally, written consent • If not, employ other methods, such as audiovisual documentation for consent • Relay understanding of potential for misuse and wider spread	• Remove individual identifiers • Black bar technique not advised • Digital editing to be used with caution • Stray away from providing captions to photographs to ensure subject's agency • Avoid sharing on social media, instead opt for a personal journal • However, if social media is desired, ensure informed consent is received before posting • Conduct a final review of the medium in which the photo is being presented to ensure accuracy, agency, privacy and dignity

References

AusAID. (2012, August). AusAID ethical photography guidelines. Retrieved from: http://social-media-for-development.org/wp-content/uploads/2014/10/ethical-photography-guidelines.pdf

Benitez, O., Devaux, D., and Dausset, J. (2002). Audiovisual documentation of oral consent: A new method of informed consent for illiterate populations. *Lancet, 359*: 1406–1407.

Berle, I. (2002). The ethical context of clinical photography. *Journal of Audiovisual Media in Medicine, 25*: 106–109.

Calain, P. (2013). Ethics and images of suffering bodies in humanitarian medicine. *Social Science and Medicine, 98*: 278–285.

Devakumar, D., Brotherton, H., Halbert, J., Clarke, A., Prost, A., and Hall, J. (2013). Taking ethical photos of children for medical and research purposes in low-resource settings: An exploratory qualitative study. *BMC Medical Ethics, 14*(1): 27.

Dysmorphology Subcommittee of the Clinical Practice Committee. (2000). American College of Medical Genetics. Informed Consent for Medical Photographs. Dysmorphology Subcommittee of the Clinical Practice Committee, American College of Medical Genetics. *Genetics in Medicine, 2*: 353–355.

Estrin, J. (2012, November 19). When Interest Creates a Conflict. *The New York Times.* Retrieved from: http://mobile.nytimes.com/blogs/lens/2012/11/19/when-interest-creates-a-conflict/?referer=

Gibson, M. J. (2011, April 1). Nursing Students Expelled for Posting Photo of a Placenta on Facebook. *Time.* Retrieved from: http://newsfeed.time.com/2011/01/04/nursing-students-expelled-for-posting-photo-of-a-placenta-on-facebook/

Lagu, T., and Greysen, S. R. (2011). Physician, monitor thyself: Professionalism and accountability in the use of social media. *The Journal of Clinical Ethics, 22*(2): 187–190.

Macintosh, T. (2006). Ethical considerations for clinical photography in the global south. *Developing World Bioethics, 6*: 81–88. doi:10.1111/j.1471-8847.2006.00142.x

Médecins Sans Frontières (MSF). (n.d.). Photographer guidelines. Retrieved from: http://www.msf.org.uk/sites/uk/files/ethics_photographers_200809231432.pdf

Murphy, T. (2016, April 27). Barbie Savior: The Parody That Makes Aid Types Feel Good, But Does Nothing. *Humanosphere.* Retrieved from: http://www.humanosphere.org/opinion/2016/04/barbie-savior-the-parody-that-makes-aid-types-feel-good-but-does-nothing/

Palacios-González, C. (2014, July 10). The ethics of clinical photography and social media. *Medicine, Health Care and Philosophy, 18*: 63–70.

Pallen, M., and Loman, N. (1998). Videos, photographs and patients consent: Medical educationalists can free themselves from constraints of 'real world' images. *British Medical Journal, 317*: 1522.

Partners in Health. (2013, August). Visual Identity Guidelines. Retrieved from: http://docplayer.net/8347806-Partners-in-health-visual-identity-guidelines-08-13.html

Pedersen, P. (1995). *The Five Stages of Culture Shock: Critical Incidents Around the World. Contributions in Psychology, No. 25.* Westport, CT: Greenwood Press.

Salter, B.J. (2008, August 19). Nurses Posts Brain Surgery Pictures on Facebook. *Telegraph.co.uk.* Retrieved from: http://www.telegraph.co.uk/news/uknews/2583411/Nurses-posts-brain-surgery-pictures-on-Facebook.html

Slue, W.E. (1989). Unmasking the lone ranger. *New England Journal of Medicine, 321*: 550–551.

Statement of Rights and Responsibilities. (2015, January 30). *Facebook.* Retrieved from: https://www.facebook.com/terms

Taub, S. (2001, April). Images of healing and learning. *Virtual Mentor.* Retrieved from: http://journalofethics.ama-assn.org/2001/04/imhl1-0104.html

United Nations Children's Fund (UNICEF). (2005). *Ethical Guidelines*, Second Edition. Retrieved from: http://www.unicef.org/ceecis/media_1482.htm

United Nations Children's Fund (UNICEF) Guyana. (n.d.). Section 2, UNICEF Photography Guidelines. Retrieved from: https://www.google.ca/url?sa=t&rct=j&q=&esrc=s&source=web&cd=1&cad=rja&uact=8&ved=0ahUKEwjmkd2Xh7bOAhVOlxQKHdR2BwEQFggcMAA&url=http%3A%2F%2Fwww.unicef.org%2Fguyana%2FTOR_Photography_Consultant_Fin(2).doc&usg=AFQjCNF_whhTdEflawErokc7N1ZuaReYfw&sig2=3Hq-yE8TnkqNlHxhespm4Q&bvm=bv.129389765,d.d24

University of Toronto, International Centre for Disability and Rehabilitation. (2016). Guidelines for Ethical Photography. Retrieved from: http://icdr.utoronto.ca/wp-content/uploads/2016/01/ICDR-Ethical-Photography-Guidelines.pdf

Ventola, C. L. (2014). Social media and health care professionals: Benefits, risks, and best practices. *Pharmacy and Therapeutics, 39*(7): 491–520.

Welsby, P. D. (1998, November 28). Digital disguising techniques need to be improved. *British Medical Journal, 317*(7171): 1522.

Chapter 7

Preparing to Go Abroad

Kevin Chan and Neil Arya

Contents

Introduction

An ideal global health experience doesn't just happen overnight. Planning a global health experience requires planning and thought. In this chapter, we outline what steps need to be thought through, what actions you need to take going abroad and what are the key things not to miss before you go on that global health journey!

Plan Well in Advance

Depending on the complexity of the global health experience, it may take up to 2 years in advance to contact a project coordinator/supervisor, process documentation for the country of elective, obtain a visa and immunizations, register for a license, secure lodging, arrange funds, approach sponsoring agencies and plan your trip abroad. Have you given yourself enough time to organize the project and given enough preparation time prior to going abroad?

Contacting a Potential Elective Supervisor

Is there a department chair in charge of a teaching program or a doctor you specifically want to work with? Send an e-mail, post a letter, fax or make a telephone call early (at least 4 months in advance). Ideally, you want to establish first contact as early as possible, to give everyone plenty of notice of your arrival. It's not uncommon to find out about last-minute paperwork that needs to be completed by your host institution, so international delivery times need to be accounted for. Don't be surprised if you need to use all four forms of contact to finally get in touch with the person and be cognizant of whether delays on reply times will become a problem later down the road. If you need something from your contact person quickly, for example 1 week before you leave, is this going to be an issue?

In conjunction with your hosts abroad, it's also important to clarify your responsibilities prior to arriving. Often, if this is not clarified, there is a period of confusion and difficulty with integration into the project/program/elective. Furthermore, you do want to identify what your skills, learning objectives and supervisory needs entail.

In your introductory letter

- Introduce yourself, what school you're from and all other vital information.
- Provide some explanation of what your level of training entails – for example, many parts of the world have 5- to 7-year medical programs beginning after high school versus the North American norm of 4 years after an undergraduate degree. Describe any previous clinical experiences, procedures, and so on. Be specific about your knowledge level, being conscientious of under/over-representing yourself and notifying your supervisors that you will not be doing procedures with less supervision than you would be allowed in Canada or than local trainees get.
- State your objectives very specifically. Explicitly state what you want to accomplish from your elective time and what skills you need to acquire. If your objective is to have your own patients and present your findings to a supervisor for a quick check before discharge, then say that. If you want to be first-assist on surgeries and learn how to do procedures independently by the end of your summer, say that too!

Who Is My Contact Person?

- **Establish your contact person** and determine what role(s) they will play. Find out who you can communicate with to get your questions answered; what sorts of help that person will be able to give you in general; how you will arrange transportation, accommodations, orientation to setting; and what you have to do yourself. Who can be your 'go-to' person? What are the administrative costs and any letters required from the university?
- **After finalizing your location,** look into airline tickets, visas and insurance early. Learn about price fluctuations, cancellation, travel medical and personal loss insurance (i.e. baggage, valuables). Find out if you need a visa and how to obtain one, whether it is available at the airport and how much time it takes (it may take weeks and leave you without a passport for some time).

Before leaving, it's important to make sure all your key documents are in place and that you register with the relevant government agency, consulate or embassy abroad. To travel outside the country, a passport is required, and it must be valid for 6 months beyond your proposed travel dates. Other key documents include any required travel or work/education visas and permits. These may require consultation well ahead of time and coordination with your host partners. Having spare passport photos is a good idea, as sometimes these are required for the visa acquired on entry. In some countries, you may need to register with the appropriate medical licensing body. This could take time and require communication and coordination with the organization in the host country. Making sure you are aware of which documents are required for a license, months in advance, may be critical.

Continue contact every 2–3 weeks. Finalize your accommodations. Determine modes of communication with your family (e.g. stock up on phone cards) and learn the logistics hospital/clinic life, water supply, question of political instability (elections, violence, foreigners), possible advance readings and possible local student contacts.

Risk Management Forms and Objective Approval Forms

Institutions now ask students or personnel to fill out health self-assessments, risk assessment and management packages, statements of responsibility, releases and identification of insurance policy forms. A faculty advisor and institutional person may need to approve the assessment and to sign off on your objectives form. You may also need to sign a waiver and an agreement of responsible conduct.

Logistics

Depending on the length of your time away from home, you may want to arrange for someone to file your income tax for you on your behalf if you will be away during the month of April. You may also want to arrange a Power of Attorney for someone you trust to carry out your banking and legal matters in your absence.

Make two photocopies of your passport (and other important documents). Leave one with a responsible friend or family member at home; carry the second copy separately from your passport.

Visit a travel clinic as soon as possible – refer to Centers for Disease Control and Prevention: Traveler's Health or Health Canada Travel Medicine Program C for more information. Vaccinations and the physician's visits may not be covered by your insurer. Check the Centers for Disease Control and Prevention, World Health Organization (WHO) and other guidelines for recommendations for the location you plan to visit. HIV prophylaxis kits may be valuable. Check local availability or plan to take your own. Attend pre-departure sessions if available or mandatory.

Packing List

There are many different things that you may want to bring abroad. Often, though, many supplies can be bought in your host country.

A unique thing to bring is a portable printer. You could take pictures with a phone or camera and print the pictures immediately to give to families. It's amazing how much joy a photo can bring to people, especially in rural areas in resource-poor countries.

Sometimes, you may need to bring specific equipment and supplies to carry out your project. If there is a lot of equipment, it is useful to communicate with your airline ahead of time, to see if they will waive some of the carriage costs for your work. Remember, some of your supplies may need special conditions such as refrigeration and planning ahead of time is required.

Donating equipment and supplies that you don't need at home may be useful to your hosts, but more often, it is not. Without proper maintenance and the appropriate electrical supplies, the equipment may be headed to the dump. Stories abound of abandoned equipment in the corridors of hospitals abroad. Have a conversation with your hosts, before you take equipment and supplies abroad. When your hosts request specific equipment and supplies, try and accommodate, if it's reasonable and feasible. Do not bring expired medicines or unsolicited donations of discarded equipment or clothing.

Packing considerations: pack light! Donations/medical supplies: *only* take these if requested/discussed ahead of time. Pack your letter of invitation and list of contents (Table 7.1). Avoid packing unnecessary items which might be stolen: Do you need your computer, jewellery, watches, camera, iPod, BlackBerry and large sums of cash?

Planning Travel

Travel may be booked through websites offering the best deals. However, travel agents may be more helpful with advice on specific travel routes or more complicated itineraries. It's helpful to share your travel itinerary with your hosts abroad well before departing and also provide them with communication contact numbers upon arriving. Adjusting to a new culture and to jet lag are real considerations. Ensure you have enough time.

Health Insurance

It is important to understand health insurance. Some policies from academic institutions may not cover you when you are on personal leave, even during an elective/practicum.

Read the fine print in your policy, especially regarding pre-existing conditions which do need to be declared. Also, look at riders that deduct your lifetime extended coverage amounts if you already have group insurance and are buying independent supplementary insurance, something known as a 'first payer' clause. For this reason, it may be better to extend your current group or individually held insurance, rather than buying supplemental insurance. If you are planning on undertaking mountaineering, diving or doing extreme sports, for example, but especially before or after, your elective, make sure your insurance company knows and that your policy covers you in such accidents. Finally, make sure you are comfortable with your insurance policy's repatriation clauses.

In Ontario, for example, if you will be out of the country for more than 7 months, you must notify the Ontario Ministry of Health. You would need to go to your local Ontario Health Insurance Plan (OHIP) office in person and show them documentation that proves you will be travelling abroad and list the dates of your placement abroad term.

Malpractice insurance: *Check with your sending institution for what is required and what coverage they provide.*

Communications

There are many ways to communicate with home today compared to even 15 years ago. Communication by cellular phone is significantly easier and cheaper, as well as texting, WhatsApp, Skype/g-chat and e-mail communications. Often, you need to purchase a SIM card and ensure that your phone is unlocked to allow for communication back home. Otherwise, prior to going abroad, discuss with your cellular company about having global access, that allows access to cellular towers in your host country.

Table 7.1 Packing List

Documents	Travel Equipment
• Airline tickets • Business cards • Cash (local, U.S.$)/travellers cheques • Credit cards/debit cards • Driver's license (international if required) • Immunization records • Itinerary • Medical license (including local license) • Money belt • Passport + additional copies • Personal travel form • Visa (if applicable, for country) • Your emergency contact card *Note:* Make sure that your passport is valid for at least 1 month after your planned return date. Some countries require passports to be valid for longer, even 6 months. The address and phone number of the Canadian or U.S. embassy/consulate that will be nearest to you.	• Adapters/converters (know the voltage!) • Air mattress • Backpack/suitcase • Cooking equipment • Day pack • Ear plugs/ear phones • Flashlight/headlamp • Garbage bags/ziploc bags • Linens • Phone (international-open) • Pillows • Sleeping bag/blankets • Tent • Umbrella • Watch/travel alarm • Water filter/iodine tablets
Clothes	Medications/Health
• Dresses/skirts/sarongs • Hat/cap • Jackets/coats (rain) • Jeans/pants/slacks • Pajamas • Scrubs, if worn at site • Shirts (long-/short-sleeve), formal clothing (shirt ± tie for men, skirts for women) • Shorts • Socks • Sweaters/sweatshirts • Swimsuits • T-shirts • Underwear • Walking shoes/sandals • Warm clothes if cold	• Acetaminophen/Ibuprofen • Antibiotic ointment • Antibiotics, antifungals • Antihistamines • Antimalarials • Band-aids/gauze • Cold/flu medication • First aid kit • HIV post-exposure prophylaxis • Hydrocortisone cream • Laxative • Loperamide • Mosquito coils/repellent • Mosquito net • Motion sickness pills – Gravol • Oral rehydration salts • Personal medical supplies, birth-control pills and prescription medications (in their original containers) • Thermometer

(Continued)

Table 7.1 (*Continued*) Packing List

Personal Items	Miscellaneous
• Batteries • Clothes pegs/laundry detergent/scrub brush • Condoms/contraceptives • Contact lenses and solution • Deodorant • Feminine hygiene products • Glasses/sunglasses • Hair clips, bands • Hairbrush/comb • Hand sanitizer • Kleenex • Lip balm • Lotion/powder • Mirror (small) • Nail clipper • Needles/sewing kit • Razors • Shampoo/conditioner • Soap • Sunscreen • Toilet paper • Toothbrush/toothpaste/floss • Towel • Tweezers	• Binoculars • Books/textbooks/iPad • Calculator • Camera and camera cards • Candy/food snacks, drink crystals, dehydrated • Computer/computer files • Donated supplies (with a letter of request from host site and a letter of permission from local government, if needed) • Elastic bands • Games/playing cards • Gifts for hosts and thank you cards • Map guides/language book • Money belt • MP3/iPod • Pictures/postcards/books from home • Portable printer • Project materials • Radio (short-wave) • Rope • Surge protector • Swiss army knife • Tape (duct, electrical) • Writing material (journals, pens) • Ziploc bags
Medical Equipment	Other
For the wards: Stethoscope, penlight, lab coat Small notebook, medical handbooks: *Lonely Planet, Where There Is No Doctor, Oxford Handbook of Tropical Medicine, Pocket Internal Medicine* formularies Teaching resources to share Consider (thermometer, reflex hammer, otoscope/ophthalmoscope, portable BP cuff, code cards, gloves sterile/non-sterile, tongue blades, fitted TB N 95 mask if appropriate or disposable masks, hand sanitizer) Phrase book	• _____ • _____ • _____ • _____ • _____ • _____ • _____ • _____ • _____ • _____ • _____ • _____ • _____ • _____

Note: This is not meant to be an all-inclusive or exhaustive list, and depending on context many of these may be unnecessary. It should be used as a guide only.

Source: Drain P et al., *Caring for the World*, University of Toronto Press, Toronto, 2009. With permission.

Orientation

Both pre-travel and in-country orientations ought to be major components of projects/programs/ electives geared towards personnel travelling abroad. Possibilities include

1. Longitudinally (throughout the year): With faculty and past participants with global health experience and diaspora from your host country.
2. Concentrated orientation (over 2 weeks or a weekend): Also with faculty and past participants.
3. Guides and orientation manuals with planning work exploring culture, customs, social, economic and political landscapes and some language training.
4. Global health courses, online orientation modules and podcasts that help broaden the global health knowledge base and provide some basic learning before travelling abroad.
5. In-country: Often, a fun activity prior to starting a project/program helps ease jet lag and helps you to get accustomed to the culture and the habits of your host country. Ideally, if you can get a local to help you orient abroad, it's immensely useful. It may involve some time in a country's capital, largest city or some tourism.
6. Learning some of the basic cultures and customs could go a long way in paying proper respect to your hosts. Gaining some prior knowledge about the community can often help foster respect and partnerships, and hopefully, friendships.

If you do not speak the local language, you may require translators to help you communicate with patients (and sometimes, colleagues/supervisors). Clarifying what is required ahead of time is helpful. Be mindful that the time it takes to provide interpretation for you may be taking them away from their own work. Don't make assumptions about who will be available to translate and try to ascertain how this will happen in advance. It's helpful to try and learn a little of the local language ahead of time. Often, a few key phrases go a long way in opening doors and spreading goodwill.

Part of the orientation should also focus on the logistics – who are your key partners, where are you staying, how are you getting there and what things you should bring abroad. Even seasoned global health professionals should spend some time orienting to a new locale (Tables 7.2 through 7.5).

Table 7.2   Twenty-Five Questions to Orient Yourself

1. How many prominent individuals, historical figures and politicians can you name from your host country?
2. What are the official languages of your host country? What are the social and political implications of these languages?
3. What are the major religions in your country? Is there an official state religion? What are the official dates of observance and/or ceremonies? Do people participate in them regularly?
4. What things are taboo in the society?
5. What is the official position of the state on HIV/AIDS? Does the community stigmatize people with HIV/AIDS?
6. What is the official position of the state on adultery? Polygamy? Homosexuality? Divorce?
7. What is the attitude towards drinking and smoking?
8. What are the major food types and dishes in this area?

(Continued)

Table 7.2 (*Continued*)   Twenty-Five Questions to Orient Yourself

9. If you're in the market, is the labelled price the final sale price or can you barter for a better price? If so, how is a sale concluded?
10. If you're invited for dinner, should you arrive early? On time? Or late?
11. Do you need to bring gifts for dinner?
12. How do people greet one another? And how do they leave one another?
13. What leisure activities are there?
14. What is a normal work schedule?
15. How many children do people have on average? What games do children play?
16. How are children disciplined? Are they expected to be part of social events?
17. How are children recognized as turning into adults?
18. What kind of local transportation is available?
19. What is the history of the relationship between the host country and the United States or Canada?
20. Is military training compulsory? Male/female? At what age and how long?
21. What health services are available? Where would the nearest location be?
22. What 'home treatments' are available for various diseases?
23. Is education free? Is education compulsory?
24. In school, how important is learning by rote? Are there libraries? Books? Science labs? Sports equipment? Equal number of boys and girls? Do children drop out?
25. How does your wealth compare with that of the majority of people in this society?

Source: Drain P et al., *Caring for the World*, University of Toronto Press, Toronto, 2009. With permission.

Table 7.3   Timelines

12–18 Months before Departure

• Explore opportunities
   • Look at timing of travel and funding opportunities
   • Look at type of work, language requirements and supervision
   • Find an advisor, mentor and/or former travellers for their experience

9–12 Months before Departure

• Finalize home country-based mentor
• Finalize site of travel
• Note key deadlines
   • Visa
   • Medical license/work permit
   • Passport
   • Key forms/elective materials

(*Continued*)

Table 7.3 (*Continued*) **Timelines**

9–12 Months before Departure
• Write out key goals and objectives • Consider language training • Converse with your host status • Begin orientation
6–9 Months before Departure
• Finalize housing and daily transport arrangements • Apply for travel visa and medical license/work permit • Make sure passport is up to date • Visit travel clinic • Check for any travel advisories or warnings • Determine what equipment and supplies are required • Identify any needs/requirements at your host site • Continue with orientation
3–6 Months before Departure
• Identify your specific responsibilities and projects at host site • Purchase airline tickets and domestic transport • Obtain travel/medical/evacuation/baggage insurance • Obtain an international driver's license, if driving • Review packing list • Look at phone coverage abroad (SIM card abroad or global access from home) • Identify on-site translators • Ensure all paperwork sent • Continue with orientation
2–3 Months before Departure
• Confirm logistics – accommodation and travel plans • List emergency contacts • Scan passport, plane tickets, insurance, medical license • Continue with orientation
1–2 Months before Departure
• Register with Foreign Affairs (Canada) or the State Department (United States) • Obtain any necessary medication • Go to bank for cash (a mixture of large and small U.S. dominations) • Schedule debriefing upon return • Check for any travel advisories or warnings
Last Month before Departure
• Arrange home care issues • Pack if possible • Confirm emergency contacts • Confirm arrival with host institution • Print or download any clinical resources • Start malaria prophylaxis • Call credit card companies to identify your travel

(Continued)

Table 7.3 (*Continued*)   Timelines

• Reconfirm your hotel, flight arrangements and contact info prior to departure.
• Provide a friend, family member or contact at the university with a copy of your itinerary and inform them of changes while you are away. • Ensure arrangements for how you can obtain additional funds if needed
Abroad
• Have time for in-country orientation • Make sure you thank your hosts and provide feedback • Have adequate time for return
Upon Return
• Rest and reflect on your experience, complete evaluation forms • Debrief with your advisor/mentor/friend • Disseminate information and provide feedback • Obtain purified protein derivative (PPD) (tuberculosis [TB] test) 3 months after you return • If required, see travel clinic if any concerns

Table 7.4   Travel Info List

Personal Name: _____ Address: _____ _____ _____ Phone #: _____ E-mail: _____ Passport number: _____ Expiry date: _____
Emergency contact
Family doctor Contact:
Host contact Address: _____ _____ _____ Phone #: _____ E-mail: _____
Medical issues **Medications with dosages** **Allergies**
Flight info
Travel insurance **Credit card** **Travellers cheques**
Name: _____ Phone #: _____ Policy #: _____

Table 7.5   Resource List

• **USAID Global Health eLearning Center**
  • http://www.globalhealthlearning.org/login.cfm
    • Self-directed learning modules in global health in a wide range of topics
    • Provides opportunities for self-assessment with quizzes
    • Earn 'certificates' for completing modules

• **Action Global Health Network**
  • http://www.actionglobalhealth.com/education/
    • Set of web-based learning modules of relevance to pre-departure preparation and also variety of topics in global health

• **Global Health eLearning modules**
  • http://ccirhken.ca/eLearning/Welcome.html
    • Global health modules based on CanMeds roles

• **Global Health Education Consortium**
  • https://www.cugh.org/resources/educational-modules
    • A very complete collection of PowerPoint presentations on an extensive number of global health topics

• **University of Minnesota Tropical and Travel Medicine Seminar Series 2012**
  • http://www.globalhealth.umn.edu/residenttraining/curriculum/tropicaltravelseries/home.html
    • A collection of various online modules and courses about global health topics

• **Johns Hopkins Center for Global Health – Travel Resources**   • A collection of links for various resources in global health

• **Centers for Disease Control and Prevention (CDC) Yellow Book for Travel Medicine**
  • http://wwwnc.cdc.gov/travel/yellowbook/2016/table-of-contents
  • Various topics in tropical medicine and health – this resource is particularly useful for preparing oneself for health concerns in specific areas of the world

• **Medecins sans Frontieres (MSF) Reference Books**
  • http://www.refbooks.msf.org/msf_docs/en/MSFdocMenu_en.htm
    • A free collection of PDF books. Titles include *Rapid Health Assessment of Refugee or Displaced Populations*, *Clinical Guidelines* and *Obstetrics in Remote Settings*

• **WHO e-Book International Travel and Health**
  • http://apps.who.int/bookorders/anglais/detart1.jsp?codlan=1&codcol=80&codcch=79
    • An electronic copy of this document can be purchased for $10. 'This book explains how travellers can stay healthy and provides WHO guidance on vaccinations, malaria chemoprophylaxis and treatment, personal protection against insects and other disease vectors and safety in different environmental settings. It covers all the principal risks to travellers' health, both during their journeys and at their destinations. It describes all relevant infectious diseases, including their causative agents, modes of transmission, clinical features and geographical distribution and provides details of prophylactic and preventive measures'.

Reference

Drain P, Huffman S, Pirtle S, Chan K. Table 8.1: 25 Questions to orientate yourself. In *Caring for the World*. Toronto, Canada: University of Toronto Press, 2009.

ASPECTS OF PRE-DEPARTURE PREPARATION

Chapter 8

Staying Safe While Abroad

David Ponka and Alison Eyre

Contents

Introduction

Guiding students about personal safety is challenging. First, what one individual considers safe may be foolishly perilous to another. Second, safety considerations are very contextual, and so we will limit our comments to general principles and a few representative cases. Specific safety guidelines and protocols of sponsoring organizations should always be followed. Instead of replacing these, we hope to provide resources and illustrative vignettes to help the learner during an independent project: indeed, travelling without the relative protection of a larger organization – still the reality for most educational electives – makes these considerations even more important.

Going overseas on an elective is a great time to learn in a new environment. Since electives are often not more than a month or two, it is important to stay safe to get the maximum experience. The good news is that overseas medical electives generally proceed without incident; however, accidents and the unexpected can happen. Road accidents present by far the greatest risk to the overseas traveller (Iverson, 2014). We will discuss this further below, but first, let us present some overarching concepts to help you stay safe.

1. **Orient yourself to your new locale.** Have your address and your contacts address on you at all times. Identify where the hospital is, where the police station is and whom you would talk to if your health or safety becomes at risk. Be sure that you know what numbers to call if you need to use your insurance. Have these in a place that you could direct someone to access if you are not able to. When you are in a precarious situation, it is not the time to start thinking of whom you could reach out to for help. Anticipatory planning is always a good idea: make sure that you have a copy of essential documents, travel itineraries, financial information and insurance. It is a good practice to scan these, e-mail them to yourself and a contact back home.

2. **Orient yourself to the local customs and culture.** We cannot emphasize this point enough: your best protection to stay safe, just like staying healthy, is to research local conditions on the ground. Make sure that you do not stand out more than you have to.

3. **Practice 'situational awareness' (Personal Safety Group, 2015): If you feel unsafe, just like when you start feeling ill, always let someone know.** Odd though it may be, healthcare workers are not good at reaching out for help when we are unwell, and perhaps because of this same sense of pride, when we fear for our safety as well. This puts us at accrued risk.

4. **Have responses ready for the unexpected.** For example, if something does not seem right, be politely inquisitive, such as 'I am sorry, I am not from here, can you please explain . . ..' If a driver is going too fast, consider feigning illness: it is OK to say 'I am very sorry, but I get terribly carsick when cars go fast. Is there any way we could go a bit more slowly?' Your safety is the most important. People are more likely to change their behaviour to help you because you think they are doing something wrong. They also do not want people to throw up in their car!

Understanding Risk and Risk Taking

Preparing yourself for travel to work in an unfamiliar locale, as any other major life decision, is all about trying to mitigate risk. There are risks to all of our everyday activities, just as there are risks in travelling. Quantifying these risks may help some, but ultimately making a decision about travelling, let alone travelling for work (with longer stays and thus accrued risk) is a very subjective decision (Shlim, 2016).

Understanding your own risk tolerance is an important part of understanding how you travel. For this elective, have you chosen to go to a similar society to your own or have you chosen to go to a place such as a remote rural community or a country where the realities make the risk of daily life higher? Each of these experiences carries different learning and growth potential as well as different levels of risk.

It is interesting to use a survey tool such as the one presented at the end of this chapter (see Box 8.4) to better understand your risk tolerance, and thus to make more informed decisions. Consider completing the online survey presented now to make the following sections more useful for you.

Understanding your risk tolerance can help you to stay safe: it is a major part of maintaining your 'situational awareness'. It is also important to understand that your risk tolerance can change or shift with time, and according to your stage of life. What may have been acceptable to you as a student may no longer be so with a partner, or as a parent (see more under the section 'Specific Considerations').

BOX 8.1   WHAT WE KNOW ABOUT GROUPTHINK

There are three dangerous patterns of thinking while assessing safety when in a group.

1. Being unduly influenced by the opinions of those close to us, dismissing any evidence to the contrary.
2. Blindly trusting the leader, regardless of his/her experience, despite any internal misgivings.
3. Being influenced by other groups. We may think 'someone has gone ahead or been here before us, so it must be fine'.

(Adapted from some of the literature on 'Groupthink'.) (Northwestern University, 2012.)

It is also important to note that as medical volunteers, we tend to be slow to ask for help. As supervisors, we have also seen visiting students display some dependency, on the other extreme. However, we are more concerned about stories where visitors become unwell or disoriented without telling anyone. In one case, an exchange health worker was in advanced stages of renal failure from acute malaria, but did not inform anyone on the ground, only reaching out to colleagues back home who assumed he was getting all the help available. Local staff became concerned after several days of his absence, and was able to locate the visitor only after calling his home university. Thankfully, he recovered fully, and he also prompted several new standard protocols.

Another pattern that is quite human is to become more complacent as the medical elective proceeds, especially over a longer period. If you are going to be in country for months, one or two days with diarrhoea may not ruin the experience. However, activities that put you at risk of serious accidents – road accidents and the like – will at best put an end to any elective experience and at worst, leave you seriously hurt, or worse (Box 8.1).

One of the hardest truths of an international learning experience is that the experience may not turn out to be what you expected. The level of supervision may be different, the patient volume or what you can or cannot participate in may not be what you anticipated. The team may not be a functioning team. When you have spent a lot of time and money to prepare for an experience, these kinds of disappointment can be hard to cope with. They challenge your flexibility and resilience.

A positive attitude is important in these situations. Review what were the global goals for the elective and see if there is a different way to achieve them: you may surprise yourself and build your leadership skills, so critical for a career in global health.

Being Prepared for the Worst

As mentioned, the single most important step in making a safety plan for yourself (see Box. 8.2) while overseas is to research the destination. This is why working for larger organizations, or with local partnerships, tends to be safer (but not universally, as explored later) – they are already established locally and can guide you as to what is appropriate, and what is not. In the absence of this, you will have to do your homework. You may be able to glean some information from travel guides and websites, but this is no replacement for speaking to those intimately familiar to the locale you will be working or studying in.

BOX 8.2   QUICK REFERENCE LIST FOR MAKING A SAFETY PLAN

1. After checking for travel warnings, register with your local embassy or consulate (see Box 8.4) and update them as to internal movements.
2. Tell friends and family where you are and what you are doing. Consider using social media, especially those functions that identify you as 'safe' after major events.
3. Be prepared in case of emergency. Identify hospitals, clinics, pharmacy and emergency contacts and phone numbers. When you are sick or vulnerable is the worst time to negotiate for yourself.
4. Do not stray from your plan. Most accidents happen when improvising.
5. 'Create safety': research local geography, customs, and seek out others in order to help you make your safety plan.

Before committing to an overseas elective, check for travel advisories and weather advisories warning against travel to your destination of interest. Also, make sure that both your sending and receiving universities have agreed to the elective, and find out how they will be able to assist you in case of emergency. This will be helpful when arranging supplementary travel and repatriation insurance (see further below).

What to Bring

We cannot be exhaustive here, but the more remote or isolate your destination, the more you should bring. Do not assume that supplies, medical or otherwise will be readily available at your host clinic or institution (see Chapter 7).

If you are debating bringing a satellite phone or SPOT® device, we feel you should be asking the question: Why am I putting myself in such an isolated situation to start with, and how much can I truly contribute or learn professionally in these situations? Perhaps it would be best to take such a venture on your own time.

What to do when hurt and alone

Most tenuous moments tend to occur when alone, without the relative safety of working within a larger organization. Perhaps the most important advice in these situations is to listen to one's inner feelings about developing situations. If you start feeling unsafe, you probably are. Demonstrations, for example, can sometimes turn violent. One of us was once peppered with an offensive chemical for not getting out of the way of a political procession. Curiosity is not usually an advantage when alone in a changing environment.

When alone, we are also more likely to wait before getting help. Perhaps out of embarrassment, we tend to retreat and isolate ourselves: doctors and medical trainees are perhaps especially apt to underestimate their injuries. Therefore, it is best to have an established protocol when hurt, in order to quickly reach trusted individuals and facilities.

Specific Considerations

Dress and Social Behaviour

As a medical practitioner, it is important to observe and respect the norms of the new country and our potential patients and co-workers. This is important for the ability to gain respect, a crucial aspect of patient care and teamwork. It also makes us less likely to stand out in public, and thus remain at less risk of becoming targets.

Gender-Based Safety and Travelling with Children

It is important to be aware of your surroundings at all times. This can be particularly true for women. While it is true that some cultures have different norms for gender interactions, it is important to be careful in all countries, even having dinner with someone of the opposite gender can convey a message which you may not intend. Social situations statistically cause the greatest risk, but being alone can clearly leave you vulnerable. If a situation feels unsafe, do not stay in it. In general, mixed gender groups are safest.

In North America and other similar cultures, it is very acceptable for women to travel alone and to wear clothing that reveals their arms, chest and legs. In countries where revealing clothing is not the norm, it is important to be aware of the reactions of others around you and adapt as necessary.

Travelling with small children always takes careful consideration, although overseas experiences can be very beneficial to a child's development. We have also refused assignments where we were not able to get enough information, or where we knew the children would have relatively little to do safely, even in the best of circumstances. One cardinal rule of working with young families in tow is to do so with other young families: other parents are the best resource on local activities that are both entertaining and safe for young children.

Gender Identity

Know the laws around general identity and sexual orientation in the country you are working in and be aware of the risks. Appreciate your comfort with who you are, and balance the need to be recognized with understanding that sharing details about your personal life could put you at risk.

Transportation

Wear your seatbelt! Over 68 million Americans travel each year, and over the past 10 years, there have been 8000 U.S. deaths from unnatural causes (Tozzi, 2015). Approximately 40% of the deaths in the United States were caused by road traffic accidents over the past decade (U.S. Department of State, 2016). More relevant to our chapter, a study looking at Peace Corp volunteers from 1962 to 1983 had 185 deaths: 70% from injury (46% motor vehicle accidents, and 18% drowning), 21% from illness, 4% from homicide and 5% from suicide (Hargarten and Baker, 1983).

Road traffic accidents are a major global burden of disease (WHO, 2009) and, as we mentioned at the outset, also the major risk to you as an overseas traveller. Again, remember to follow your instincts. Remember this when you are tempted to 'go local' and hop onto an over-packed bus or as the third passenger on a motorcycle. These situations put you at great risk to add to the local statistics for road accidents (Box 8.3).

Working with Larger Organizations

These guidelines presuppose that you are volunteering in relatively stable geopolitical circumstances, and therefore feel relatively safe to go on a smaller scale or even independent elective.

BOX 8.3   OTHER ESSENTIALS TO STAY SAFE IN TRAFFIC

1. Don't assume that traffic will follow the rules. Always follow 'defensive' pedestrian or driving principles.
2. Always wear a helmet on a bicycle or motorcycle. Avoid motorcycles or mopeds if possible; they carry a statistically higher risk to travellers.
3. Always wear a seatbelt. If renting a car, make sure that all belts work, and that basic safety equipment is supplied.
4. Drive with doors locked and windows closed when driving slowly through the city, and watch out for purposeful 'accidents' that are a ploy for a robbery.
5. Avoid driving at night, especially alone in foreign circumstances.

BOX 8.4   ONLINE RESOURCES

- Registering while overseas, travel alerts (for Canadians): www.travel.gc.ca
- Other travel alerts: www.cdc.gov
- Online training for NGO volunteers and other travelling abroad: www.disasterready.org
- Comparing travel insurance options, including repatriation: www.squaremouth.com
- Canadian Federation of Medical Students Pre-departure Training Handbook: http://www.old.cfms.org/downloads/Pre-Departure%20Guidelines%20Final.pdf
- Understanding your own risk tolerance: http:/www.humanmetrics.com/rot/rotqd.asp (with thanks to Humanmetrics Inc. for permission to include)

Some will choose to aid those affected by conflict or natural disasters, through the logistics of major humanitarian organizations. In this case, your organization will provide more or less extensive training and briefing on safety and what rules to follow in your assignment. It may be tempting to bend the rules, but don't: just because the immediate context seems secure, does not mean that your area is not at risk of incursion. If you disregard the rules, you are potentially putting many of your colleagues at risk, not just yourself.

One special comment about international aid organizations is that they do not always share information seamlessly between them. We have witnessed one NGO become victim to a kidnapping but subsequently not inform a sister organization of that fact, even though they shared a hospital. The moral of the story might be: follow your organization's rules but feel free to say something if something does not seem right. An organization cannot force you to do something that does not feel safe.

In conclusion, personal safety must be at the forefront of your consciousness when you are travelling. It involves forethought, planning and flexibility. Awareness of the actual and perceived risks and actions to mitigate them as well as a plan for how to respond if things go wrong are crucial. Our risk perception and risk tolerance varies according to stages of our lives, and external and internal responsibilities. Remember that plans that are well thought pre-travel preparation, in a time of clarity and calm, should be changed in travel only if new information can positively affect the outcome.

References

Hargarten SW, Baker SP. Fatalities in the Peace Corps. A retrospective study: 1962 through 1983. *JAMA*. 1985; 254 (10): 279–287.

Iverson KV. *The Global Healthcare Volunteer's Handbook*. Tucson, AZ: Galen Press; 2014.

Northwestern University. School of Education and Social Policy. Groupthink: The Role of Leadership in Enhancing and Mitigating the Pitfall in Team Decision-Making. 2012. http://www.sesp.northwestern.edu/masters-learning-and-organizational-change/knowledge -lens/stories/2012/groupthink-the-role-of-leadership-in-enhancing-and-mitigating-the-pitfall-in-team -decision-making .html (accessed April 3, 2016).

Shlim D. *Centers for Disease Control Yellow Book*. Atlanta: CDC; 2016.

The Personal Safety Group. Situational Awareness. 2015. http://www.personalsafetygroup .com/about/situational-awareness-training/ (accessed April 3, 2016).

Tozzi J. How Americans Die Abroad. *Bloomberg News*: July 27, 2015 (updated July 29, 2015).

U.S. Department of State, Bureau of Consular Affairs. U.S. Citizen Deaths Overseas. 2016. https://travel .state .gov/content/travel/en/statistics/deaths.html (accessed May 18, 2016).

WHO. *Global Health Risks: Mortality and Burden of Disease Attributable to Selected Major Risks*. Geneva: WHO; 2009.

Chapter 9

Travel Health Considerations

Andrea Hunter and Anne McCarthy

Contents

Introduction

Students and healthcare workers travelling to low-resourced settings are at particular susceptibility to unique health hazards. These result both from their potential exposures in healthcare work as well as from the geographic context itself. Risks vary depending on the destination as well as the role of the student or healthcare worker and the practice setting. There are multiple potential work-related factors that may increase the health risk. There may be increased prevalence of pathogens such as human immunodeficiency virus (HIV), tuberculosis (TB), chronic hepatitis, with limited resources to deal with inadvertent exposure. There may also be outbreaks of uncommon infectious disease that can be spread in healthcare settings, such as viral hemorrhagic fevers (e.g. Ebola) or Middle East respiratory syndrome (MERS). In many countries, there are less stringent safety regulations or infection control standards, as well as limited ability to adhere to appropriate infection control practices due in part to the realities of practicing in a resource-limited setting where there may not be readily available personal protective equipment (PPE) or safety-engineered devices. To compound things, trainees and medical professionals may be faced with unfamiliar medical procedures, practice conditions and/or equipment. In addition, travellers may experience increased psychological stress resulting from practicing in resource-limited settings, isolated areas and long-term assignments.

Travel Health Consultation

All trainees and healthcare workers engaging in electives, work or travel in low- and middle-income countries (LMICs) are highly encouraged to seek personalized travel medicine consultation, ideally 6–8 weeks prior to the planned departure. The dynamic nature of global infectious disease epidemiology, drug resistance patterns, available prophylactic and treatment agents and the availability of medical care at geographic destinations all add complexity to personal health recommendations to global travel and further warrant professional travel medicine advice for each trip.

Individuals with underlying health conditions should ensure stability of those conditions prior to travel and should discuss the planned travel with their primary healthcare provider. Practical considerations, including ample supply of medications for travel, accessibility in carry-on luggage and planning for potential complications should be considered.

The pre-travel consultation should address all aspects of health risk. Travel in itself is stressful both physically and emotionally, and this is compounded by working in healthcare and living in countries daily affected by the social determinants of health. It is important to adequately prepare for these experiences and have resources available for debriefing and mitigating issues as they arise.

Travel Health Preparation and Travel Insurance

Many health- and occupation-related risks can be anticipated and planned for – this includes prevention strategies as well as plans for treatment in the event of occupational exposure or of illness. As with all travellers, students and healthcare providers should ensure that they have the necessary health and evacuation/repatriation coverage for their planned trip. Most basic medical insurance does not have coverage outside the United States or Canada. Some policies may not be valid for health workers or those participating in 'adventure' activities, including whitewater sports or riding on a motorcycle for transport, and therefore it is important to read the 'fine print' of any policy purchased. The single most important component of travel health insurance is evacuation insurance for medical emergencies, including transport to the nearest medical facility.

In addition to health/evacuation insurance, all travellers should investigate healthcare services in destination countries. Much of this information is available through the Government of Canada's website (www.travel.gc.ca) or U.S. Department of State – Consular Affairs site (https://travel.state.gov) providing extensive information about the travel destination as well as visa requirements and potential health concerns. In addition, International Association for Medical Assistance to Travellers (IAMAT, www.iamat.org) provides travel medicine resources, including a medical directory of healthcare providers around the world that are available to travellers, and particularly able to provide guidance towards English-speaking providers.

Resources

There are many resources available to help travellers find additional information about the areas they plan to visit. Most bookstores and libraries have travel sections with resources containing facts on climate, geography, political conditions, disease risks, and other concerns. There are also many websites where travellers can find free, detailed and current information. Some of the most evidence-based include the following:

- TripPrep.com: www.tripprep.com
- Public Health Agency of Canada (PHAC): https://travel.gc.ca/travelling/health-safety
- Centers for Disease Control and Prevention (CDC): www.cdc.gov/travel
- NathNAC (National Travel Health Network and Centre): www.nathnac.net
- Travel Health Pro: www.travelhealthpro.org.uk
- World Health Organization: www.who.int
- International Society of Travel Medicine: www.istm.org
- U.S. Department of State: www.travel.state.gov

Vaccines

Students and healthcare workers, like all travellers to LMICs should be up to date on all their routine vaccines, vaccinations specific to healthcare workers, and those specific to travel.

Routine Vaccinations

For all travellers, the following vaccines should be up-to-date according to their home country guidelines:

- Measles, mumps, rubella (measles is very common in many LMIC settings)
- Tetanus, pertussis, diphtheria
- Varicella
- Influenza (occurs year round in the tropics)
- Polio – Outbreaks are still occurring in limited locations. An adult booster dose of inactivated polio vaccine may be warranted for those travelling to regions with particularly high prevalence or outbreaks (e.g. Pakistan, Equatorial Guinea, Cameroon, Syria, Afghanistan, Ethiopia, Iraq, Israel, Somalia and Nigeria) (CATMAT, 2014b)

Healthcare workers are at higher risk for some vaccine-preventable diseases due to potential occupational exposure, including influenza, varicella, pertussis and hepatitis B. All those working in healthcare should ensure immunity to varicella and hepatitis B.

Vaccinations Specific to Travel

Yellow fever vaccination is unique in that international health regulations outline the requirements for proof of vaccination when travelling between countries of yellow fever risk. It is important to consider the whole travel itinerary, since travel to a non-yellow fever endemic country with transit, even only at the airport, through a country designated as having yellow fever vaccine requirements, such as Kenya, will require proof of vaccine. In Canada and the United States, this vaccination is only available at centres designated by Public Health Agency of Canada and Centers for Disease Control, respectively, in order to meet the requirements of the International Health Regulations (PHAC, 2012). World Health Organization (WHO) updated yellow fever vaccination guidelines in 2011, including classification of geographic areas of risk and revisions of maps to illustrate vaccination recommendations rather than yellow fever risk (CATMAT, 2013). It is important for each traveller to ensure that they are compliant with the requirements for yellow fever vaccine at their destination, and that they also include any transit through yellow fever designated countries. Failure to have properly documented vaccine may result in denial of entry or vaccine administration at the destination.

Hepatitis A vaccine is recommended for all travellers to lower resource areas since hepatitis A virus infections are moderately to highly endemic in nearly all LMICs (CATMAT, 2013).

Quadravalent **meningococcal** vaccine should be considered for travellers departing for areas of high endemicity (e.g. sub-Saharan Africa, Saudi Arabia during the Hajj and Umrah pilgrimages) or places with current outbreaks or heightened disease activity (McCarthy, 2015).

Typhoid vaccine (Ty21a or Vi polysaccharide vaccine) is recommended for most visitors to South Asia, in addition to basic hygiene precautions (Greenaway et al., 2014).

Oral cholera vaccine in Canada (Dukoral®) is also marketed for protection against travellers' diarrhea. It should be considered for those working in refugee camps where cholera outbreaks are a risk. It is not, however, routinely recommended for the prevention of travellers' diarrhea (CATMAT, 2015). General considerations for the prevention and treatment of travellers' diarrhea are presented below.

Rabies vaccine should be considered for those going to countries with rabies risk, and the risk assessment should consider the availability of safe and effective post-exposure prophylaxis at the destination (CATMAT Guidelines, 2002).

Japanese encephalitis is a risk in South and Southeast Asia and consideration for use should be considered in high-risk travel (CATMAT, 2011).

Travellers' Diarrhea

Evidence-based prevention options for travellers' diarrhea include: hand hygiene (hand washing or hand sanitizer use), careful food and beverage choice and preparation. Management can be supported with bismuth subsalicylate, fluoroquinolones or rifaximin (not licensed in Canada for travellers' diarrhea), as needed.

The risk of adverse drug reactions and development of resistance needs to be weighed against the benefit of antimicrobial drugs for prevention. In general, travellers should plan a management strategy for travellers' diarrhea. Many travel medicine providers recommend carrying antiemetics as well as antimotility agents for self-treatment of diarrhea, with use of an antimicrobial (usually a fluoroquinolone or azithromycin) for more severe cases. Those with severe or bloody diarrhea, or with high fever associated with diarrhea should seek medical attention (Connor, 2016).

Malaria Prevention

Malaria is a common and serious infection worldwide, caused by five different *Plasmodium* species: *falciparum, ovale, vivax, malariae and knowlesi*. Malaria is transmitted by the bite of a female *Anopheles* mosquito and characterized by fever and generalized symptoms, including myalgias, headaches, malaise and abdominal pains. Microscopy of blood film or rapid antigen detection test is required for diagnosis due to the non-specific nature of symptoms. Since the development of rapid diagnostic tests (RDTs) for malaria in the 1990s, the availability of accurate testing in remote areas of LMICs has increased dramatically (WHO, 2011). *P. falciparum* infections carry the highest associated mortality, but all types have potential to cause significant disease. Non immune travellers are at particular risk of morbidity and mortality, with higher rates often resulting from delays in diagnosis or treatment (CATMAT, 2014a).

The risk of acquiring malaria depends on a number of exposure factors (endemicity in destination area, presence of *P. falciparum*, and duration of exposure) as well as host factors (general health, potential drug–drug interactions, access to medical care, risk tolerance of individuals). All those travelling to areas of malaria risk are advised to use personal protective measures in the form of physical and chemical barriers to prevent mosquito bites: ensure, wherever possible, that screening on doors, windows, eaves are intact; sleep under bed nets treated with insecticide; and consider wearing long, loose fitting light-coloured clothing treated with insecticide for additional protection. Use of topical insect repellents containing 20–30% DEET or 20% icaridin is recommended for exposed skin and impregnation of bed nets and clothing (Bogglid et al., 2014).

In addition to the primary preventative measures above, malarial chemoprophylaxis is recommended for students and healthcare workers engaging in electives, work or travel in regions of malarial risk. There are multiple drug options available, and the choice should be based on an individual risk assessment with a provider familiar with malaria risk and prevention. The ultimate choice of therapy should take into consideration a number of factors, including the following:

■ Travel itinerary, including areas of malaria risk and regional drug resistance patterns.
■ Potential contraindications to specific drugs, including allergies, drug–drug interactions, and likelihood of adverse reactions. In addition, cost of the drugs as well as potential for adherence with frequency of drug administration should be considered.

Chloroquine or hydroxychloroquine resistance rates are significant, but these medications can still be considered effective prophylaxis in Haiti, Dominican Republic, Central America north of the Panama Canal, parts of Mexico, parts of South America, North Africa, parts of the Middle East and west/central China (Bogglid et al., 2014). Most of sub-Saharan Africa, South America, Oceania and Asia are chloroquine resistant and therefore require other malaria prophylaxis, including atovaquone-proguanil, doxycycline or mefloquine. Areas with chloroquine and mefloquine resistance have also emerged, particularly in rural, wooded regions where Thailand borders with Myanmar (Burma), Cambodia and Laos, and in southern Vietnam (Bogglid et al., 2014); in such areas choice of chemoprophylaxis is limited to doxycycline and atovaquone-proguanil.

Students and healthcare workers are advised to discuss with their travel medicine practitioner prior to departure the alternative options in the event of drug adverse reactions, or consider a drug trial prior to departure to ensure tolerance. Discontinuation of malaria chemoprophylaxis while in an area of malaria risk is not a reasonable option. Travellers embarking on international electives or work are advised to secure all their antimalarials prior to departure as medications available in other areas of the world not only may be cheaper but also may be less effective, may be associated with serious adverse effects or may not be manufactured to HIC standards (Bogglid et al., 2014).

It is important for travellers to seek immediate medical attention if experiencing fever during or within particularly 3 months of travel to a malaria endemic area. The medical assessment should include blood testing to rule out malaria (CATMAT, 2014a).

Special Considerations for Healthcare Providers

Many healthcare workers in LMICs do not have access to North American standards for infection control, or occupational safety. In many instances, there are not supplies of personal protective equipment such as N95 masks, latex or similar gloves, or ready access to drugs for post-exposure prophylaxis against HIV in the event of blood or body fluid exposure. It is up to the individual healthcare provider to investigate and anticipate health risks related to their planned activities. Many involved in international global health activities advocate that visiting healthcare providers should bring their own personal protective equipment and also a supply of antiretroviral therapy for potential post-exposure prophylaxis (PEP). The latter can be quite expensive, and some individuals choose to bring just a one-week supply. This provides a safety net to start effective antiretroviral therapy and time to secure the remainder of the 28 days of therapy.

Other Travel-Related Risks

Travellers can be faced with many physical and emotional situations of risk and include management of that are covered in a travel medicine consultation, including strategies to mitigate the risk of trauma, environmental risks such as altitude illness, and management of illness while away.

Altitude-Related Illness

During travel to high altitude (>1500 m/4900 ft), due to barometric pressure and partial pressure of oxygen decrease, travellers incur increasing risk of hypoxia. This can be associated with hyperventilation, headache, light-headedness, fatigue, altered perceptions, decreased exercise tolerance and disordered sleep. There are a number of specific altitude illnesses, including acute mountain sickness (AMS), high-altitude pulmonary edema (HAPE), high-altitude cerebral edema (HACE), snow blindness as well as risk of aggravating any underlying illnesses, particularly cardiopulmonary compromise or thromboembolic risk (CATMAT, 2007).

Guidelines exist for prevention and treatment of these specific altitude-related illnesses; however, travellers should be aware that risk of altitude illness increases directly with the rate of ascent and the altitude reached (CATMAT, 2007). Ascent rapidly to altitudes >5500 m (18,000 ft) are at risk of severe or fatal illness, as the barometric pressure at this altitude is one-half that of sea level. Increased UV exposure, decreased temperature, along with hypoxia from decreased barometric pressure contribute to risk of illness. Acclimatization, through slow ascent to altitude, and careful attention to any symptoms of altitude-related illness are recommended for all travellers.

Guidance from CDC Health Information for International Travel *Yellow Book* 2016 indicates that travellers should consider the following precautions for acclimatization:

- Ascend gradually, if possible. Avoid going directly from low altitude to more than 9000 ft (2750 m) sleeping altitude in 1 day. Once above 9000 ft (2750 m), move sleeping altitude no higher than 1600 ft (500 m) per day, and plan an extra day for acclimatization every 3300 ft (1000 m).
- Consider using acetazolamide to speed acclimatization, if abrupt ascent is unavoidable.
- Avoid alcohol for the first 48 hours.
- Participate in only mild exercise for the first 48 hours.
- Having a high-altitude exposure at more than 9000 ft (2750 m) for two nights or more, within 30 days before the trip, is useful (Hackett and Shlim, 2016).

Summary of the Guidance Often Offered to Health Professionals and Trainees Embarking on Work in LMICs

• Book a travel medicine consultation at least 6–8 weeks prior to travel to consider local epidemiology, preventative strategies, treatment options and management of underlying health issues.
• Find out from pre-travel research or local colleagues where to go for medical treatment if needed and secure comprehensive health and evacuation insurance ahead of time.
• Wash your hands!

• Be careful what you eat and drink.
  • Check on the safety of local water – boiling all drinking water is necessary in some areas. Avoid ice that may have been made with impure water.
  • Peel, boil or cook all foods. Avoid uncooked foods (including salads).

• Take your malaria prophylaxis as directed when travelling to endemic areas. Sleep under a mosquito net, wear protective clothing after dusk, and buy your malaria medications before travel.
• Bring and use personal protective equipment (PPE) such as masks, gloves, as much as possible. Do not recap needles!
• To learn and care for patients while away, you need to look after your own physical and mental health.

Conclusion

Travelling to LMICs can incur some personal health risks that can be largely mitigated by careful preparation and diligence to basic precautions while working in a new context.

References

Bogglid A, Brophy J, Charlebois P, Crockett M, Geduld J, Ghesquiere W, McDonald P, Plourde P, Teitelbaum P, Tepper M, Schofield S and A McCarthy. 2014. Summary of recommendations for the prevention of malaria by the Committee to Advise on Tropical Medicine and Travel (CATMAT). *Canada Communicable Disease Report (CCDR)*. 40(7). April 3, 2014. http://www.phac-aspc.gc.ca/publicat/ccdr-rmtc/14vol40/dr-rm40-07/dr-rm40-07-prev-eng.php

Committee to Advise on Tropical Medicine and Travel (CATMAT). 2002. Statement on travellers and rabies vaccine. *Canada Communicable Disease Report (CCDR)*. 28(4). March 1, 2002. http://www.collectionscanada.gc.ca/webarchives/20071116023105/http://www.phac-aspc.gc.ca/publicat/ccdr-rmtc/02vol28/28sup/acs4.html

Committee to Advise on Tropical Medicine and Travel (CATMAT). 2007. Statement on High Altitude Illness. *Canada Communicable Disease Report (CCDR)*. 33(5). April 2007. http://www.phac-aspc.gc.ca/publicat/ccdr-rmtc/07vol33/acs-05/index-eng.php

Committee to Advise on Tropical Medicine and Travel (CATMAT). 2011. Statement on Protection Against Japanese Encephalitis. *Canada Communicable Disease Report (CCDR)*. 37(1). April 2011. http://www.phac-aspc.gc.ca/publicat/ccdr-rmtc/11vol37/acs-1/index-eng.php

Committee to Advise on Tropical Medicine and Travel (CATMAT). 2013. Statement for travellers and yellow fever. *Canada Communicable Disease Report (CCDR)*. 39(2). March 2013. http://www.phac-aspc.gc.ca/publicat/ccdr-rmtc/13vol39/acs-dcc-2/index-eng.php

Committee to Advise on Tropical Medicine and Travel (CATMAT). 2014a. Canadian recommendations for the treatment and prevention of malaria: Advisory committee statement. http://publications. gc.ca/collections/collection_2014/aspc-phac/HP40-102-2014-eng.pdf

Committee to Advise on Tropical Medicine and Travel (CATMAT). 2014b. Statement on polio and the international traveller. Canada Communicable Disease Report (CCDR). 40(13). July 10, 2014. http:// www.phac-aspc.gc.ca/publicat/ccdr-rmtc/14vol40/dr-rm40-13/dr-rm40-13-com-eng.php

Connor B. A. 2016. Travelers' diarrhea. In *CDC Health Information for International Travel (Yellow Book)*. Edited by Gary W. Brunette. Oxford: Oxford University Press. http://wwwnc.cdc.gov/travel /yellowbook/2016the-pre-travel-consultation/travelers-diarrhea

Greenaway C., Schofield S, Henteleff A., Plourde P., Geduld J. Abdel-Motagally M. and Bryson M. 2014. Summary of the statement on international travellers and typhoid by the Committee to Advise on Tropical Medicine and Travel (CATMAT). *Canada Communicable Disease Report (CCDR)*. 40(4). February 20, 2014. http://www.phac-aspc.gc.ca/publicat/ccdr-rmtc/14vol40/dr-rm40-04 /dr-rm40-04-tropmed-eng.php

Hackett P. H., Shlim D. R. 2016. Altitude illness. In *CDC Health Information for International Travel (Yellow Book)*. Edited by Gary W. Brunette. Oxford: Oxford University Press. http://wwwnc.cdc.gov/travel /yellowbook/2016/the-pre-travel-consultation/altitude-illness

McCarthy, A. On behalf of Committee to Advise on Tropical Medicine and Travel (CATMAT). 2015. Statement on meningococcal disease and the international traveller. *Canada Communicable Disease Report (CCDR)*. 41(5). May 7, 2015. http://www.phac-aspc.gc.ca/publicat/ccdr-rmtc/15vol41/dr-rm41 -05/com-2-eng.php

Public Health Agency of Canada (PHAC). 2012. Yellow Fever Vaccination Centres in Canada. Last updated: June 8, 2012. http://www.phac-aspc.gc.ca/tmp-pmv/yf-fj/index-eng.php

Public Health Agency of Canada (PHAC). Travel Health. http://www.phac-aspc.gc.ca/tmp -pmv/index-eng.php

World Health Organization (WHO). 2011. *Universal Access to Malaria Diagnostic Testing: An Operational Manual*. http://apps.who.int/iris/bitstream/10665/44657/1/9789241502092_eng.pdf

Chapter 10

Chapter 10

Seeking Cultural Competence

Jill Allison and Melissa Whaling

Contents

Introduction

Global health opportunities, whether they involve training, working or researching, have tremendous transformative potential for personal and professional development. In order to maximize this potential, it is important to develop a measure of what is called cultural competence. Cultural competence is an awareness of the importance of lifelong learning and an emerging critical consciousness necessary to be effective partners in intercultural contexts. In this chapter, we aim to provide guideposts for preparation as a key to being sensitive, responsive, humble and receptive to the importance of cultural context. The information in this chapter is informed by two important points. The first is the need to be responsive and respectful of culture as a factor in shaping the experience of giving and receiving care in all domains of practice. The second is the knowledge that cultures change, adapt, shift and are taken up and experienced very differently by individuals and families within a particular community.

Defining Culture

Culture is a complex web of shared values, concepts and beliefs that are transmitted through symbols, social relations and practices that shape worldview and influence our behaviours (Goode et al., 2006). Elements of life that both shape and are shaped by culture include language, spirituality, social values, gender roles, family and kin relationships, politics, economies and history. Geography and climate also exert an influence. Expressions of culture include manner of dress, ways of interacting and showing respect, living arrangements and community organization. Some of these elements constitute what is referred to as ethnicity, which is an aspect of culture but links to shared set of practices and values. Because culture is dynamic and interactive, it is a living construct and never static (Kleinman and Benson, 2006). We all interact with and take up variations of social practice within our own cultures and in response to opportunities to learn and participate in new social experiences. In other words, there is no singular representation of any culture and we can never assume that people will share exactly the same ideas or behave in exactly the same way. Such assumptions are called essentialism and reduce culture to a set of simplified practices rather than appreciating the richness and complexity that is central to the very notion of culture. Spend a few moments thinking about what social practice you would identify as a universal aspect of Canadian or American 'culture'.

What Is Cultural Competence?

Cultural competence is a key component of preparation for intercultural or cross-cultural experiences in healthcare delivery, research or training. It is not exclusively related to the movement of students or professionals across geographical borders since intercultural contexts often occur within the healthcare domains of our own communities. Thus the concept of cultural competence transcends local and global contexts and has been taken up by many disciplines, particularly in social work, psychology and psychiatry. The term 'competence' has been critiqued for its achievement-oriented associations (Eichbaum, 2015) and its potential for neo-colonial assumptions and essentialism (Pon, 2009; Kleinman and Benson, 2006). In this chapter, the term includes the need for self awareness and reflection on one's own cultural background and influences and the need for humility in approaching life situations that we do not fully understand. As a component of competence, cultural humility is a modest, unassuming way of assessing oneself, reflecting, recognizing limitations in one's knowledge and opening one's self up to new ideas, information and ways of being and doing. It is important for people undertaking learning, clinical or research projects to understand the role that cultural context and cultural background play in shaping the process and outcomes. Cultural competence enables us to acknowledge the admixture of what we bring into the experience and what we engage with as we work in a cross-cultural setting.

Cultural competence relates to humility, responsiveness and critical consciousness (Hook et al., 2013; Kirmayer, 2012). It is an awareness of self and a willingness to be reflexive and reflective, exploring fully the influence of our own cultural values and background. This takes practice, courage and a willingness to change our way of thinking about the world.

ACTIVITY BOX

There are a number of activities that can be used to encourage participants in a pre-departure training program to think about the impact of culture. One of these is the card game Barnga. People at different tables are given the same game to play but certain key rules are different at each table. After a couple of rounds, participants move tables so that they are suddenly playing by a different set of rules. The key is that there is no talking allowed as play progresses. People have to communicate by gesture. Debriefing allows participants to consider how they felt when the internalized 'rules of the game' suddenly changed. The game provides an excellent opportunity for discussing the need for examining our own cultural backgrounds in the process of understanding what we think we know (Pittenger and Heimann, 1998).

Instructions for Barnga are available at: http://pt.educationforsocialjustice.org/file .php/1/Bargna_Game.pdf

One way to consider this point is to reflect upon and explore our own cultural values and influences. Beginning with what constitutes our own 'culture', acknowledging that we belong to a cultural context of our own will lead us to examining the multiplicity of elements that shape our worldview. It will also help to point out that we do not ascribe to the views and influences of just one 'culture' but rather, are influenced by many cultural intersections within our social lives. Our views may differ from our neighbours and friends and colleagues because of our experiences and opportunities in life. Considering the complexity of culture in our own lives provides a platform for recognizing the same nuanced impact that culture plays in shaping the attitudes and practices of our colleagues, patients, teachers and friends.

Historical Context: Power and Politics

History and political structures influence not only cultural context but also the way we are received and perceived within various communities. This is especially true in LMICs with a colonial past. Vestiges of uneven power structures, economic exploitation and systematic racism contribute to interactions on the ground. Pon (2009) argues that simplistic perspectives on cultural competence can participate in 'an ontology of forgetting' that obscures racism and complex colonial pasts. This occurs because discrete and essentialized views of culture fail to acknowledge how cultures have been historically constructed in relation to one another. Scholars have argued that this constitutes a form of new colonialism by locating power in the Global North while making our partners in the south the recipients of assistance (Baskin, 2006; Gross, 2000; Sakamoto, 2007; Yee and Dumbrill, 2003).

As part of a deeper awareness of the context in which we are going to study, work or conduct research, it is valuable to know the political history of the host country. Has the country you are visiting been colonized by another nation in the past? This may shape current politics, social relationships and perceptions of visitors like ourselves.

ACTIVITY: REFLECTION ON POWER AND PRIVILEGE

Think about the work, project or learning context in the host country. Do you see yourself in a position of leadership and authority? What does that look like? Do you see yourself as having a greater or less amount of knowledge compared to your peers in the host country? Do you see yourself as having more or less advantages in comparison to your peers in the host country? Consider what has contributed to that vision of your role and social position. Now think about this in reverse. If a peer from the county you are visiting came to your community, would they answer the questions the same way you did? Consider the importance of partnerships and being a peer even if you have come from an advantaged high-income country. It is important to think about the role of power and privilege as you prepare for an experience in a different context. We are often unconscious of the many social and structural contributions we have enjoyed and that have enabled us to have choices, be successful and our views of our own leadership capacity are shaped by these sometimes invisible attributes (see Bourdieu, 1993; McIntosh, 1989; Shiffman, 2014, 2015). Power, like culture, can be an elusive concept. As Michel Foucault argues, it is in the exercise of power that we understand that we are both vehicle and mechanism for the circulation (Foucault, 1980). We are often unaware how power is exercised within a cultural context and it is only in unpacking our own sense of our social position that we come to understand the relationship with privilege.

Stereotypes and Essentializing

It is important to consider where and how we get information and concepts about culture and cultural practices. Are our ideas shaped by popular culture or representations in news media? Making assumptions about groups of people based on religious practices or language or ethnicity leads to misconceptions. A number of scholars point out that culture is often essentialized in discussions and training involving cultural competence aimed at practice (Carpenter-Song et al., 2007; Kirmayer, 2012; Kleinman and Benson, 2006; Kumaş-Tan et al., 2007; Taylor, 2003; Willen et al., 2010). Kirmayer argues that it is important to recognize and acknowledge 'the ways in which ethnoracial categories are themselves culturally constructed and contested' (2012:251). In other words, what we decide constitutes a cultural difference or cultural domain is based on categories that we have decided are meaningful in some way. Consider for a moment how our perception of cultural difference would be altered if we included as a single culture everyone who speaks French? What if we considered everyone who is lactose intolerant as a single cultural or racialized category? While this is obviously contrived, we can see how arbitrary the categories of race and culture can become.

Ethnocentrism/Ethnorelativism/Cultural Relativism

Our worldview and personal construction of reality have a dramatic impact on intercultural interactions. Being able to identify our own cultural and personal lens is key in becoming a more culturally sensitive individual. Varying experiences, thoughts, and attitudes about people, places and cultures can place individuals along a continuum that ranges from ethnocentrism to ethnorelativism. Ethnocentrism entails a view of the world in which one's own group/ culture is at the centre of everything, and all others are scaled and rated with reference to it (Borden, 2007). The attitudes of ethnocentric persons tend to view their own group or culture as superior or more legitimate than others and sometimes do not acknowledge the existence of other worldviews or perceptions. Generally, there are three stages of ethnocentrism: denial, defence and minimization. Those in the denial stage discard the existence of cultural differences, those in the defence stage demonize them, and those in the minimization stage diminish differences (Perusek, 2007). Within a cultural competence framework, there is a focus on reducing ethnocentric views, thereby improving intercultural competence.

On the other hand, ethnorelativism recognizes difference in cultures, worldviews and perceptions while accepting that all are equal and valid, avoiding judging others according to their own cultural and personal viewpoints (Bennett, 1993). Stages of ethnorelativism include acceptance, adaptation and integration. Ethnorelativists are open to learning, difference and are quite adaptable. Their values include tolerance empathy, open-mindedness, and appreciation for diversity, meaning and context. Culturally competent individuals tend to be ethno-relativists who are interculturally sensitive, open, accepting, tolerant and adaptable to change.

Cultural relativism locates social practices in relation to culture and can provide a frame through which you accept certain practices in a different cultural context that you would not find acceptable at home. It can be part of cultural humility and respect. Relativism can also be a way of sidestepping moral dilemmas. When confronted with a challenging issue, it is important to remember that culture is not superficial and it helps to try to understand the deeper historical, political, spiritual, social or economic reasons behind a practice, such as wearing particular clothing or cutting the body, rather than thinking of culture as an excuse for abusive or unsettling practices (Abu Lughod, 2002). We can be more effective advocates for equality and justice if we understand the structural impact of change.

Gender and Sexuality

Cultural competence also means being aware of gender roles, expectations for modesty, attitudes around sexuality and social norms around relationships between people in the workplace and socially. It is sometimes culturally inappropriate for men and women who are not related or married to be seen together in a social situation. Think about how often this occurs in our own daily social activities and try to imagine what you would have to do in order to avoid making a cultural error. Choosing where you will sit in a meeting room, deciding whether to get into an elevator, deciding who you will have lunch or dinner with, study with or walk home with – all these simple activities are visible acts with cultural connotations.

Relationships with local people can also present opportunities for miscommunication and the risk of unanticipated expectations. The meaning of a sexual relationship is also culturally shaped and laden with power dynamics that are not always evident. It is always safest to avoid a relationship during a short-term experience in a community where we do not know with certainty that sexual encounters are viewed the same way as we view them or where it is not obvious what expectations they have. People may feel exploited, hurt or angry when the relationship ends.

Another point to be aware of is the challenge of negotiating safety around sexuality in many cultural contexts. In many countries, homosexuality is illegal or persecuted to the point of extreme danger. It is important to know the social and legal norms and rules around sexual behaviour for our own safety and for that of our friends, colleagues and partners in another cultural context. We never want to put ourselves or anyone else at risk. It is especially important to remember that while we can leave a community where we are engaged in short-term training, research or project work, our local partners do not have that opportunity. If someone is inadvertently 'outed' by our actions and behaviours, they may be in danger.

Food, Drink and Clothing

Eating seems simple enough, but this basic activity is culturally laden with meaning and important to many relationships. When we eat, what we eat and with whom we eat are all products of our cultural background. Trying new foods and being willing to share food with people is one of the most fundamental ways of gaining social insights. You can prepare in advance by reading about food traditions so you know what you are eating, what its cultural significance is and how this food fits into the broader economic, agricultural or social relationships of the community. Some of this information is available on websites or is easily discovered through conversations with people. Refusing food can be problematic but explanations about allergies, dietary practices such as vegetarianism, and so on, will generally be accepted if presented in a matter of fact way before a meal begins. *Always compliment the cook!*

Alcohol consumption is a complex issue. It may or may not be part of traditions in the community. It may be prohibited or it may be consumed freely with expectations that guests also consume while visiting. Know the general rules about alcohol consumption and be aware of penalties for breaking laws or cultural norms. In many Islamic communities, alcohol is forbidden for religious reasons and this translates into national laws. This is both a cultural and a legal issue. In some cultures, alcohol is produced in people's homes and served regularly to guests. It can be difficult to refuse but finding respectful ways to explain that your culture or values prohibit consumption will generally be accepted without question.

Clothing is an expression of culture and conveys many meanings. The most practical approach to making decisions about how to dress in a new cultural context is to do some reading about the community you are going to work in and look at the types of clothing people wear. Remember that ceremonial dress is often quite different than day-to-day clothing. Modesty is a good policy and being prepared to have shoulders and knees covered is a good starting point. In some places, it may be expected that long sleeves, long trousers for men and long skirts for women are the cultural norm. Dressing inappropriately not only offends our hosts, it reduces our credibility in the professional domain in which we want to work.

Worldview, Religion and Belief Systems

Worldview is based on how we perceive ourselves in the world. It is part of a complex set of beliefs and practices that include spirituality but are not exclusively part of a religious domain.

Religious viewpoints have an impact on healthcare delivery and care seeking. Religion shapes people's views on life, health illness and death. In Japan, people who are dying are sometimes considered to be in the process of becoming an ancestor. Such views shape the way people grieve as the individual continues to have a presence within the family but now has a new role. Belief in reincarnation, afterlife or ancestor worship have a profound effect on the way people view life and death. While you may not be able to grasp fully, all the nuances of religious views in the host country or among your peers and patients, it is important to be respectful of the importance people may place on religious activities in their daily lives.

CASE EXAMPLE

Think about how you make a decision in your professional or personal life. If you are offered a new job, for example, who would you consult, what factors would you weigh into the decision and what values would be most important? Your list probably includes family, location of the job, professional opportunities, income and perhaps the status that might be associated with the position. If you are from a country like Nepal, your deliberation will include all of those things as well, but the ultimate decision about whether you take the job will probably either be made or be largely determined by the eldest man in your household. Many people live in extended family circumstances where the eldest male holds the decision-making authority. Such decision making affects workplace hierarchies as well and in many instances, decisions will be deferred to people considered to be more senior or in a position of power. Such hierarchies can be difficult to understand when we come from circumstances where we are used to a more autonomous approach to decision making.

Communal versus Individual Values

Worldview is also bound with key values around the communal or collective versus the individual as the site of moral and social decision making. Much like our discussion above about family hierarchies, the way that many people consider their place in the world is as part of an organic social collective such as family, community or other network (Ward et al., 2005). Decisions are thus never considered from the position of a single individual. Family values and relationships, social hierarchies and education all contribute to this perspective. The way we make decisions about healthcare, family issues, marriage and finances are deeply embedded in whether we are accustomed to communal or individual approaches. A decision about the surgical options for a patient in a clinic or hospital in which we are training, working or researching may be made by a number of family members rather than the individual patient, especially if the patient is a woman. The expectations and norms that apply in this situation are valid just as autonomy in decision-making is the norm in most Global North contexts. It is important to recognize the difference in perspective but not allow it to create a barrier to providing the care someone needs, continuing to learn and developing collegial relationships.

Space, Privacy and Confidentiality

The meaning and importance of space, privacy and confidentiality are culturally influenced. Structural conditions like population density and urban housing conditions, socio-economic circumstances and public transport systems contribute to the way people are organized in social space. However, comfort with and notions of personal space are often varied. People may have a different view of privacy and confidentiality, listening actively to conversations between strangers, looking over shoulders to read newspapers, letters and even computer screens and e-mails. Consultations in medical facilities may be sources of community discussion and entertainment for others in the waiting room. While this can pose an ethical dilemma for those of us who are trained to respect confidentiality, it is equally important to respect the social conditions in which we are working. It is important to take the advice of your colleagues rather than assume that individuals are comfortable with confidentiality. In many contexts, people are not given bad news directly but are told by elders in their community. Telling an individual something devastating about their health directly could have profound emotional consequences for them and the family. Ask your colleagues how to negotiate conversation about people's health and medical care.

Time Perception

Some aspects of our culture are so ingrained in our minds and so commonplace to us that we begin to feel they are universally accepted. One of the most challenging aspects of working and/ or living in a culture other than our own is the meaning of time. In fact, for most of the world, the rigidity of a time clock is much less important than it is in the Global North. The timing of meetings, events and travel arrangements may be contingent, flexible and unpredictable. This is not a sign of disrespect as might be interpreted in the Global North. It is part of social dynamic in which time is not measured by the clock but rather, by who has arrived or is participating, what conditions are necessary for starting and how events traditionally unfold in any particular context. Watching colleagues, leaving space in schedules and being respectful of processes ensure that our participation is not marked by tension or frustration. Perceptions of time may be visible in various ways, through different behaviours such as walking speed, work pace, the abundance or lack of public clocks and punctuality for appointments or meetings.

Expectations (Productivity, Progress and Customer Service)

Just as the concept of time should not be presumed to be understood the same by all, neither should the ways in which social, economic and cultural systems function and operate. We must recognize that our own expectations are culturally derived and stem from deeply rooted beliefs and values that have evolved over time through our own lens. We can therefore not assume that everyday concepts such as productivity, progress and customer service will be viewed and constructed in the ways to which we are accustomed. Customer service interactions can also be influenced by general societal structures and hierarchies, management structures, protocols, policies, laws, communications styles, logistical capacities and needs, and measurement systems to name a few. While in the Global North, we are accustomed to standing in orderly queues for services; in other countries, individuals may be used to a less structured system of service and may be influenced by customer social status, the nature of their needs, or the availability of services. Quietly observing or asking for help along the way are recommended strategies for knowing where to go, who to talk to and how to interact. Patience, humility, flexibility and open-mindedness will go a long way in respectfully interacting with individuals and in navigating new environments.

Culture Shock/Cultural Adjustment

Culture shock is a sense of disorientation we may feel when we enter into a cultural environment which is different from our own. It is precipitated by the anxiety that results from losing all our familiar signs and symbols of social relations (Ward et al., 2005). It can include confusion, uncertainty and anxiety and can affect people in any context but is often increased in an under-resourced community where we might be confronted with poverty and illness on a scale that is overwhelming.

You may initially experience a brief period of elation and excitement when you enter into a new and unfamiliar cultural context. This is often followed by a period of growing frustration, an awareness of difference and a sense of loneliness or longing for the familiar. Most people overcome this sensation and steadily gain the comfort and competence to begin enjoying experiences that open new opportunities (UCLA Study Abroad Center, http://www.cie.uci.edu/prepare/shock .shtml). Being aware of the potential for feeling lonely, disconnected, frustrated and impatient in the new context can be balanced with knowledge that a strong social network is one of the most important mechanisms for reducing culture shock (Pantelidou and Craig, 2006). Being active participants in the experience abroad helps minimize culture shock (Zhou et al., 2008). Reading prose and poetry by local writers, going to arts performances and galleries and attending local celebrations can provide deeper insights into the way people live in the community.

Preparation in advance is key. First, consider how you manage stress under normal conditions. Music and photos, a few favourite treats from home as well as a plan for communicating with family are important. Keeping a reflective journal is helpful both for recording thoughts, feelings, questions and experiences and for processing the meaning of experiences and enhancing learning on return home. Second, have a plan in place for getting support for anxiety and extreme adjustment difficulties. This will reduce the likelihood of saying or doing something that is inappropriate or overly critical of your hosts and the community.

Conclusion

Cultural competence and gaining a deeper understanding of other ways of living and being are essential in opening up our interactions to be more mutually beneficial. Making assumptions based on a little bit of information about individuals within a particular culture can limit our experiences and ability to gain a more holistic understanding of the world around us, and thus may limit our ability to assist and understand others. What we are urging people to develop is a sense of cultural humility that enables us to be not only competent but receptive and collaborative. Practicing cultural humility means taking into account both the larger, systemic cultural context while recognizing that each individual has their own worldview, their own viewpoints and their own lens through which they see the world. At the same time, as individuals we are not obligated to accept risk, disrespectful treatment or abuse under the guise of cultural relativism. Cultural competence recognizes power imbalance, privilege and vulnerabilities, variation in experience due to gender, sexual orientation, race, ethnicity, religion, and so forth. Competence provides us tools to make respectful decisions knowing that each social interaction is approached with the recognition that we all have our own bias and prejudices but we must remain open, respectful and ready for a focus on person-centred interaction. It entails lifelong learning, change, reflection and critique and a deep knowledge of self-awareness. It allows for both the recognition of individual difference as well as cultural context.

References

Abu Lughod, L. 2002. Do Muslim women really need saving? Anthropological reflections on cultural relativism and its others. *American Anthropologist* 104(3):783–790.

Baskin, C. 2006. Aboriginal worldviews as challenges and possibilities in social work education. *Critical Social Work* 7(2).

Bennett, M. 1993. A developmental model of intercultural sensitivity. Derived from: Bennett, Milton J. Towards a developmental model of intercultural sensitivity in R. Michael Paige, ed. *Education for the Intercultural Experience*. Yarmouth: Intercultural Press.

Borden, AW. 2007. The impact of service-learning on ethnocentrism in an intercultural communication course. *Journal of Experiential Education* 30(2):171–183.

Bourdieu, P. 1993. *The Field of Cultural Production*. New York: Columbia University Press.

Carpenter-Song, E., Nordquest Schwallie, M., and Longhofer, J. 2007. Cultural competence reexamined: Critique and directions for the future. *Psychiatric Services* 58(10):1362–1365.

Eichbaum, Q. 2015. The problem with competencies in global health education. *Academic Medicine* 90(4):414–417.

Foucault, M. 1980. *Power/Knowledge: Selected Interviews and Other Writings 1972–1977*. London: Harvester Press, p. 98.

Goode, T., Sockalingam, S., Brown, M., and Jones, W. A. 2000. A Planners' Guide, Infusing Principles, Content and Themes Related to Cultural and Linguistic Competence into Meeting and Conferences. Washington, DC: Georgetown University Centre for Child and Human 3.0 Development, National Centre for Cultural Competence. http://nccc.georgetown.edu/documents/Planners_Guide.pdf

Goode, T.D, Dunne, M.C., and Bronheim, S.M. 2006. The evidence base for cultural and linguistic competency in health care. The Commonwealth Fund. http://www.commonwealthfund.org/usr_doc/Goode_evidencebasecultlinguisticcomp_962.pdf

Gross, GD. 2000. Gatekeeping for cultural competence: Ready or not? Some post and modernist doubts. *Journal of Baccalaureate Social Work* 5(2): 47–66.

Hook, JN., Davis, DE., Owen, J., Worthington, EL., Jr., and Utsey, SO. 2013. Cultural humility: Measuring openness to culturally diverse clients. *Journal of Counseling Psychology* 60(3):353–366

Kirmayer, L. 2012. Cultural competence and evidence-based practice in mental health: Epistemic communities and the politics of pluralism. *Social Science and Medicine* 75(2):249–256.

Kleinman, A., and Benson, P. 2006. Anthropology in the clinic: The problem of cultural competency and how to fix it. *PLoS Med* 3(10): e294. doi:10.1371/journal.pmed.0030294

Kumaş-Tan, Z., Beagan, B., Loppie, C., MacLeod, A., and Frank, B. 2007. Measures of cultural competence: Examining hidden assumption. *Academic Medicine* 82(6):548–557. doi:10.1097/ACM .0b013e3180555a2d

McIntosh, P. 1989. White privilege: Unpacking the invisible knapsack. *Peace and Freedom Magazine*. July August:10–12.

Pantelidou, S., and Tom, KJ. Craig.2006. Culture shock and social support: A survey in Greek migrant students. *Social Psychiatry and Psychiatric Epidemiology* 41(10):777–781.

Perusek, D. 2007. Grounding cultural relativism. *Anthropological Quarterly* 80(3):821–836. Retrieved May 29, 2008 from EBSCO online database, SocINDEX http:// search.ebscohost.com/login .aspx?direct=true&db=sih&A N=26466793&site=ehost-live

Pittenger, K., and Heimann, B. 1998. Barnga: A game on cultural clashes. *Developments in Business Simulation and Experiential Learning* 25: 253–254

Pon, G. 2009. Cultural competency as new racism: An ontology of forgetting. *Journal of Progressive Human Services* 20:59–71.

Sakamoto, I. 2007. An anti-oppressive approach to cultural competence. *Canadian Social Work Review* 24(1):105–118.

Shiffman, J. 2014. Knowledge, moral claims and the exercise of power in global health. *International Journal of Health Policy Management* 3(6):297–299.

Shiffman, J. 2015. Global health as a field of power relations: A response to recent commentaries. *International Journal of Health Policy Management* 4(7):497–499.

Taylor, J. 2003. The story catches you and you fall down: Tragedy, ethnography, and "Cultural competence." *Medical Anthropology Quarterly* 17(2):159–181.

Ward, C., Bochner, S., and Furnham, A. 2005. *The Psychology of Culture Shock,* 2nd Edition. Philadelphia, PA: Taylor Francis.

Willen, S., Bullen, A., and Good, MD. 2010. Opening up a huge can of worms: Reflections on a "cultural sensitivity" course for psychiatry residents. *Harvard Review of Psychiatry* 8:4. doi:10.3109/10673229 .2010.493748

Yee, JY., and Dumbrill, G. 2003. Whiteout: Looking for race in Canadian social work practice. In A. Al-Krenawi and JR. Graham (eds.), *Multicultural Social Work in Canada* (pp. 98–121). Don Mills, ON: Oxford University Press.

Zhou, Y., Jindal-Snape, D., Topping, K., and Todman, J. 2008. Theoretical models of culture shock and adaptation in international students in higher education, Studies in Higher Education, 33:1:63–75. doi:10.1080/03075070701794833

Chapter 11

Communicating Effectively

Melissa Whaling and Carolyn Beukeboom

Contents

Effective communication skills allow people not just to clearly understand one another, but to respect each other's culture and differences and develop meaningful relationships. Although cultural and language competence are strongly intertwined, this chapter strives to discuss the importance of verbal and non-verbal communication in another country, learning key words in a local language, preparation for language learning, prior to departure and while in-country and effective strategies to work with interpreters. We'll use examples of our own experiences in learning languages while working in South America and Africa.

Language competence can at first seem like a pretty simple concept of retaining linguistic or grammatical competence but in fact, the term is much more holistic, including aspects of sociolinguistic/sociocultural competence and contextual competence whereby understanding, meaning and practical application play key roles in acquiring language competence (Mede and Hasan, 2015). Language competence includes an ability to utilize knowledge to interpret and produce both theoretical and practical insights into expressive and meaningful communication that is in line with the present situation and circumstance (Scarino and Liddicoat, 2009; Good, 2000). It is an ability that should continually develop and flourish with changing context and communication.

Context, culture and meaning all play an integral role in the comprehension and production of discourse. Language competence is an integrative process combining language instruction with cultural and contextual practice (Goode, 2000; Unite for Site, 2015). It is best developed in context, where all aspects of the language are heard, seen and represented in real-life situations. When learning, speaking, reading, writing, listening to and communicating in a new language, it is best for one to apply one's knowledge of discourse and how it is organized, how the language is structured and sequenced to interpret and produce text and to apply one's knowledge of the sociocultural context (Goode, 2000).

Why Learn Another Language?

Many international learning programs and experiences are quite short in duration (less than 6 weeks), catering to those with demanding schedules, causing many participants to question the benefits of acquiring language competence in terms of learning the host language(s). Linguistic and cultural learning require a certain mental, emotional and physical time commitment (Unite for Site, 2015). That being said, there are substantial benefits in committing to learning (even if in part) a host language, even if the international experience is short in length.

Building language competence often increases cultural sensitivity as individuals are more aware of and are better able to understand communication, beliefs, values and behavioural systems of their host community, creating a broader empathy and tolerance of difference. Acquiring new language skills opens up opportunities for truer, deeper and more meaningful interactions which greatly broadens our ability to learn and accumulate knowledge, especially of other practices, traditions and ways of life. In the same way, it also allows for others to learn from us and interact with us and allows all parties to become more comfortable interacting with each other. It demonstrates one's interest, respect and openness for the host culture and ways of life. It is an avenue that allows us to break down communication barriers that separate us such as negativism, prejudice, cultural generalization and ethnocentrism.

Learning a local language can build social capital and both personal and professional relations, opening up opportunities for meaningful, mutually beneficial and long-lasting connections, friendships and camaraderie. It provides an avenue to access social resources which often have a positive impact on health, well-being and security. It greatly eases the social integration process and helps us to navigate a foreign environment to better understand and cope with problematic, potentially harmful contexts.

For instance, even some familiarity with the local language makes it much easier to appreciate what is going on around you and how to handle a dangerous situation. Being able to communicate effectively can also increase the number of local allies you attain and enhance social and professional networks. Although your ability to learn a new language can be limited by factors such as time, exposure and so on simply being able to greet those in your neighbourhood and surrounding area can have a huge impact on safety. As you make your presence known by interacting with others around you, they will be better able to recognize that you are a foreigner and will make an extra effort to protect or warn you when necessary.

Solid long-term friendships expand sociocultural opportunities to experience the authentic local way of life, the more you engage in learning a local language. For instance, you may be able to get the 'insider's view' on where to eat, what to buy, places to visit and may be allowed inclusion in events, activities or experience of popular local entertainment. It may create long-lasting relationships that expand your global network of supports and experiences. In many cultures, many business relationships are often formed through and sustained by personal friendships, connections and camaraderie. In East Africa and the Arab world, business meetings and interactions always begin with personal banter and inquiry around families before delving into business matters. Greater communication therefore can be a professional advantage, opening up greater opportunities for learning, networking and connectivity.

Achieving linguistic facility can result in personal growth and overcome obstacles and challenges related to intercultural immersion. It is a process that promotes higher levels of self-awareness, interpersonal development and insight into one's own culture, values, behaviours and life direction. Language competence can, and often is, enjoyable and pleasurable as it leads to new pathways of discovery and leaves us with a feeling of accomplishment. It increases our confidence in our work and daily interactions and empowers us in navigating a new environment. In addition, it can reduce a sense of shock, loneliness, isolation and homesickness, often associated with cultural immersion.

Non-Verbal Communication

Both non-verbal and verbal communication vary from culture to culture. Many gestures that seem like common sense in your own culture may be quite foreign and even impolite in other cultures. Non-verbal communication includes people's body language in the form of facial expressions, head movements, hand and arm gestures, physical space, touching, eye contact and physical postures (Management Sciences for Health [MSH], 2007).

When first entering a new culture, it is important to quietly observe people's mannerisms, body language and informal ways of communicating. A basic understanding of when to shake someone's hand or only slightly bow to the other person with hands together will come a long way in showing respect within another culture. It will help facilitate communication and connections with others. As children develop, the cultural dynamics, norms, values, beliefs and practices of their own society are often learnt unconsciously over time. Often, a person only becomes aware of these unconsciously learnt cultural aspects when exposed to unfamiliar cultural and linguistic systems.

A few examples: Head movements nod for yes and shake of the head for no, are reversed in some countries. Hand movements – in North America gesturing someone to come is with palms up and movement of the fingers towards you, in some cultures this gesture is done with palms are down. The universal sign of choking is to put one's hands up to the neck, in one community the sign was to hit the top of one's head. Sitting with your feet over one knee, or putting your feet up on another chair or bench is considered rude or impolite in many cultures, as seeing the bottoms of your feet is unclean. Eye contact varies from culture to culture as well, in some cultures women must keep their eyes lowered when speaking to a man, in other cultures not using eye contact with another is considered impolite.

Long pauses or a tendency to stay quiet may be interpreted in many different ways. In some instances, a lack of verbal communication or 'silence' is a component of respectful communication. Definition of and importance of lack of punctuality, may be perceived differently across cultures.

Verbal Communication

Verbal communication encompasses a broad range of topics. The way in which you are expected to interact through language with others can depend on who is being engaged. The tone and topic of discourse may vary depending on who that person is, what they do for a profession, their seniority within a larger hierarchy, their social status, age, gender or education level to name a few. In East Africa, when engaging in conversation with an elder or in passing them on the street, you must greet them with a particular term of respect that symbolizes appreciation. In addition, when speaking to elders, you will use more formal, traditional language instead of slang.

In many Global South countries, asking personal questions to another is considered normal polite conversation. Thus, on a bus, in a taxi, at work or shopping at the local market do not be surprised to have people ask you 'How old are you?', 'Are you married?', 'How many children do you have?' or 'How much income do you make?' and so on.

It is important to be aware of the time, place and context of discursive interactions as certain conversations will have a 'time and a place' in different cultures. Both in East Africa and South America, it is considered impolite to enter in a conversation, even in a work context, with someone before greeting them extensively.

Differences in opinions related to medical knowledge, skills or treatment options should be treated with respect and open, honest discussion. Western trained healthcare providers often feel that their methods and ways may be superior to their counterparts in other countries. Often, open discussion of differences in opinion regarding treatment can result in an appreciation for the rationale of each approach. Terminology used by patients may also be different than what you are accustomed to. In South America, it was noted that the patients would often talk about their kidney, ovarian or heart pain rather than location of their pain – lower pelvic, chest or right-sided abdomen. It is important to be aware of the local perspectives on different medical issues. In some countries in Africa, writing an actual diagnosis of HIV or AIDs on a patient's chart was considered taboo.

Regardless of language or cultural differences, it is vital that healthcare students specifically ask patients what their needs and preferences are. Try asking short and open-ended questions when unsure, rather than reacting quickly. Providing patient-centred care means viewing patients as individuals with unique experiences and not simply as members of one group or another. Although it is important to learn about culture-specific healthcare beliefs that may be common in your patient populations, it is equally important to understand the risk of stereotyping and believing that members of one population are all alike.

Learning a New Language

Learning the basic elements of your host country's local language should start prior to going abroad. Prior to embarking on your overseas experience try to connect with local people from that country who live near you. Vital information can be learned about culture, language and pronunciation from these people. Part of being able to learn a new language is being able to access various learning resources such as language guide books, various teaching materials such as Rosetta Stone, websites, apps, use of recordings, getting in touch with the host community, and so on. That being said, not all languages have accessible teach yourself learning materials and resources, as some languages have not been as extensively documented. When this is the case, it may seem difficult to start learning a language. There are various ways in which you can initiate their language comprehension which include contacting host participants and asking for learning materials, utilizing Internet resources (e.g. dictionaries, translation tools, websites), contacting those in your own community who may speak the desired language (prior to departure), arranging for online lessons, prior to departure with host contacts (via Skype, Whatsapp or videoconference) and accessing language lessons directly upon arrival.

It would also be prudent to find out what the language expectations of the host community and healthcare professionals with whom you will be working are, and to be realistic in terms of your own language abilities.

Learning basic phrases in the language of the country or region where you are going will create a positive relationship with the community, as they will be happy that you are trying and willing to learn their language. Create a list of helpful phrases include greetings, thank you, what is your name, where are you from, good bye, numbers, basic verbs, and so on. If you are working in a medical environment, medical terminology such as knowing body parts and basic questions – such as, Do you have fever? Diarrhea? Vomiting? Pain? Open your mouth? Take a big breath? – will be useful phrases and certainly make patients feel at ease.

Keeping an open mind, listening to others speak and having the ability to laugh at yourself are important qualities when learning a new language. The bond of laughter among different cultures keeps learning a language fun and relaxing within various settings. While trying to learn Spanish, CB asked a patient who had injured her leg about the use of crutches, 'muletas', using instead the word 'maletas', which means suitcases. Another time with a waiting room full of patients, she called out the next patient, 'Señora Ramera', a slang term for prostitute instead of 'Señora Ramero'. The whole waiting room burst into laughter, embarrassing CB but easing the tension caused by overcrowding. These types of mistakes can often reduce power differentials as well.

While in the country of your work or educational placement seek out opportunities to speak with the locals. Go to the local market on your own and buy fruits and vegetables, talk to the person beside you on the bus, play soccer with the children, look through children's school books or go to the local pub. Many people will express a desire to learn English and thus a language exchange can occur, whereby you help the locals and they in turn can teach you. Each of these opportunities will allow you to become part of the community and learn about the culture in various ways making your experience so much more rewarding.

Race Relations and 'Othering' in Language

In some cultures, race relations, power inequalities and 'othering' are quite notable and extensive in everyday linguistic interactions. Racial and ethnic inequalities, mythologies and stereotypes have historical roots and neocolonial implications in the use of everyday language. If you are not well versed in the sociocultural and historical background of a place you are visiting, use of particular racialized terms may be alarming or misunderstood in its context. For example, in many East African countries, the term 'mzungu' ('wazungu' pl.) is used extensively to identify someone who is Caucasian (white). The term 'mzungu' originated from the root word -zungu, meaning 'wondrous' or 'to go in circles' and is now frequently used to acknowledge white economic privilege. It is quite common as a white person walks down the street for people to yell 'mzungu' or for people to often refer to them as 'mzungu', similar to other pejorative terms such as 'Gringo-Green go home' and 'guilo' – meaning Chinese ghost. Within the Swahili language, multiple words are used commonly to identify individuals or groups based on power inequalities, segregation and stereotypes. It is common for people to identify 'Wazungu' (all white people), 'Wahindi' (i.e. people of Indian, Pakistani or other South Asian identities), 'Warabu' (those of Middle Eastern Background) and 'Wafrika' (all black people) as distinct races based on their visual appearance, despite vast cultural variation within each group. For example, it may be difficult for local people to stereotype someone who is Japanese-Canadian as they may be referred only as 'Mchina'. This does bring about a great opportunity to use conversation to break down existing stereotypes and barriers. It is recommended that you be aware of the historical context of the use of such terms in order to understand linguistic interactions that are racialized. It is important to note that such terms, although rich in historical meaning are sometimes identified simply as a process of identification by many. You may feel inclined to challenge the stereotypes by having a respectful conversation about assumptions and individual difference. This could include asking more questions in order to understand the contextual meaning behind such terms.

Navigating Multilingual Societies

In many countries, multiple languages exist and it may be difficult to learn one new language, let alone many. In some African countries, tribal languages are spoken, in addition to the national language. For example, in Tanzania, a country considered unique with one national language, Kiswahili, after Ujamaa of Nyerere half a century ago, in addition to the colonial language English there are over 120 tribal languages that are spoken, some of which are the first and only known language of many people.

Identify languages spoken by patients in the area that you will be working in advance of your elective. Local language used may be different from the official language of your host country. You may think you are going to a Spanish-speaking country such as Ecuador or Peru, only to learn that the main language of the people spoken in the rural areas of the Andes is Quechua and that will also differ considerably between and within the countries.

It is recommended that you first learn the national spoken language and then explore the various regional languages or dialects of the areas in which you will be based. That being said, there can be issues when translating from English to a national language to a local language and back as pieces may be lost in translation. It is beneficial to contact your host partners to inquire about which languages are spoken in the particular regions which you will visit. You can also utilize the aforementioned language learning strategies to focus on two or a few languages that they will be using the most. Realistically it may be difficult to learn more than one language prior to or during your stay so the use of an interpreter can also be considered.

Working with Interpreters

In many cases, particularly short-term experiences, it is not feasible to develop proficiency in the language of your host country. If you are not already fluent in the language, communicating with patients, without an interpreter will be a difficult. Working with interpreters is a unique experience offering many challenges.

Within medical settings, various people could act as interpreters, including medical professional interpreters, professional general interpreters, other healthcare professionals, family members and friends or strangers. There are pros and cons to working with each, depending on the setting. Health professionals who already have their own roles within the healthcare system may not have time to interpret for students who are coming from abroad and do not know the local language. It is important to be mindful of the time it takes away from the activities of other professionals, especially since most healthcare professionals are already taxed in terms of their workloads. Many of these people will take on this role for you, even if they are taken away from their regular roles and responsibilities. Sometimes, the role of interpretation will fall on the local medical or nursing students who may resent the increased workload or will expect gifts or monetary rewards.

Be very careful of the use of family members and friends, asking permission and trying to maintain patient confidentiality at all times. Family members and friends may not interpret everything exactly as said (Queensland Government, 2007). In some cultures, it is proper to withhold a serious diagnosis, such as cancer, from the sick family member. And one must be careful using children to interpret for parents, especially on sensitive topics such as domestic violence and women's gynecological issues. Gender, age and even ethnicity of the interpreter can affect the therapeutic relationship between healthcare provider and patient (Unite for Site, 2015). In some countries where tribal conflicts are common, having one person from one tribal group assist with interpretation for a patient in a rival tribal group may cause tension in the relationship. Men interpreting for female medical issues in some countries may not be allowed or preferred.

Working with interpreters requires a specific skill set of which many students and even professionals are not aware. Those who know the language may not fully understand the culture. Most people who serve as interpreters are not highly qualified, and most healthcare providers are not well trained to work with them (Queensland Government, 2007). There are clear differences between the skill sets of general translators, medical interpreters and cultural interpreters. The quality of the medical interaction depends on several factors relating to the student, interpreter and the patient.

Finding 'competent' medical interpreters who are objective parties and who take into account cultural terms, concepts and expressions in order to convey information accurately to both the patient and the provider is optimal. A well-trained interpreter will have taken a course that involves interpretation skills and techniques, ethical issues during healthcare encounters, key medical terminology, basic clinical concepts, workings of the medical system, cultural issues and professionalism. This is uncommon in many countries, although you could ask your host community about local language agencies, community colleges and/or universities, immigration programs and non-governmental organizations (NGOs). It is also important to think about fair compensation for the interpreter. Often, this is best discussed with the host community. Even in settings with highly qualified interpreters and healthcare providers who are well trained to work with them, the mere presence of a 'middle person' in a healthcare provider–patient interaction can have a negative impact.

Differences in culture and how questions are asked may also cause challenges within the relationship. As is common practice in the intake interview in North America, healthcare providers will often ask about alcohol intake. However, for some cultures who for the most part do not drink alcohol, this question can be considered very rude. Thus, one interpreter indicated that it was best if the question was prefaced with 'We ask everyone this question, but do you drink any alcohol?' The same can be done with questions around sexuality practices, orientation, HIV testing, pregnancy, and so forth. However, you must keep in mind that in the context of an elective, it is the student who is the guest and needs to be careful about how questions are phrased for interpretation.

A few guidelines for interacting with interpreters that can help make the interaction easier (Hillard, 2013; Osborne, 2000):

1. Use proper seating arrangement – place the interpreter to one side, or slightly behind the patient, so that you can maintain eye contact and watch their body language throughout the interaction.
2. Introduce yourself and the interpreter.
3. Make sure the patient is aware that all information will be kept confidential.
4. Allow for extra time when working with interpreters.
5. Make every effort to know greetings and introductions in the local language.
6. Speak directly to the patient, not the interpreter, and converse as if talking to an English-speaking person (in the first person).
7. Speak slowly and in 2–3 sentences at a time, allowing for pauses and interpretation to occur.
8. Avoid conversing with the interpreter, and if speaking directly to them, explain to the patient the nature of the conversation.
9. Pay attention to non-verbal cues – facial expressions, gestures and posture.
10. Repeat questions as necessary and have patients repeat instructions so you know the patient understands what you are trying to explain to them.
11. Avoid jargon and technical terms.
12. Treat the interpreter with respect.

Conclusion

Language is one of the most important forms of communication and social interaction. Learning the language(s) of our host partners is not only beneficial to the individual but it can also create a foundation for meaningful interactions and mutually benefitting relationships. You can expand your knowledge, understanding, opportunity and ability to grow and connect simply by engaging in language learning. Language competence empowers us to become more globally competent and eases the complexity of navigating new environments. It helps us to further understand intercultural components of the human experience and opens up more avenues for self-awareness and awareness of others. Although a seemingly simple concept of language acquisition, learning a new language is quite complex in its process and value, as it reaches into the depths of sociocultural, economic and historical ways of being and interacting. You must continue to be mindful that language shapes thoughts and your vision of life as a whole. As Ludwig Wittgenstein explains, 'the limits of our language are the limits of our world'.

References

Goode, T., Sockalingam, S., Brown, M., and Jones, W. A. 2000. *A Planners' Guide, Infusing Principles, Content and Themes Related to Cultural and Linguistic Competence into Meeting and Conferences.* Washington, DC: Georgetown University Centre for Child and Human 3.0 Development, National Centre for Cultural Competence. http://nccc.georgetown.edu/documents/Planners_Guide.pdf

Hillard, R. 2013. The use of interpreters with immigrant and refugee families. *Paediatric Child Health,* 18 (9): 457.

Management Sciences for Health (MSH). 2007. Providers guide to quality and culture – Non-verbal communication. http://erc.msh.org/mainpage.cfm?file=4.6.0.htm&module=provider&language=English

Mede, E., and Hasan, D. 2015. Teaching and learning sociolinguistic competence: Teachers' critical perceptions. *Participatory Educational Research (PER),* 2(3): 14–31. http://dx.doi.org/10.17275/per.15.29.2.3

Osborne, H. 2000. When you truly need to find other words: Working with medical interpreters. *Boston Globe's On Call Magazine.* http://healthliteracy.com/2000/07/01/medical-interpreters/

Queensland Government. 2007. Guide to working with interpreters in health service settings. http://www.health.qld.gov.au/multicultural/health_workers/work_interp.pdf

Scarino, A., and Liddicoat, A. J. 2009. A Guide: Teaching and Learning Languages. Australian Government. Department of Education Employment and Workplace Relations Teaching and Learning Languages. http://www.tllg.unisa.edu.au/lib_guide/gllt.pdf

Unite for Sight. 2015. Cultural competency online course. *Unite for Sight.* http://www.uniteforsight.org/cultural-competency/

Chapter 12

Ethics: Four Key Questions You Need to Ask

Kelly Anderson and Matthew DeCamp

Contents

Short-term global health training programs – whether in research, service or both – continue to increase in popularity among health science trainees. The thrill that comes with taking off on a trans-continental flight is palpable for many global health enthusiasts. This can be especially true for gung-ho trainees embarking on a first global health experience. For many, the momentum of this excitement runs head-on into the sometimes difficult reality of the experience and reflections upon it, following their return flight home. Uncomfortable questions such as, 'Did I cause unintended harm?' or 'What was the long-term impact of what I did?' may cause emotional or moral distress for you upon re-entry.

Fortunately, a rapidly growing body of literature emphasizes on how pre-departure training in ethics can help you anticipate and manage these questions. Preparing through exposure to the types of situations, issues and challenges you may face abroad can achieve several overlapping aims. First, pre-departure training should sharpen your awareness of the diverse ethical issues inherent in short-term global health experiences. Second, it should improve your skills in managing these issues and help us all maintain appropriate humility towards this work. Third, pre-departure concepts should help alleviate the distress caused by morally problematic situations. Finally, in some circumstances, training in ethics should aim not only to alleviate moral distress but also to cause us all to recognize morally problematic situations, which we otherwise might not.

Properly construed, pre-departure training in ethics shares the same overarching goals as short-term work itself: to benefit host communities through sustainable, culturally sensitive partnerships to alleviate gross inequalities in global health. Recognizing this, many academic institutions now offer pre-departure courses (Anderson et al., 2012). In this chapter, we briefly describe progress made in our thinking about ethical issues in short-term global health electives over the past two decades. We introduce two complementary ways in which you as a trainee can think about ethical issues. From these, we describe four core questions that you should ask during pre-departure training. We close by describing work that lies ahead.

In this chapter, we use 'trainee' in the broadest possible sense. In the global health setting, 'trainees' may include anyone with no or limited experience in global health, from the undergraduate student to the seasoned practitioner.

A Story of Progress

Understanding recent progress made regarding ethics and short-term global health is not just an intellectual enterprise. It can help you realize that you are not alone in experiencing ethically troublesome situations or moral distress while abroad and that others have developed ways to identify and manage these situations. Indeed, the idea that short-term global health experiences raise ethical issues is not new (Montgomery, 1993).

However, burgeoning attention to global health in the early years of the 2000s – a development fuelled by increased funding for global health and the development of global health centres and institutes in high-income countries – arguably contributed to a concomitant increase in short-term global health programs. For example, some surveys suggest that two-thirds of medical students in the United States now expect to go abroad during their medical studies (and about one-third actually do) (AAMC, 2015).

During these early years, ethical issues in short-term global health received attention largely through anecdotes experienced and shared by trainees (see Roberts, 2006; Wolfberg, 2006; DeCamp, 2007; Shah and Wu, 2008; Al-Samarrai, 2011). Trainees wrote rich descriptions of distressing experiences abroad. They recognized ethical issues in short-term global health training and advocated for systematic guidance related to them.

In the late 2000s, this unmet need was filled by two events. One was the development of Global Health Essential Core Competencies by the Joint U.S./Canadian Committee on Global Health (Joint U.S./Canadian Committee on Global Health, 2010). These competences explicitly note the need for trainees to demonstrate understanding of the ethical issues involved in short-term global health training. Also in 2010, the Working Group on Ethics Guidelines for Global Health Training (WEIGHT; see Crump, Sugarman and WEIGHT, 2010) published ethics and best practice guidelines for training experiences in global health. Created by an international group inclusive of individuals from the North and South, the guidelines address ethical issues of relevance to trainees, institutions and sponsors.

Two Complementary Approaches to Ethics

The transition from recognition of ethical issues to concrete guidance represents progress. Indeed some programs have used this guidance to inform real-world global health programs (see Dasco, Chandra and Friedman, 2013). Foundational to this progress are two approaches to conceptualizing these ethical issues.

One approach arguably (though not explicitly) derives somewhat from the principle-based approach to bioethics widely employed in the United States (Beauchamp and Childress, 2012). The principle-based approach sees as foundational the moral principles of respect for persons, beneficence, non-maleficence and justice (or fairness). These principles are to some extent reflected in the WEIGHT guidelines, which emphasize respect for community needs and priorities, ensuring mutual and reciprocal benefit (and avoiding undue burden) and protecting equity in the distribution of costs and benefits, among others.

Another approach represents what may be more an orientation to global health than a set of discrete principles to balance (Pinto and Upshur, 2009). This approach emphasizes humility, introspection, solidarity and social justice. In this approach, questions such as 'Why am I participating in a short-term program?' are just as important as 'What will I do?' To that end, Pinto and Upshur present 10 questions for individuals to ask prior to engaging in global health work.

In our view, these two approaches are complementary and accomplish similar or overlapping ends via slightly different means. You may find that one or the other is more helpful as conceptual tools to prepare for and manage ethical issues that arise in your global health training.

Pre-Departure Preparation: Four Core Questions

A fully comprehensive examination of how to teach global health ethics is beyond the scope of our chapter. (See "Additional Resources for Students and Teachers" for a list of web resources available for teaching global health ethics.) Here we draw upon these complementary approaches to highlight what we see as the four core ethically relevant questions that you should ask in advance of a training experience.

What Are My Motivations?

There are many well-documented benefits of short-term global health experiences for learners, and electives are often reported as representing times of memorable personal and professional development. For many altruistic learners, it can be difficult to admit, or even imagine, that some reasons for pursuing a global health experience may be self-serving. Understanding one's motivations is a crucial first step in preparing for an abroad experience because these motivations may affect how one behaves or responds to the experience itself.

Along these lines, Pinto and Upshur (2009) invite learners to take an introspective approach to their motivations. Not all motivations may be equal; for example, exploring 'an exotic part of the world' (Pinto and Upshur, 2009, p. 8) is insufficient motivation and may even be wasteful. To understand motivations, they recommend you ask yourself questions such as 'Why do you hope to do this work?' and 'What are your objectives, both personal and structural, short- and long-term?' The answers to these questions should then be compared to the knowledge and practice needs of the local community to ensure a good fit.

Philpott (2010) also offers another way for learners to frame their motivations, suggesting there are (1) those to aspire to, (2) those to tolerate and (3) those to suppress in global health work. Examples of motivations to suppress include the glamour and heroism associated with transcontinental travel and the frequent flier points thereby gained. Instead, she advocates for motivations that aspire towards understanding the challenges of others and developing a global state of mind. In our view, a useful activity could be to have students create these lists, in either a private or group activity, during pre-departure training.

What If My Elective Could Cause Harm to Patients?

Understanding motivations alone, however, is not enough because even well-meaning trainees and programs can violate the ethical principle of non-maleficence and cause harm (Crump and Sugarman, 2008). Surprisingly, there has been little research on the potential harm trainees and programs pose to host communities and patients (Bhat, 2008).

Although there are many possible unintended harms of global health programs, one of particular relevance to trainees relates to provision of care or service above their level of training (Abedini, Gruppen, Kolars and Kumagai, 2012; Elit et al., 2011; Petrosoniak, McCarthy and Varpio, 2010). The WEIGHT guidelines (2010) provide clear guidance that trainees should not provide care above their level of training and that they should be adequately supervised.

However, for individual trainees, the decision to not act above one's training is neither easy or without consequence. As Petrosoniak, McCarthy and Varpio (2010) report, trainees may experience significant pressure to impress supervisors abroad, and humiliation can result if they do not perform a specific procedure above their skill level. They may also find themselves in situations where they are not formally qualified to perform a needed task, but there is no one available who is and they legitimately feel they can safely help with a patient's needs. While this is a judgment call that few medical faculty are comfortable with, it is a reality for which students should be prepared for (and be ready to accept the consequences).

Preparing you for such situations is an important part of pre-departure training. One way to do so is to simply raise the issue (DeCamp et al., 2013; see also Humanitarian Health Ethics at http://humanitarianhealthethics.net/). Another would be to use role-play and case-based learning modalities that place trainees in hypothetical scenarios where they are being asked to do something above their level of training. Participating in these role plays develops the strategies (or even the language) to both proactively describe trainees' skills to their advisor and decline to perform such tasks when asked (Petrosoniak, McCarthy and Varpio, 2010).

Will I Be a Burden on the Community?

A third critical question for trainees relates less to directly causing harm and more to indirectly and unintentionally being a burden on the host community. Although there is little formal research published on effects on host communities receiving global health trainees (Sykes, 2014; Caldron, Impens, Pavlova and Groot, 2015), ample anecdotes and expert opinion exist to suggest trainees can present burdens to the host community. When those burdens alter how local resources are used and distributed, they can be seen as issues of justice.

Trainees, for example, can distract local advisors from their own clinical or research work by asking them to spend time teaching them or orienting them to the community. Trainees might also require tangible resources, such as food, housing, transportation or interpreters. While direct compensation of host personnel or institutions for the training and opportunities provided to trainees has not been routinely expected or provided, awareness that they are usually learning far more than contributing should be at the forefront of their consciousness in clinical settings.

A poignant example of this is the situation of a particular trainee as described in Huish (2012). The trainee, Dave clearly describes a situation where he felt he became a burden:

> The clinic could hardly handle the demand of incoming patients, let alone meet their primary care needs once admitted. Dave said that there is an ethical problem with this: This clinic can barely function, and now it has to act as a teaching centre for wealthy and privileged medical students from Canada . . .. In the middle of the bustle two guys brought in a woman severely dehydrated . . . I was in the ward wearing my white coat. The local nurses, overwhelmed, turned to me figuring that I had the appropriate knowledge and skills and they said, 'Fix her up with a saline drip'. I found the saline and the needle, but when I got to the woman I didn't know what to do. Here is someone dying in front of me from something as basic as dehydration, and I have no idea how to properly insert the needle into her collapsed veins…The nurse had to quit attending to someone else, come over and complete the job that I couldn't do, which took her away from someone else's needs. I was no help to anyone in that moment.

Due to various and complex power imbalances – of education, resources, rank and social status – between host personnel, visiting trainees and patients in the global health setting, such burdens may be difficult to identify. In the context of the Consortium of Universities for Global Health (CUGH), for example Crane (2011) reported that individuals from 'Southern' communities felt that their institutions 'often had little decision-making power in international collaborations' (Crane, 2011, p. 1388) and were left out of the process to define global health itself.

As a trainee, you must be aware that you may not know if/when you are a burden – it may be invisible to you, particularly when host communities are reluctant to raise such issues. Sometimes, the existence of such burdens can be recognized accidentally. For example, sitting in a café in a central African country years ago, one of us (Anderson) found herself next to a table of local medical students. In conversation, it came up why they were not at school: they did not have enough teachers or clinical resources for them all to attend. Recalling the dozens of Northern students I knew who had done medical electives here, I wondered, 'Were these local students being hedged out by outsiders? Who is shouldering the burden of these clinically inexperienced Northern learners?'

Therefore, the key question, 'Will I be a burden?', includes a second question, 'How will I know if I am?' Pre-departure training can open a discussion of the potential for being such burdens and the power imbalances that may hide them. At the same time, responsibility does not lie with you alone. Northern universities continuing to send learners must fully account for the resource allocation effects that could be otherwise unexplored (Crump, Sugarman and WEIGHT, 2010), including any implicit participation in potential resource drain from the local community.

When We Do Not Have 'The Answers' for Communities in Need, How Will I Respond?

A final key question often emerges for trainees during and after their experience. Eager learners may develop an overwhelming urge to change the systems and/or cultures they encounter. While well-intentioned and with a commitment to beneficence, these plans may lack understanding of institutional practices, resource scarcity, political history, cultural norms and the inherent strengths and belief systems of communities. If so, they may also inadvertently violate the principle of respect.

Well-intentioned though they may be, such urges should be restrained. Long-standing implicit biases among inhabitants of wealthy nations portray much of the Global South as impoverished and dysfunctional, necessitating remediation via foreign aid and expertise. In fact, anthropologists are quick to remind us that other societies, peoples and communities (and their beliefs) are not inherently antiquated or their practices ineffective for their circumstances (Davis, 2009). Others remind us that poverty is relative because 'everyone under the sun could be labelled as poor, in one way or another' (Rahnema, 2010, p. 174). Finally, the term 'low-resource setting' itself overemphasizes financial or material circumstances, and may inadvertently belittle non-monetary, community resources that may be the foundation upon which solutions to health can be built.

The appropriate role of a trainee or learner is a commitment to humility (Pinto and Upshur, 2009). Humility can, in some circumstances, compel trainees to respond to their desire to 'do something', by acting in quite the opposite way: by doing nothing, at least for a time. Humility compels us to listen more deeply, to further try to understand the context we are observing. Therefore in pre-departure training, it becomes important to prepare trainees to potentially act in ways that may be counterintuitive to how they are otherwise being trained – that is the beneficence and respect can require remaining a humble listener and learner.

Future Directions

The four core questions we propose can help frame pre-departure ethics education in short-term global health programs. Online modules may be convenient, free and time efficient for trainees and teachers. Ideally, given the nature and complexity of the questions involved, such resources should be used with face-to-face, small-group discussion and mentorship. Simulation training to prepare students for ethical issues may be an exciting method for future teaching (Logar, Le, Harrison and Glass, 2015).

More work lies ahead. The fundamental ethical principles behind short-term global health training remain active areas of scholarship (see Lahey, 2012; Melby et al., 2016; Stone and Olson, 2016). Systematic, explicit ethical review of short-term programs is not yet universally done (DeCamp, 2011). As attention has turned to evaluation of the (presently scant) evidence of health outcomes from short-term global health programs (Sykes, 2014), so too has attention turned to evaluation of ethically salient outcomes (Caldron, Impens, Pavlova and Groot, 2015). Finally, the evidence behind pre-departure training's ability to change knowledge, skills, attitudes and behaviours of trainees remains similarly scant (Rahim et al., 2016).

Unfortunately, pre-departure training may be at present unable to mitigate the breadth of ethical issues encountered by trainees. A recent study, for example, found that although most students had participated in pre-departure training, most also felt that their training was inadequate and that it did not prevent 'frustration, anxiety and even emotional trauma' (Dell et al., 2014, p. 67). Some have suggested that only by teaching the relevant concepts of power, privilege, humility and so on within traditional medical or pre-medical curricula will progress be made in the global health setting (Huish, 2012).

Pre-departure training in ethics may not be a panacea; some might even suggest it ought not be. Perhaps its goal should be more modest, that is to give you the language, concepts and skills to first recognize and then manage the dilemmas and circumstances you encounter, not completely relieve the complex emotions you may have in response – emotions that may be an intended effect of the programs in the first place.

References

Abedini, Nauzley C., Larry D. Gruppen, Joseph C. Kolars, and Arno K. Kumagai. 2012. Understanding the effects of short-term international service-learning trips on medical students. *Academic Medicine* 87:820–828.

Al-Samarrai, Teeb. 2011. Adrift in Africa: A U.S. medical resident on an elective abroad. *Health Affairs* 30(3):525–528.

Anderson, Kelly C., Michael Slatnik, Ian Pereira, Eileen Cheung, Kunyong Xu, and Timothy F. Brewer. 2012. Are we there yet? Preparing Canadian medical students for global health electives. *Academic Medicine* 87(2):206–209.

Association of American Medical Colleges (AAMC). 2015. Medical School Graduation Questionnaire. https://www.aamc.org/download/440552/data/2015gqallschoolssummaryreport.pdf

Beauchamp, Tom L., and James Childress. 2012. *Principles of Biomedical Ethics.* 7th edition. New York: Oxford University Press.

Bhat, Suneel B. 2008. Ethical coherency when medical students work abroad. *Lancet* 372(9644):1133–1134.

Caldron, Paul H., Ann Impens, Milena Pavlova, and Wim Groot. 2015. A systematic review of social, economic and diplomatic aspects of short-term medical missions. *BMC Health Services Research* 15:380. 10.1186/s12913-015-0980-3.

Crane, Johanna. 2011. Scrambling for Africa? Universities and global health. *Lancet* 377(9775):1388–1390.

Crump, John A. and Jeremy Sugarman. 2008. Ethical considerations for short-term experiences by trainees in global health. *JAMA* 300(12):1456–1458.

Crump, John A., Jeremy Sugarman, and the Working Group on Ethics Guidelines for Global Health Training. 2010. Ethics and best practice guidelines for training experiences in global health. *American Journal of Tropical Medicine and Hygiene* 83(6):1178–1182.

Dasco, Matthew, Amit Chandra, and Harvey Friedman. 2013. Adopting an ethical approach to global health training: The evolution of the Botswana – University of Pennsylvania partnership. *Academic Medicine* 88:1646–1650.

Davis, Wade. 2009. *The Wayfinders: Why Ancient Wisdom Matters in the Modern World.* Toronto: Anansi Press.

DeCamp, Matthew. 2007. Scrutinizing global short-term medical outreach. *Hastings Center Report* 37(6):21–23.

DeCamp, Matthew. 2011. Ethical review of global short-term medical volunteerism. *HEC Forum* 23(2):91–103.

DeCamp, Matthew, Joce Rodriguez, Shelby Hecht, Michele Barry, and Jeremy Sugarman. 2013. An ethics curriculum for short-term global health trainees. *Globalization and Health* 9:5. 10.1186/1744-8603-9-5.

Dell, Evelyn M., Lara Varpio, Andrew Petrosoniak, Amy Gajaria, and Anne E. McCarthy. 2014. The ethics and safety of medical student global health electives. *International Journal of Medical Education* 5:63–72.

Joint U.S./Canadian Committee on Global Health. 2010. Core Competencies. http://globalhealtheducation.org/resources/Documents/Primarily%20For%20Faculty/Basic%20Core_Competencies_Final%202010.pdf

Elit, Laurie, Matthew Hun, Lynda Redwood-Campbell, Jennifer Ranford, Naomi Adelson, and Lisa Schwartz. 2011. Ethical issues encountered by medical students during international health electives. *Medical Education* 45(7):704–711.

Huish, Robert. 2012. The ethical conundrum of international health electives in medical education. *Journal of Global Citizenship and Equity Education* 2(1):1–19. http://journals.sfu.ca/jgcee/index.php/jgcee/article/viewArticle/55/30

Lahey, Timothy. 2012. A proposed medical school curriculum to help students recognize and resolve ethical issues of global health outreach work. *Academic Medicine* 87:210–215.

Logar, Tea, Phuoc Le, James D. Harrison, and Marcia Glass. 2015. Teaching corner: 'First Do No Harm': Teaching global health ethics to medical trainees through experiential learning. *Bioethical Inquiry* 12:69–78.

Melby, Melissa K., Lawrence C. Loh, Jessica Evert, Christopher Prater, Henry Lin, and Omar A. Khan. 2016. Beyond medical "missions" to impact-driven short-term experiences in global health (STEGHs). *Academic Medicine* 91(5):633–638.

Montgomery Laura M. 1993. Short-term medical missions: Enhancing or eroding health? *Missiology* 21:333–341.

Petrosoniak, Andrew, Anne McCarthy, and Lara Varpio. 2010. International health electives: Thematic results of student and professional interviews. *Medical Education.* 44(7):683–689.

Philpott, Jane. 2010. Training for a global state of mind. *Virtual Mentor* 12(3):231–236.

Pinto, Andrew D. and Ross E.G. Upshur. 2009. Global health ethics for students. *Developing World Bioethics* 9(1):1–10.

Rahim, Anika, Felicity Knights, Molly Fyfe, Janagan Alagarajah, and Paula Baraitser. 2016. Preparing students for the ethical challenges on international health electives: A systematic review of the literature on educational interventions. *Medical Teacher* 38(9):911–920. doi:10.3109/0142159X.2015.1132832.

Rahnema, Majid. 2010. Poverty. In: *The Development Dictionary: A Guide To Knowledge As Power.* 2nd edition, edited by Wolfgang Sachs, pp. 174–94. London: Zed Books.

Roberts, Maya. 2006. Duffle bag medicine. *JAMA* 295(13):1491–1492.

Shah, Sural and Tina Wu. 2008.The medical student global health experience: Professionalism and ethical implications. *Journal of Medical Ethics* 34(5):375–378.

Stone, Geren S. and Kristian R. Olson. 2016. The ethics of medical volunteerism. *Medical Clinics of North America* 100:237–246.

Sykes, Kevin. 2014. Short-term medical service trips: A systematic review of the evidence. *American Journal of Public Health* 104(7):e38–e48.

Wolfberg, Adam J. 2006. Volunteering overseas – Lessons from the surgical brigades. *New England Journal of Medicine* 354:443–445.

Additional Resources for Students and Teachers

Books

Evert, Jessica, Paul Drain, and Thomas Hall. 2014. *Developing Global Health Programming: A Guidebook for Medical and Professional Schools.* 2nd edition. San Francisco, CA: Global Health Collaborations Press.

Lasker, Judith N. 2016. *Hoping to Help: The Promises and Pitfalls of Global Health Volunteering.* Ithaca, NY: Cornell University Press.

Seager, Greg. 2012. *When Healthcare Hurts: An Evidence Based Guide for Best Practices in Global Health Initiatives.* Bloomington, IN: AuthorHouse.

Online Media

Consortium of Universities for Global Health (CUGH) Educational Modules. https://www.cugh.org/resources /educational-modules

Ethical Challenges in Short-term Global Health. http://ethicsandglobalhealth.org

The Ethics of International Engagement & Service Learning. (University of British Columbia) http:// ethicsofisl.ubc.ca/

Global Ambassadors for Patient Safety (University of Minnesota). https://www.healthcareers.umn .edu/courses-and-events/online-workshops/global-ambassadors-patient-safety

Global Health Clinical Ethics (Association of American Medical Colleges). https://www.mededportal .org/publication/10232

Global Service Learning. http://globalsl.org/

Humanitarian Health Ethics. http://www.humanitarianhealthethics.net/

The Practitioner's Guide to Global Health (Boston University). https://www.edx.org/course/practitioners -guide-global-health-part-1-bux-globalhealthx-1

SPECIFIC PROFESSIONS

Chapter 13

Emergency Medicine

Rahim Valani

Contents

Emergency medicine is a relatively new speciality across the globe and its work may differ significantly within and between countries. Undertaking electives in low- to middle-income contries (LMICs) presents unique and variable challenges with respect to resources available and competencies of local medical practitioners in this field. Being cognizant of the determinants of health assists understanding at a meta level of the inequalities that surround access and provision of care. What you might expect to find in a relatively high-resourced city teaching hospital will differ from a rural area staffed only by a nurse or midwife with limited medications.

In addition to the geopolitical and economic landscape, the utilization of care can differ. Lacking the adequate financial resources may preclude these people from seeking medical care until later in the course of the disease process. Thus, rare findings in the developed world with access to care may be more common and knowledge of late symptoms and disease complications will be beneficial.

Finally, the differential diagnosis changes based on the region of practice. While common things are common, one needs to include pathology that is also unique to that area. For example, tuberculosis (TB) osteomyelitis is in the differential in a patient who presents with thoracic back pain in an endemic area. Be aware of the neglected tropical diseases.

Differences in Clinical Presentation

Knowing how death and disease differ in low-income countries and the most common causes of emergency room (ER) visits is helpful to any student considering a health elective in a LMIC. While the leading causes of death are from ischemic heart disease, cerebrovascular disease and chronic obstructive pulmonary disease (COPD) when looking at worldwide statistics, the burden changes by country and region (Institute for Health Metrics and Evaluation, [IHME] 2013), as can be seen in Table 13.1.

Not surprisingly, the largest burden of disease in Africa and South East (SE) Asia is due to infections. However, in Africa the most common infectious culprits are human immunodeficiency virus (HIV)/ acquired immunodeficiency syndrome (AIDS), diarrheal disease and malaria, whereas in SE Asia it is diarrheal disease, TB and childhood cluster diseases (pertussis and measles).

It is important to recognize that Emergency medicine entails a spectrum of clinical presentations. There are common presenting problems that are seen everywhere – headaches, back pain, and so on. Common things are common across the globe. However, the important part is to recognize common presenting problems that have a unique differential diagnosis. Some of these are discussed below.

Common Presentations

Infection and Fever

In North America, a well appearing child who is fully immunized has about a 2% chance of an occult bacteremia, and less than 5% of those proceed on to a serious bacterial infection (Chancey

Table 13.1 Mortality-Based Stratification by Region and Cause

	Africa	SE Asia	Americas	Eastern Mediterranean	Europe	Western Pacific
Infectious/ parasitic	43.1%	17.5%	5.7%	16.6%	2.3%	5.7%
Respiratory infections	12.8%	9.3%	4.2%	9.8%	2.6%	3.9%
Maternal conditions	2.3%	1.1%	0.3%	1.4%	0.0%	0.1%
Perinatal conditions	8.7%	7.8%	2.4%	9.7%	0.9%	2.9%
Nutritional deficiency	1.4%	1.2%	0.9%	1.2%	0.1%	0.2%
Cardiovascular disease	10.4%	25.4%	32.0%	27.0%	50.2%	33.6%
Unintentional injuries	4.4%	8.7%	5.6%	7.5%	5.9%	6.9%

Source: Adapted from WHO, *The Global Burden of Disease – 2004 Update*, World Health Organization, Geneva, 2008.

and Jhaveri, 2009; Jhaveri et al., 2011). Fever is common everywhere, but the etiology and differential diagnosis of life-threatening diseases need to be extended. The usual culprits are still common etiological agents for urinary tract infection (UTI), pneumonia and meningitis. However, in places where children are not immunized the causative organism may not be commonly seen in the developed world. For example, vaccines are available for *Haemophilus influenzae* type B and *Neisseria meningitidis* serotype A/C/Y/W-135. Infections from these organisms can be seen in areas where routine vaccination is either not available or affordable. Furthermore, malaria, TB and other neglected tropical diseases would enter the picture. A broader and more thorough differential must be considered (malaria and diarrhea are also addressed in more detail in Chapter 14):

1. *Malaria*: Malaria is common in sub-Saharan Africa where over 600,000 people died from this infection in 2012 (Centers for Disease Control and Prevention [CDC], 2016). Endemic areas are aware of the symptoms and lab technicians are experts at diagnosing it on a smear. Patients can present with any of the following:
   a. Cerebral malaria: This can have variable presentation, but any neurological symptoms/signs or altered mental status is considered cerebral malaria until proven otherwise. Hypoglycemia is a poor prognostic factor.
   b. Severe anemia: Check for the size of the spleen, as splenomegaly can result in rupture.
   c. Sepsis and septic shock: Along with renal failure and acute respiratory distress syndrome (ARDS) – type picture.
   Knowing the local resistance patterns to common drugs such as chloroquine and mefloquine helps with effective treatment. Chemoprophylaxis is also important for you as the traveller.
2. *Diarrhea*: Each year, diarrhea is responsible for the death of over 2000 children/day (Liu et al., 2012). Diarrhea causes may be bacterial, viral or parasitic. Lack of appropriate therapy and clean water supplies makes treatment very difficult. While dehydration is the underlying cause of mortality, especially in children, the concomitant malnutrition and lack of proper therapy exacerbates their clinical course. Furthermore, invasive bacterial and parasitic diseases causing bloody diarrhea (dysentery) are more common and carry an even higher morbidity and mortality.
   Therapy should be with the World Health Organization (WHO) recommended oral rehydration salts made from clean water. In cases of severe dehydration, intravenous fluids may be required. For severe dehydration, getting intravenous (IV) access may be difficult and intraosseous access or hypodermoclysis should be considered. Patients also need nutrition to help develop enough metabolic reserves to fight off the offending agents. As a traveller, ensure clean water sources and take appropriate therapy if you develop diarrhea.
3. *Tuberculosis*: Over 95% of deaths caused by TB occur in developing countries, with SE Asia and Western Pacific regions accounting for most of the new cases (WHO, 2016b). TB should not be thought of as only a respiratory disease – extrapulmonary TB can affect all of the other organ systems. Miliary TB constitutes 10% of extrapulmonary TB, often seen as generalized nodules that are <2 mm in size. Lymphadenitis is the most common form of extrapulmonary TB and any person with lymphadenopathy should be suspected of having TB until proven otherwise. The most important risk factor for having TB is HIV, and concomitant infection is the norm rather than the exception. The use of protease inhibitors also worsens the clinical symptoms of TB.
   The Bacillus Calmette–Guérin (BCG) vaccine is used in countries with a high prevalence of TB meningitis in the pediatric population and miliary TB. The issue with treatment of

TB is ensuring adequate duration of therapy, recognizing multi-drug-resistant TB and being cognizant of the high risk of prevalence among patients with HIV.

4. *HIV*: HIV is transmitted through unprotected intercourse, blood/blood products transfused from an HIV-positive donor, parenteral inoculation (sharing needles) and perinatally. The WHO estimates 36.7 million people with HIV globally, with 2.1 million new cases/year and 1.1 million HIV-related deaths annually (Joint United Nations Programme on HIV/AIDS [UNAIDS], 2016). The acute infection occurs within days to weeks after exposure and presents as nonspecific viral-type illness. Progressive decrease in CD4 counts is the hallmark of this infection, and a count of <200 cells/mL requires Pneumocystis jiroveci pneumonia (PCP) prophylaxis, and patients should not be given any live virus vaccines. For those with a CD4 count less than 50 cells/mL, Mycobacterium avium complex (MAC) prophylaxis should be initiated.

A new diagnosis of HIV is often devastating to the patient and their families. The stigma associated with it along with lack of information about the disease and its transmission leads to alienation. Also, with poor resources, there may not be access to antiviral medications. There are major ethical and cultural issues to tackle based on the local beliefs behind HIV, and appropriate counselling for patients and their families is crucial.

Secondary infections are common in patients who are HIV positive, and some are pathognomonic for defining those with AIDS. The most common ones are

a. PCP: This is usually seen when CD4 counts are <200 cells/mL. Staining of induced sputum is reasonable in making the diagnosis. Treatment is with trimethoprim-sulfamethoxazole for 21 days. Adjuvant steroid therapy may be beneficial.

b. Tuberculosis: See the section 'Tuberculosis'.

c. MAC: Seen when the CD4 counts are <50 cells/mL. Typical anti-TB drugs do not work well for these organisms and multidrug therapy is the key.

d. Cryptococcal disease: The spores of this yeast are usually inhaled, resulting in pneumonia. It can also disseminate, usually to the central nervous system (CNS) causing cryptococcal meningitis (usually when the CD4 counts are <50 cells/mL).

e. Cytomegalovirus (CMV) infection: Again seen in those whose CD4 counts are <50 cells/mL and presents as chorioretinitis.

In addition to opportunistic and coinfections, patients with HIV are also prone to several malignancies. Kaposi's sarcoma is the most common malignancy seen in this patient population which is due to infection with human herpesvirus 8. Lymphoma is the other common malignancy.

Management of HIV is through antiviral medications. There are six classes of drugs, and treatment is usually with the use of drugs from more than one class:

a. Nucleoside/nucleotide reverse transcriptase inhibitors

b. Non-nucleoside/nucleotide reverse transcriptase inhibitors

c. Protease inhibitors

d. Fusion inhibitors

e. Integrase inhibitors

f. Chemokine co-receptor antagonists

There are combination drugs available that improve compliance for patients taking multiple medications. The WHO is working with other groups to improve access to medications globally, and an estimated 17 million people are on retroviral therapy (HIV/AIDS, 2016).

5. *Protozoan infections*: Protozoan infections are from ingestion of contaminated food/water. The cysts are ingested, and excystation occurs in the bowel lumen. The resulting trophozoites then form more cysts, which then cause the symptoms and are also excreted, thus repeating the cycle. A summary of the common protozoan infections is provided in the following table, including common presentations, complications to be aware of and treatment (the medications listed may not be available where you are working, so check with local resources who will have a better idea of what can be used) (Guerrant, 2011) (Table 13.2).

6. *Other infections*: There are a multitude of other infections you need to be aware of. However, having a handy resource is helpful as you may not be familiar with the signs and symptoms that are common to a tropical disease or one that is seen more frequently in resource-poor nations (an excellent resource is the global health training modules by the Consortium of Universities for Global Health [CUGH, 2016]).

Schistosomiasis, for example, can present with hematuria and pruritus. The infection can also cause non-cirrhotic periportal fibrosis with resultant hepatosplenomegaly and the stigmata of chronic liver disease. Knowing the plethora of presentations and having a broad differential diagnosis is the key. Praziquantel is the recommended therapy for schistosomiasis.

Seizure is usually a late manifestation for most of the infections mentioned above and carries with it a poor prognosis. Acquired epilepsy, however, is most commonly from neurocysticercosis, which is caused by the tapeworm *Taenia solium*. Management is with cysticidal therapy (praziquantel and albendazole are the agents of choice, but therapy is debated if needed for dead cysts) and antiepileptic drugs (Abba Ramaratnam, and Ranganathan, 2010).

Sickle Cell Disease

Sickle cell disease is caused by a mutation in the hemoglobin moiety such that under stress, the erythrocyte changes its morphology to a sickle shape. The adherence of these sickle cells and associated inflammation result in various complications. Symptoms and complications are not seen before the age of 5–6 months, when the hemoglobin F is at the nadir.

Increased complications are associated with higher mortality. Therefore, managing these patients in the community through education and primary care is crucial. A list of several complications follows; the management guidelines are based on the National Institute of Health publication 02–2117 (National Institutes of Health [NIH], 2002):

1. *Pain crisis/vaso-occlusive crisis:* This is the most common complication. Patients are usually aware of what to do, so if they are presenting to the clinic or healthcare facility, aggressive therapy is the key.
   Management:
   a. Fluid therapy: *Per os* (PO) or IV but make sure they continue to drink. IV fluids often 1.5 times maintenance.
   b. Analgesia: Any route to start getting the pain under control. If the pain is severe, start with morphine. Titrate accordingly.
   c. Remove the offending stressor if possible. For example cold weather, dehydration, hypoxia and infection.

Table 13.2   Common Protozoal Infections

Infection Organism	Clinical Presentation	Complications	Treatment
Amebiasis *Entamoeba*	Diarrhea, dysentery, liver abscess	Liver abscess is the most common extraintestinal manifestation Dissemination into the pulmonary system (usually right-sided) and cardiac abscess (liver, brain)	Iodoquinol Paromomycin Diloxanide furoate Metronidazole
Giardiasis *Giardia*	Foul-smelling diarrhea, malaise, abdominal cramps Usually not enterotoxigenic	Malnutrition due to malabsorption	Metronidazole
Cryptosporidiosis *Cryptosporidium* Completes life cycle in one host	Watery explosive diarrhea that is foul-smelling, vomiting, malaise	Usually in those with AIDS – severe, protracted diarrhea, cholangitis, cholecystitis and chronic malabsorption Is chlorine resistant, making this more difficult to eradicate	Self-limiting disease in healthy people Issue is with patients with no humoral immunity
Sleeping sickness *Trypanosoma*	Transmitted via tsetse flies Seen only in Sub-Saharan Africa Lymphadenopathy (classically posterior cervical) seen early on and regresses with time Trypanids (cutaneous lesions) Splenomegaly without hepatomegaly Anemia Asymptomatic phase – nonspecific malaise, myalgias, headaches, weight loss and pruritus CNS involvement results in headaches, somnolence, psychosis	Meningoencephalitis Secondary bacterial infection (aspiration pneumonia)	Pentamidine
Leishmaniasis *Leishmania*	Cutaneous ulcers with raised borders Erosion of nasal and oral mucosal surfaces Hepatosplenomegaly	Mucosal erosion may result in ulceration and perforation Malnutrition	Amphotericin B

2. *Fever*

This is the second most common complication. Patients with sickle cell disease have difficulties fighting off infections to begin with due to their immunocompromised state (they have functional asplenia or may have had a splenectomy) and encapsulated organisms are particularly concerning. In addition to the usual culprits and sources of infection, also consider osteomyelitis and acute chest syndrome in patients with fever. Check their immunization status, if available, to help guide treatment:

a. Obtain blood and urine cultures.

b. Broad-spectrum antibiotics: Ceftriaxone agent of choice when the organism or source is unknown.

c. IV fluids: Make sure they do not go into septic shock.

3. *Acute chest syndrome*

Any sickle cell patient complaining of chest pain, fever and cough should be considered to have acute chest crisis until proven otherwise. The diagnosis requires the presence of a new infiltrate on chest X-ray; the lack of imaging in resource-poor areas should not preclude one from being cautious by managing the patient as such. Causes can be infectious (virus, bacteria), respiratory conditions (asthma), cold weather and other causes of hypoxemia. Management should include the following:

a. Broad-spectrum antibiotics and hydration as previous

b. Oxygen therapy

c. Incentive spirometry – simple, helps recruit alveoli and prevent atelectasis

4. *Aplastic crisis*

This is usually caused by Parvovirus B19 that is cytotoxic to erythroid progenitor cells. Temporary suppression of erythrocytes can cause a profound anemia. Tissue hypoxia and precipitation of sickle pain crisis follows.

These patients appear pale and lethargic. Treatment is largely supportive with oxygen, fluids and blood transfusions (if the patient has reticulocytes on the blood count, you may hold off on the transfusion as they are starting to produce red cells). Also review other family members since they may be infected as well.

Trauma

Road traffic accidents and violence are a major burden apart from disease and a cause of mortality in developing countries (see Table 13.3). While most of the trauma is preventable and predictable, the difficulty lies in prevention due to the socio-economic costs (WHO, 2004). Infrastructure repair may not be a high priority item for the government. Care is also often delayed due to access

Table 13.3 Road Traffic Accidents and Violence as a Proportion of Total Injuries Stratified by Region

	Africa	SE Asia	Americas	Eastern Mediterranean	Europe	Western Pacific
RTA	26.7%	15.7%	25.9%	30.1%	16.3%	28.1%
Violence	23.7%	5.9%	26.5%	5.2%	8.2%	4.8%

Source: Adapted from WHO, *World Report on Road Traffic Injury Prevention*, edited by Peden et al., World Health Organization, Geneva, 2004.

to care and cost/affordability issues. In order to take care of these patients, following the principles of ATLS is helpful, with the caveat that care should be provided in keeping with resources available (American College of Surgeons [ACS], 2016).

How to Prepare

Medical trainees are choosing to incorporate global health experiences by undertaking learning opportunities in developing countries. In 2010–2011, 74% of American programs had at least one resident participate in a global health experience, of which 40% of programs had no pre-departure preparation prior to going abroad (Havryliuk, Bentley, and Hahn, 2014). Furthermore, the possibility to get an international experience is impacting residency choice among medical students who are interested in emergency medicine (Breyer, Sadosty, and Biros, 2012; Dey et al., 2002).

Emergency medicine is relatively recent in its recognition as a specialty in and of itself. For example, in Africa, there are 13 African country representatives within the African Federation of Emergency Medicine, with eight societies representing individual countries (AFEM, 2016). The burden of emergency conditions and emergency care usage is large, yet the emergency medical services (EMS) infrastructure may also be poor or lacking, triaging is inconsistent or non-existent and wait times are highly variable based on local resources (Chang et al., 2016). These differences arise from lack of resources and can impact the learning experience. Furthermore, the imposition of foreign trainees, especially those that don't speak the language, and the lack of reciprocity in opportunity are seen as barriers and need to be considered (O'Donnell et al., 2014).

From a learning perspective, there are also concerns regarding appropriate opportunities. Most of the ERs in non-urban areas are staffed by house-staff trainees who are either moonlighting or fulfilling their time so as to meet the requirements for other training programs. Also, in regions where emergency medicine is not recognized, the urban centres may not have consultants available in the ER to foster a structured learning program or evaluation.

Planning is key when undertaking any global health elective. The pre-departure requirements are covered in Section II of this volume. With emergency medicine, specific risk of exposure to infections and blood-borne pathogens may be greater than in an outpatient clinic and consideration of relevant immunizations, prophylaxis and personal protective equipment is extremely important. For example, in South Africa, interpersonal violence and road traffic accidents account for over 70% of injury-related mortality (Norman et al., 2007). Many centres are resource-poor and may not have the suitable equipment or prophylactic medications needed should it be required. Taking additional equipment (gloves, masks) as well as medications such as antibiotics should strongly be considered.

When visiting TB endemic areas, take along a few N95 masks for personal protection since respiratory isolation precaution availability is limited in resource-poor settings. When working in regions that have a high burden of HIV infection (Africa followed by SE Asia), additional safety precautions must be adhered to. Needlestick injuries or exposure to blood products increases the risk of infection. Use of gloves, safety needles and avoiding high-risk procedures is key. Having access to post-exposure prophylaxis is important so as to begin therapy immediately after exposure.

Differences in Clinical Practice

Anyone considering an elective in emergency medicine should be aware of these important issues:

1. *Delayed clinical presentation*: In many countries, healthcare is costly and patients come to the ER late in the disease process. There are three kinds of delays that are recognized to cause these delayed clinical presentations: (1) deciding to seek care; (2) identifying and reaching a health facility and (3) reaching adequate and appropriate treatment (Calvello et al., 2015). No longer is an infection a simple abscess but rather a septic patient with multi-system organ failure. Extremes of presentation are the norm and learning how to recognize and treat early is critical.

2. *Standard of care*: Resource-poor countries may not have the same equipment, diagnostic tests and personnel available as available back home. Being cognizant of this beforehand can prepare for any frustrations or sense of hopelessness. For example, not all areas have access to an X-ray or a computed tomography (CT) scanner, yet these are common in North America. The same with bloodwork. Basic blood panels may or may not be available in small centres, at least not in a timely fashion, and some tests such as a D-dimer or troponins may be completely unavailable. The same goes for access to medications and equipment. The WHO has created a model list of essential medications for adults and children that help guide what should be available (WHO, 2016a). Adhering to the best practice of the region is critical so as to optimize care.

3. *ER teams*: Most developed countries have well-functioning ERs with nurses and physicians working side-by-side. Allied healthcare workers such as respiratory therapists, physician assistants and nurse practitioners may also be involved in patient care. In comparison, there is limited staff in resource-poor areas. The nursing scope of practice may not be as comprehensive as we are used to in North America. For example, starting an intravenous line or drawing blood may not be in their skill set and you might be required to perform these tasks. The lack of high-tech equipment requires a reliance on strong clinical skills and the physician skills are usually at a high level. Furthermore, nurses in some regions are trained in a focused area of practice, such as maternity or anesthesia, to help with the lack of healthcare personnel.

4. *Shiftwork*: Most ERs in developed countries function on a shift rotation. However, with lack of human resources, some resource-poor ERs allocate 24-hour shifts which makes it exhausting. The added physiological changes of time difference, climate change, availability of food and transportation logistics compound this risk, making clinical errors a high risk. Adequate hydration and nutrition is key.

5. *EMS and transport*: Infrastructure can be a major hurdle to accessing care. There may not be an ambulance service or the road conditions may be terrible to transport patients safely and effectively. Some patients travel long distances to get access to care since healthcare facilities may be sparsely populated.

6. *Consent and end-of-life care*: Differences in beliefs and cultural practices are the strength of a community. It is harder in emergency care to always get consent in the case of limb or life-threatening emergent care. The same holds for end-of-life care. You may be faced with patients whom you feel can be resuscitated given the right access to resources. Many places do not have an intensive care unit (ICU), a ventilator or oxygen for that matter. Knowing what resources are available early in the rotation is important so that you have realistic expectations.

As a trainee, be cognizant of the local resources and expertise. For example, ultrasound competency may be seen in junior doctors who have learnt to use an old machine during obstetrical care; or they may have better skills at IV insertion, as it is part of their job. Asking for help and instruction is always helpful. Some remote areas may also have access to telemedicine which can be a great resource.

Learner Issues

1. *Medical students*

   At the medical student level, ER electives may pose a challenge. While residency electives generally have structured learning objectives and mentors attuned to trainee needs, learning needs and outcomes at the undergraduate level are often less formally defined and less closely supervised – partly due to the limitations that location, training needs and local resources impose on global electives.

   The Society for Academic Emergency Medicine's Global Emergency Medicine Academy has come up with a code of conduct (Hansoti et al., 2013). Armed with limited knowledge, there may be difficulties in having appropriate supervision. Furthermore, they may be asked to perform procedures for which they have little or no training (lumbar puncture or C-sections) and without supervision. The push comes from making them feel guilty about not doing it as the outcome of the patient could potentially change. Being aware of one's limitations is key. You are there as a learner and observer. Knowing where to draw the line is difficult and complex in these challenging environments. However, knowing your capabilities and what you are there for is paramount.

   Ways to avoid such situations are to avoid rural settings, work in a setting where there is appropriate medical supervision (ideally under an emergency-trained doctor) and let the team know at the start what your role is as a medical student.

2. *Residents and fellows*

   Residents, especially more senior ones, would benefit from the unique exposure of emergency medicine in the global setting. There are still logistic issues related to supervision, evaluation and appropriate experience. However, there are collaborative programs and international ER electives that are formalized to help overcome this obstacle. In addition, there are also fellowships in international emergency medicine (EM) that are available from several schools that also incorporate a master's in public health as part of the training (Society for Academic Emergency Medicine [SAEM], 2016).

   In order to appreciate the context and have a worthwhile learning experience, the recommended duration is a minimum of 4–6 weeks. There are no formal studies to show what duration would be ideal, but the minimum recommended would provide a good opportunity to learn the local healthcare system, see a wide variety of pathology and appreciate ER practices in those settings.

Other Resources

Society of Academic Emergency Medicine (www.saem.org) – Great resource showing all the fellowship programs available. Also includes resources for accreditation of fellowships.

Canadian Association of Emergency Medicine (www.cape.ca) – The international EM section has some great contacts where students and residents can connect.

International Federation of Emergency Medicine (www.ifem.cc) – Both for general EM as well as subspecialty areas such as pediatric EM.

References

Abba, K., S. Ramaratnam, and L. N. Ranganathan. 2010. Anthelmintics for people with neurocysticercosis. *Cochrane Database Syst Rev* 1:Cd000215. doi:10.1002/14651858.CD000215.pub3.

American College of Surgeons (ACS). 2016. Advanced Trauma Life Support. American College of Surgeons. https://www.facs.org/quality programs/trauma/atls.

African Federation of Emergency Medicine (AFEM). 2016. http://www.afem.info/members/current-members/?id=35.

Breyer, M. J., A. Sadosty, and M. Biros. 2012. Factors affecting candidate placement on an emergency medicine residency program's rank order list. *West J Emerg Med* 13 (6):458–62. doi:10.5811/westjem.2011.1.6619.

Calvello, E. J., A. P. Skog, A. G. Tenner, and L. A. Wallis. 2015. Applying the lessons of maternal mortality reduction to global emergency health. *Bull World Health Organ* 93 (6):417–23. doi:10.2471/blt.14.146571.

Centre for Disease Control and Prevention (CDCP). 2016. Malaria Worldwide. http://www.cdc.gov/malaria/malaria_worldwide/index.html.

Chancey, R. J. and R. Jhaveri. 2009. Fever without localizing signs in children: A review in the post-Hib and postpneumococcal era. *Minerva Pediatr* 61 (5):489–501.

Chang, C. Y., S. Abujaber, T. A. Reynolds, C. A. Camargo, Jr., and Z. Obermeyer. 2016. Burden of emergency conditions and emergency care usage: New estimates from 40 countries. *Emerg Med J.* doi:10.1136/emermed-2016-205709.

CUGH. 2016. Consortium of Universities of Global Health – Global Health training modules. Consortium of Universities of Global Health. https://www.cugh.org/resources/educational-modules.

Dey, C. C., J. G. Grabowski, K. Gebreyes, E. Hsu, and M. J. VanRooyen. 2002. Influence of international emergency medicine opportunities on residency program selection. *Acad Emerg Med* 9 (7):679–83.

Guerrant, R. L., D. H. Walker, and P. F. Weller, eds. 2011. *Tropical Infectious Diseases*. 3rd ed. New York, NY: Elsevier.

Hansoti, B., S. G. Weiner, I. B. Martin, S. Dunlop, A. S. Hayward, J. P. Tupesis, T. K. Becker, and K. Douglass. 2013. Society for academic emergency medicine's global emergency medicine academy: Global health elective code of conduct. *Acad Emerg Med* 20 (12):1319–20. doi:10.1111/acem.12264.

Havryliuk, T., S. Bentley, and S. Hahn. 2014. Global health education in emergency medicine residency programs. *J Emerg Med* 46 (6):847–52. doi:10.1016/j.jemermed.2013.11.101.

Institute for Health Metrics and Evaluation (IHME). 2013. *The Global Burden of Disease: Generating Evidence, Guiding Policy*. Edited by IHME. Seattle, WA: Institute for Health Metrics and Evaluation.

Jhaveri, R., C. L. Byington, J. O. Klein, and E. D. Shapiro. 2011. Management of the non-toxic-appearing acutely febrile child: A 21st century approach. *J Pediatr* 159 (2):181–5. doi:10.1016/j.jpeds.2011.03.047.

Liu, L., H. L. Johnson, S. Cousens, J. Perin, S. Scott, J. E. Lawn, I. Rudan, H. Campbell, R. Cibulskis, M. Li, C. Mathers, and R. E. Black. 2012. Global, regional, and national causes of child mortality: An updated systematic analysis for 2010 with time trends since 2000. *Lancet* 379 (9832):2151–61. doi:10.1016/s0140-6736(12)60560-1.

National Institutes of Health (NIH) NIH Publication No. 02-2117. 4th Edition. Revised June 2002. Bethesda. 2002. *The Management of Sickle Cell Disease*. 4th ed. Bethesda, MD: NIH. https://www.nhlbi.nih.gov/files/docs/guidelines/sc_mngt.pdf

Norman, R., R. Matzopoulos, P. Groenewald, and D. Bradshaw. 2007. The high burden of injuries in South Africa. *Bull World Health Organ* 85 (9):695–702.

O'Donnell, S., D. H. Adler, P. C. Inboriboon, H. Alvarado, R. Acosta, and D. Godoy-Monzon. 2014. Perspectives of South American physicians hosting foreign rotators in emergency medicine. *Int J Emerg Med* 7:24. doi:10.1186/s12245-014-0024-5.

Society for Academic Emergency Medicine (SAEM). 2016. Society for Academic Emergency Medicine fellowship directory. SAEM. http://www.saem.org/membership/services/fellowship-directory?Fellowship_Type=Global+International+Emergency+Medicine.

Joint United Nations Programme on HIV/AIDS (UNAIDS). 2016. Global AIDS update 2016. Switzerland: UNAIDS.

WHO. 2004. *World Report on Road Traffic Injury Prevention*. Edited by Peden, M, Scurfield, R, Sleet, D, Mohan, D, Hyder, A. A, Jarawan, E, and Mathers, C. Geneva: WHO.

WHO. 2008. *The Global Burden of Disease – 2004 Update*. Geneva: WHO.

WHO. 2016a. Essential Medicines and Health Products. WHO, Geneva. http://www.who.int/medicines/publications/essentialmedicines/en/.

WHO. 2016b. Tuberculosis – Fact Sheet 104. WHO, Geneva. http://www.who.int/mediacentre/factsheets/fs104/en/.

Chapter 14

Pediatrics and Child Health

Andrea Hunter and Kevin Chan

Contents

One in twenty children born worldwide do not survive until their fifth birthday. In some parts of the world, this climbs to 1 in 12 children (United Nations Children's Fund [UNICEF], 2015b). It is a stark reality often forgotten by those who work exclusively in high-income countries or high-resourced healthcare settings. Medical learners planning to work in low- to middle-income countries (LMICs) or low-resourced settings will inevitably encounter a high proportion of childhood disease. This chapter outlines some of the major causes of morbidity and mortality to children and youth worldwide, as well as some key topics of relevance in caring for this population.

Global Burden of Childhood Disease

Globally, child mortality rates have fallen substantially – particularly, during the late twentieth century, with approximately 2.5% per year decline from 1960s to 1990s and 3% per year decline from 1990 onwards. Under-five deaths worldwide have declined from 12.7 million in 1990 to 5.9 million in 2015 (global under-five mortality rate of 43 deaths/1000 live births) (UN IGME, 2015; You et al., 2015). These reported trends are based on statistical models from the best available

Table 14.1 Mortality Rate Definitions

	Definition	Worldwide (1990)	Worldwide (2015)	Canada (2015)	United States (2015)	United Kingdom (2015)
Under-five mortality rate	Deaths in the first 5 years of life/1000 live births	91	43	5	7	4
Infant mortality rate	Deaths in the first year of life/1000 live births	63	32	4	6	4
Neonatal mortality rate	Deaths in the first 28 days of life/1000 live births	36	19	3	4	2

Source: United Nations Inter-Agency Group for Child Mortality Estimation (UN IGME). 2015. Levels and Trends in Child Mortality. Accessed on Oct 15, 2016, http://www.childmortality .org/files_v20/download/IGME%20report%202015%20child%20mortality%20final.pdf.

data, recognizing that accurate data is often fragmented and inconsistent. In the setting of sparse data, frequent absence of birth and death registration, reliance on verbal autopsies and extrapolation of cause of death models, many efforts have been made to renew cause of death modelling strategies and use of improved tools for ensuring internal consistency of mortality and epidemiological estimates by the World Health Organization (WHO) (WHO, 2013b).

Life remains riskiest in the first few hours and days of life. Early neonatal (first 7 days of life) and neonatal (first 28 days of life) mortality rates comprise a substantial proportion of under-five mortality rates, with each of these demonstrating significant decline in the last 25 years. Worldwide neonatal mortality rate fell by 47% between 1990 and 2015 (UNICEF, 2015a).

Child mortality continues to vary significantly and increasingly by region, with the greatest rates in sub-Saharan Africa (81 deaths per 1000 live births) and South Asia (53 deaths per 1000 live births). Inequalities continue to exist in the survival of children – not only regionally, but also between countries, within countries, by urban/rural divide and most notably between income levels across the world (UN IGME, 2015; You et al., 2015). The most common causes of childhood mortality worldwide remain acute respiratory illnesses, diarrheal disease and neonatal causes (including birth asphyxia, infection and prematurity), with undernutrition overlying at least one-third of childhood mortality (WHO, 2013).

As we depart the era of the Millennium Development Goals and enter the even more ambitious era of Sustainable Development Goals, we are reminded by UNICEF that 'too many children remain excluded from the progress of the last 25 years'. A few examples are provided in UNICEF's 2015 State of the World's Children report (UNICEF, 2015a):

■ The poorest 20% of the world's children are twice as likely as the richest 20% to be stunted by poor nutrition and to die before their fifth birthday. Children in rural areas are at a similar disadvantage compared to those who live in urban areas.

■ The richest 20% of the world's women are 2.7 times more likely than the poorest 20% to have a skilled attendant present at delivery. In South Asia, the richest women are nearly four times more likely than the poorest to have this benefit.

The shift towards focus on the financial, political, institutional and cultural barriers that stand between children and their right to health and well-being broadens the lens of our approach and reminds healthcare providers of the key importance that social determinants play in childhood morbidity and mortality both at home and away (UNICEF, 2015a) (Table 14.1).

Care of Neonates

Given that 40% of under-five mortality arises during the neonatal period, care of neonates within their first month of life should be a critical consideration of any healthcare professional or learner participating in an global health experience (GHE) involving children.

In LMICs, many births occur at home or in under-resourced local clinics leading to nearly half of all mothers and newborns not receiving skilled care during and immediately after birth (WHO, 2011). Multiple programs have resulted in significant reduction in neonatal mortality. As one key example, Helping Babies Breathe (HBB) is an evidence-based educational program to teach essential skills of newborn resuscitation in resource-limited areas worldwide, targeting birth attendants in LMICs. It was an initiative of American Academy of Pediatrics (AAP) in collaboration with the WHO, U.S. Agency for International Development (USAID) and a number of other global health organizations, launched in 2010.

These educational programs and many others highlight the goal of having at least one person who is skilled in newborn resuscitation present at the birth of every baby. They also assist in identifying factors that would signal a higher risk birth context and may necessitate further intervention, including the following:

■ Limited antenatal care
■ Maternal health or pregnancy conditions (HIV, substance use, TORCH infections, pregnancy-induced hypertension or pre-eclampsia, gestational diabetes)
■ Premature delivery (<37 weeks gestation)
■ Intrapartum complications (maternal fever, premature or prolonged rupture of membranes >18 hours, fetal distress, prolonged labor, meconium-stained amniotic fluid)

Every newborn requires good routine care immediately after birth, which includes the following:

■ Drying baby with a clean towel, replacing wet cloths and placing skin-to-skin with mother ideally as soon as possible.
■ Maintain warmth: Cover the exposed parts of the baby to prevent heat loss, particularly the head and keep with mother. Kangaroo Mother Care has been demonstrated to have equal efficacy to incubator or external heating device (Conde-Agudelo et al., 2011).
■ Encouragement and support for breastfeeding within the first hour of life, and on demand.
■ Administration of injectable vitamin K with clean needle (to prevent hemorrhagic disease of the newborn) and antibiotic or antiseptic eye ointment (to prevent ophthalmia neonatorum)– though in higher resource settings with routine access to maternal and infant testing for chlamydia and gonorrhea may not be necessary.

Skills in providing appropriate breaths with a self-inflating bag and mask are essential for any learners participating in care of newborns or attending births.

Any health professional or learner embarking on a GHE should be able to recognize the signs of a seriously unwell newborn and work to develop an approach to outlining comprehensive differential diagnosis and management principles in each of these cases.

Unwell newborns may present simply with an inability to breastfeed, quickly leading to hypoglycemia and often inability to maintain appropriate thermoregulation. Others may have respiratory presentations: apnea (>15 seconds), bradypnea (<20 respirations/minute) or tachypnea (>60 respirations/minute), chest in-drawing or grunting. Although mild chest in-drawing, transient grunting and mild tachypnea can be a part of a normal transition to extrauterine life, these newborns should be monitored closely with mother for any signs of progression. Newborns demonstrating signs of deep jaundice, convulsions, mottled or dusky appearance, central cyanosis, intolerance of feeds or significant abdominal distention require more immediate and comprehensive assessment and monitoring, ideally in a neonatal care unit or by an experienced provider.

Learners embarking on GHEs may wish to consider further exploration of topics that are commonly encountered in the broad differential diagnosis of an unwell newborn, including the following:

- Neonatal sepsis including meningitis/encephalitis
- Respiratory: Transient tachypnea of the newborn, respiratory distress syndrome, meconium aspiration syndrome, pneumothorax/pneumomediastinum or other air leak syndromes
- Congenital cardiac defects, particularly cyanotic types
- Hypoglycemia and other fluid/electrolyte disturbances
- Congenital issues (i.e. inborn errors of metabolism, congenital hypothyroidism, genetic syndromes/malformations, teratogenic effects of medications, *Toxoplasma*, other, rubella, CMV, HSV [TORCH] infections)
- Delivery-related trauma (i.e. brachial plexus injury, subgaleal hemorrhage)

In addition, the multiple short- and longer-term complications of prematurity will be frequently encountered in LMICs, as approximately 15 million births annually are complicated by preterm birth (<37 weeks gestation) and it remains the leading cause of neonatal mortality (Blencowe et al., 2012). Common complications of prematurity in the short term include hypothermia, hypoglycemia, feeding difficulties, infection, jaundice, respiratory distress syndrome, apnea of prematurity, intraventricular hemorrhage, patent ductus arteriosus, necrotizing enterocolitis, inguinal hernia, and anemia and in the long-term chronic lung disease such as bronchopulmonary dysplasia, hearing impairment, retinopathy of prematurity or vision impairment and cerebral palsy or other neurodevelopmental impairment.

Over 60% of preterm births occur in LMICs, and in many resource-constrained settings, conditions known to be risk factors for preterm birth (such as urinary tract infections, malaria, undernutrition and hypertensive disorders) are frequently underdiagnosed, undertreated or both (Katz et al., 2014; Vogel et al., 2014).

Emergency Management of Sick Children

In 2005, the World Health Organization (WHO) and United Nations Children's Fund (UNICEF) released combined guidelines for *Integrated Management of Childhood Illness (IMCI)* – these promote evidence-based assessment and treatment of common illnesses in children in contexts with limited resources using a syndromic approach (WHO, 2005a). The clinical guidelines are designed mostly for use in outpatient clinical settings with limited diagnostic tools and limited medications although they allow adaptability to each country, regional educational methods and also contain some hospital care guidelines (WHO, 2005b). These are designed for the management of children 1 week to 5 years of age by a trained health worker, integrating improved management of childhood illness with aspects of nutrition, immunization and other important elements of health promotion.

The hospital care guidelines contain an essential component outlining Emergency Triage, Assessment and Treatment (ETAT) principles for rapidly screening and treating sick children. These contain principles that some learners may recognize from resuscitation courses that are taught in high-resource countries (e.g. Basic Life Support, Pediatric Advanced Life Support) but are adapted appropriately to a health worker in a more remote and/or limited resource setting. Knowledge of normal vital signs in children by age, is essential basic information for learners embarking on GHE in pediatrics, to begin applying these ETAT principles (Table 14.2).

Dehydration, Diarrheal Disease and Fluid Management in Children

Despite the progress made in reduction in child mortality rates worldwide in the last few decades, diarrheal disease and the resulting dehydration is the second leading cause of death in children under 5 years old, killing approximately 760,000 children annually (WHO, 2013a). This is also a leading cause of malnutrition in the same age group, as children under 3 years of age living in LMICs experience an average of three episodes of diarrhea each year. Each of these illnesses results in nutritional deprivation as well as increased susceptibility to future infection with progressive undernutrition (Walker et al., 2013).

Table 14.2 Normal Vital Signs for Children, by Age

	Heart Rate (HR) Beats/ Minute Awake	*Heart Rate (HR) Beats/ Minute Sleeping*	*Respiratory Rate (RR) Breaths/ Minute*	*Systolic Blood Pressure (SBP) mmHg*	*Diastolic Blood Pressure (DBP) mmHg*
Neonate (<28 days)	100–205	90–160	30–60	67–84	35–53
Infant (1 month to 1 year)	100–190	90–160	30–53	72–104	37–56
Toddler (1–2 years)	98–140	80–120	22–37	86–106	42–63
Preschool (3–5 years)	80–120	65–100	20–28	89–112	46–72
School age (6–11 years)	75–118	58–90	18–25	97–115	57–76
Adolescent (12–15 years)	60–100	50–90	12–20	102–130	61–83

Source: American Heart Association, *Pediatric Advanced Life Support Provider Manual,* American Heart Association, Dallas, 2016.

Diarrhea, the passage of three or more loose or liquid stools per day, usually results from a viral, bacterial or parasitic infection of the intestinal tract. These infections are spread more commonly in LMICs or low-resourced settings, particularly where sanitation measures and hygiene resources are often limited, either through contaminated food, drinking water or person-to-person. The most common etiologic agents of diarrheal disease of children in LMICs are rotavirus, adenovirus, norovirus, *Giardia, Cryptosporidium* (in immunocompromised host), *Campylobacter, Shigella,* enterotoxigenic *Escherichia Coli* (ETEC) and *Salmonella* (WHO, 2013a; Walker et al., 2013) though in one recent large cohort of sub-Saharan African children *Campylobacter, Shigella* and ETEC were found without the traditionally expected bloody stools (dysentery) (Pernica et al., 2015).

Although prevention measures including safe drinking water, improved sanitation and handwashing with soap, the so-called WAter, Sanitation, Hygiene (WASH) interventions, seem simple in a high-income setting, these remain lacking worldwide for many: 750 million who lack access to clean drinking water and 2.5 billion who lack improved sanitation (WHO, 2013a). More recent introduction of rotavirus and cholera vaccines have demonstrated effectiveness in preventing hospitalizations (by 47%, rotavirus) and infection (by 52%, cholera) (Bhutta et al., 2013).

Most illnesses in infants and young children, particularly those with fever, tachypnea or other mechanisms for increased insensible losses, as well as vomiting or diarrhea put children at risk of dehydration through loss of water and electrolytes (sodium, chloride, potassium and bicarbonate) due to liquid stools, vomit, sweat, urine and breathing. Table 14.3 outlines classifications of severity of dehydration in children with diarrhea.

Table 14.3   Classification of Severity of Dehydration in Children with Diarrhea

	Signs or Symptoms	*Treatment*
No dehydration	Not enough signs to classify as some dehydration or severe dehydration	Give fluid and food to treat diarrhea at home (Plan A) Advise caregiver on when to return immediately Follow-up in 5 days if not improving
Some dehydration	Two or more of the following signs: • Restlessness, irritability • Sunken eyes • Drinks eagerly, thirsty • Skin pinch goes back slowly	Give fluid and food for some dehydration (Plan B) After rehydration, advise mother on home treatment and when to return immediately Follow-up in 5 days if not improving
Severe dehydration	Two or more of the following signs: • Lethargy/unconsciousness • Sunken eyes • Unable to drink or drinks poorly • Skin pinch goes back very slowly (≥2 seconds)	Give fluid for severe dehydration (Plan C) and admit to hospital

Source: Adapted from World Health Organization (WHO), *Handbook: Integrated Management of Childhood Illness,* WHO Press, Geneva, Switzerland, 2005a.

Treatment of children with diarrheal disease involves rehydration, zinc supplementation and ensuring that nutritional intake is maintained or restarted whenever possible.

Oral rehydration salts (ORS) solution is a mixture of clean water, salt and sugar, that can be made at home from basic ingredients (1 L of clean water + 6 teaspoons of sugar + ½ teaspoon of salt) or prepared from a pre-packaged sachet in clean water. Continuing to breastfeed or provide food-based fluids such as rice-water soup and yogurt drinks at home is advised for children with little apparent dehydration. For a comprehensive view of plan A, B, C rehydration methods, please see the Integrated Management of Childhood Illness (WHO, 2005a, pp. 95–100).

Oral supplementation with zinc has been demonstrated to be effective both for preventative complications from diarrhea and reduction in all-cause mortality (Mayo-Wilson et al., 2014) as well as for the treatment of acute diarrhea disease (Bhutta et al., 2013). Antibiotics are indicated in only a few specific circumstances: infection with *Shigella*, *Vibrio cholerae* or cryptosporidiosis but otherwise may worsen diarrhea in young children or contribute to resistance. Other agents such as antimotility agents, adsorbents, antisecretory agents demonstrate either harm from delayed transit time and prolonged course of illness or toxicity or limited effectiveness in children with gastroenteritis or acute diarrheal illness – none should be used routinely (Galeao Brandt, 2015).

Acute Respiratory Infections/Pneumonia

Pneumonia (often categorized more broadly as acute respiratory infections) is the leading cause of death in children younger than 5 years of age, resulting in 1.3 million deaths in 2011, with the highest burden of disease in sub-Saharan Africa and Southeast Asia (Bhutta et al., 2013). Eighty-one percent of these deaths occur in the first 2 years of life, suggesting that an increased emphasis on early prevention and treatment is critical in contributing to further reductions in global childhood mortality (Walker et al., 2013).

Young children presenting to healthcare with fever and cough are most often found to have an acute respiratory infection: viral bronchiolitis/pneumonia or suspected bacterial pneumonia but these clinical signs may also herald malaria, bacteremia/sepsis, tuberculosis or other infections. Given that most serious acute respiratory infections are bacterial in etiology, the IMCI approach emphasizes the use of early antibiotics if clinical signs lead to a suspicion of pneumonia – quite a different approach from the judicious use of antibiotics that learners likely have encountered in high-resourced settings, where chest X-ray is readily accessible to rule out the consolidation of bacterial pneumonia, and most acute respiratory infections are of viral etiology. Table 14.4 outlines the IMCI approach to classification of severity and treatment approach for pneumonia in a lower resourced setting.

Most bacterial pneumonia in young children is caused by *Streptococcus pneumoniae*, *Staphylococcus aureus* (often causing very severe presentations), non-typhoidal *Salmonella* species (particularly in regions of Africa where malaria is endemic), *Klebsiella* pneumonia (especially in context of undernutrition), *Mycoplasma pneumoniae*, *Chlamydia pneumoniae* (in children >3 years of age) and *Mycobacterium tuberculosis* (particularly in HIV-positive children). The most common viral cause of acute respiratory infections necessitating seeking healthcare assistance is respiratory syncytial virus, which does not undergo the typical seasonal variation of the northern hemisphere but is a year-round issue in the tropics. Less frequently, respiratory viruses including parainfluenza, metapneumovirus, adenovirus, coronavirus and bocavirus can lead to cough and respiratory distress, often with fever (Walker et al., 2013).

Table 14.4 Classification of the Severity of Pneumonia and Treatment Suggested by IMCI

	Signs or Symptoms	*Treatment*
Very severe pneumonia	Cough or difficulty breathing plus at least one of the following: • Central cyanosis • Severe respiratory distress • Not able to drink	Admit to hospital Give recommended antibiotic Give oxygen Manage the airway Treat high fever, if present
Severe pneumonia	Cough or difficulty breathing plus: • Chest in-drawing	Admit to hospital Give recommended antibiotic Manage the airway Treat high fever, if present
Pneumonia	Fast breathing • ≥60 breaths/min in <2 months • ≥50 breaths/min in child 2–11 months • ≥40 breaths/min in child 1–5 years • Definite crackles on auscultation	Outpatient treatment Give appropriate oral antibiotic for 5 days Soothe the throat and relieve cough with safe remedy Advise the caregiver when to return Follow-up in 2 days
No pneumonia: cough or 'cold'	No signs of pneumonia or severe or very severe pneumonia	Outpatient treatment Soothe the throat and relieve cough with safe remedy Advise the caregiver when to return Follow-up in 5 days if not improving If coughing for more than 30 days, follow separate chronic cough instructions

Source: Adapted from World Health Organization (WHO). *Pocketbook of Hospital Care for Children: Guidelines for the Management of Common Illnesses with Limited Resources.* WHO Press, Geneva, Switzerland, 2005b.

Prevention of pneumonia, similar to diarrheal disease, begins with environmental measures of WASH interventions, reducing overcrowding and household air pollution and the promotion of breastfeeding and appropriate childhood nutrition (Bhutta et al., 2013). Multiple causes of pneumonia are vaccine preventable, including *Haemophilus influenzae* type b, *S. pneumoniae* and measles.

Treatment involves early administration of antibiotics, oxygen as needed and the decision to follow as inpatient or outpatient is made based on severity of initial symptoms as well as other risk factors (including age and immunocompromised status) of the child.

Management of critically unwell children with suspected sepsis or poor perfusion has typically involved significant isotonic fluid resuscitation. However, the results of the recent Fluid

Expansion as Supportive Therapy (FEAST) trial, involving more than 3000 critically ill children (excluding those with malnutrition or gastroenteritis) with poor perfusion at six sub-Saharan African hospital sites demonstrated *increased* 48-hour mortality with fluid bolus compared with no-bolus controls (Maitland et al., 2011). These results have begun to change the approach to fluid management in children with critical illness both in the tropics and possibly in high-resourced settings as well.

Malaria

Children under-five, along with pregnant women and non-immune travellers, are the most vulnerable groups affected by malaria. Approximately 300,000 children under 5 years of age died of malaria infection in 2015, making it an important cause of childhood morbidity and mortality in affected global regions (WHO, 2016a).

There are five species of plasmodia parasite that cause malaria, *Plasmodium falciparum* (most severe form), *Plasmodium ovale, Plasmodium vivax, Plasmodium malariae and Plasmodium knowlesi*. Malaria is transmitted through the bite of the nocturnal-feeding female *Anopheles* mosquito, with rare cases reported from congenital, transfusion-related or travel-related (mosquitos on flights/packages from endemic areas) transmission.

Malaria should be suspected in any child with fever, vomiting, generalized weakness, change in behaviour/level of consciousness or signs of being unwell. Although well known in adults, the regularly recurring fever is an uncommon presentation in a child. Diagnosis is *not* clinical, although a high index of suspicion is warranted in any endemic or epidemic region (or in fever in any returned traveller from an affected region): it requires a specific, rapid, monoclonal antibody test or traditional thin/thick smears for microscopy (WHO, 2016a). Malaria is an important risk factor for bacteremia in African children, and therefore a blood culture should also be drawn, where available, in children with suspected or documented malarial infection (Scott et al., 2011).

Complications in children commonly include hypoglycemia, splenomegaly, moderate thrombocytopenia, severe hemolytic anemia sometimes leading to congestive heart failure and respiratory distress, metabolic acidosis, cerebral malaria, vascular collapse and shock (with hypothermia and adrenal insufficiency). The non-cardiogenic pulmonary edema, renal failure secondary to acute tubular necrosis ('black-water fever') and jaundice that are well described in adults are much less common in children (WHO, 2015).

Treatment of uncomplicated falciparum malaria in children is with oral combination medications including an artemisinin derivative, by regional or country specific guidelines to ensure resistance pattern is considered. Parenteral therapy is warranted in young children who are unable to tolerate oral medication, have severe (>5% parasitemia), complicated or cerebral malaria (WHO, 2015), and recent data support the use of artesunate over quinine (WHO, 2016a).

Although a number of trials demonstrate promise with vaccines, these are not yet available outside research trials (RTS,S Clinical Trials Partnership, 2015). Prevention strategies target the elimination of the *Anopheles* mosquito and its breeding areas (reducing standing water repositories, indoor and outdoor spraying programs), as well as the avoidance of bites to individual children (avoiding exposure from dusk to dawn where possible, sleeping under a permethrin-impregnated bed net). WHO has recently recommended, in areas with highly seasonal transmission such as the Sahel sub-region of Africa, seasonal malaria chemoprevention (SMC) for children aged 3–59 months as part of a package of interventions for the prevention and treatment of malaria in children (WHO, 2016a).

Malnutrition

Severe acute malnutrition remains a major cause of under-five childhood mortality worldwide. Approximately 19 million preschool age children, mostly from sub-Saharan Africa and South East Asia, have severe wasting, the hallmark of severe acute malnutrition. While infections such as diarrheal disease or pneumonia are often 'the final steps in the pathway' and therefore incorporated into epidemiologic data as the causes of death, undernutrition is thought to account for approximately 35% of under-five mortality and 4.4% of deaths have been shown to be specifically attributable to severe wasting (WHO, 2013b).

Malnutrition in children typically develops between 6 and 18 months of age, when growth velocity and brain growth are particularly high and increasing reports highlight severe acute malnutrition in infants less than 6 months of age. Infants and young children are susceptible to undernutrition if complementary foods are offered/available infrequently, are of low nutrient density, have low bioavailability of micronutrients, if introduced too early or too late, or are contaminated (WHO, 2013b). The complex 'spiral of malnutrition' refers to the interplay between inadequate intake (whether from scarcity or poor nutrient quality) and disease processes including the decreased absorption, increased metabolic needs and decreased intake that are seen in many infectious diseases and particularly those prevalent in LMICs (HIV, TB, diarrhea, malaria, measles, etc.). These are further compounded by the underlying and many social factors contributing to food insecurity. (Black et al., 2008)

In children who are 6–59 months of age, severe acute malnutrition is defined as the following:

- Weight-for-height ≤ –3 Z-score (using WHO growth standards)
- Mid-upper-arm circumference (MUAC) <115 mm
- Presence of bilateral edema

MUAC has been found to be a reliable measure of severe acute malnutrition in young children, as this measurement is reasonably stable from 6 to 59 months of age. This is a valuable, easily performed marker (see Figure 14.1), that in addition to examination for bilateral pitting edema can be assessed by a trained community health worker or community member, facilitating early identification and referral to treatment centres.

Children identified to have severe acute malnutrition should have a full assessment for medical complications as well as presence/absence of appetite. WHO has provided a 10-step guideline for children with severe acute malnutrition (WHO, 2013b). Those who have appetite and are clinically well and alert can be treated as outpatients. Those with medical complications, generalized edema, poor appetite or with one or more of the IMCI 'danger signs' (convulsions, significant vomiting, lethargy/unconscious state) should be treated as inpatients initially (WHO, 2013b).

Those requiring admission to hospital should be assessed for presence of dehydration and rehydrated slowly (5–10 mL/kg/hour) with low-osmolarity oral rehydration solution with added potassium and glucose, unless there is presence of cholera or profuse watery diarrhea. Broad-spectrum antibiotics and treatment with vitamin A daily also are also indicated in the initial stages of inpatient treatment (WHO, 2013b).

Refeeding syndrome is a significant concern in children with severe acute malnutrition, as this can result in potentially fatal shifts in fluids and electrolytes in children receiving parenteral or enteral nutritional support early in the course of their treatment. The hallmarks are hypophosphatemia, hypokalemia and hypomagnesemia but can also feature changes in sodium and fluid balance, as well as fat, protein and glucose metabolism (Mihanna et al., 2008). As these electrolytes are often impossible to monitor frequently in LMICs or lower-resourced settings, care is taken in clinical guidelines to introduce nutrition in a careful, stepwise manner.

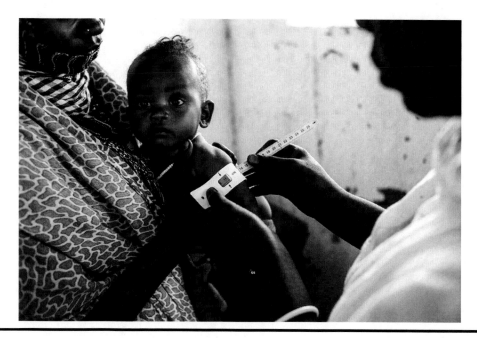

Figure 14.1   Mid-upper-arm circumference measurement. (Courtesy of C. Fohlen.)

Ethical and Cultural Issues When Working with Children Abroad

There are many issues that may arise when working with children abroad. It is important to understand the cultural and ethical issues, and doing so respectfully remains a challenge, as you want to do what is in the best interest of the child, while at the same time, respecting the culture and customs around family autonomy.

In this section, we take a look at five specific examples and highlight the challenges.

The first example is female genital mutilation (FGM), which is the practice of intentionally altering or causing injury to the female genital organs in infants and children for non-medical reasons. It is a common practice affecting 200 million girls throughout Africa, the Middle East and Asia (WHO, 2016b). The practice has no health benefits and can cause health harm including complications in childbirth (WHO, 2016b). The process of FGM is seen as a violation of human rights. However, as someone undergoing a GHE, arriving and appearing judgmental is unlikely to make you welcome and unlikely to change the practice.

It isn't that as an individual shouldn't be concerned about the practice, but realize that what we deem as 'norms' at home may be quite different when working abroad. We need to take into consideration that changing cultural values doesn't occur overnight and requires diligence and dialogue to affect change. Groups that have worked with communities and used health professionals working with religious leaders over lengthy periods have successfully changed FGM practices (Johansen et al., 2013).

Acute humanitarian emergencies are common contexts where we see significant challenges, especially in pediatric populations. Sometimes, children are separated or abandoned while families are fleeing crises. In high-resource countries, the approach to treatment would require consent from the parents. But often, these children are unwell, but not in life-threatening conditions and require care and help in a timely manner. Who provides the permission for you to act in the child's best interest? Most of us would tend to do what's in the best interest of the child, but sometimes these processes may cause pain to the child (e.g. an insertion of an intravenous or a nasogastric tube for hydration). But in this context, are we the best people to judge the best interest of the child? These are difficult questions to answer.

Working on a hospital ward may lead to other ethical challenges. The reality in many resource-poor countries is that there are only a few doctors and nurses available. As an outsider with the expectation of very minimal childhood mortality, we ask for or expect interventions to be performed and for investigations and treatments that aren't necessarily customary locally. They may or may not be practical. It's important to remember that some countries and regions may not have the same resources (human, financial and infrastructure) support that you would expect at home and that your orders and frantic attempts to save one child, may be affecting the well-being of other children more likely to survive. These ethical questions are important to consider when making daily clinical decisions.

Orphanages are common in many parts of the world, and many students on GHE may work in an orphanage. It's easy to get attached with children, as you may be the only ones providing the care and stimulation they require. It is important to provide the best care possible, but also realize that real change occurs when you help in improving the system: supporting the education and training of staff, working with the community to find longer-term acceptable solutions and providing sustainable solutions.

No matter where you work in the world, there is enormous variation in practice. You'll see places such as East Asia where the parents are heavily involved in decision making and care. In other parts of the world, a lot of the decision making is deferred to the healthcare practitioner, and discussion of treatment options aren't really practiced – 'You're the doctor, do what's best for my child'.

Remember when going abroad – be open to learn the cultures and customs of the individual locale and adapt your practice accordingly!

Other Key Topics for Self-Study

Healthcare providers or learners participating in a clinical elective experience in global child health may also want to consider seeking learning resources around a number of other topics, in addition to those outlined in the previous section:

- Child maltreatment
- HIV (addressed briefly in Chapter 13 but should include prevention of mother to child transmission)
- Infections more common in the tropics including *Salmonella*, tuberculosis, brucellosis, borreliosis, rheumatic fever
- Immunizations and preventative care
- Adolescent health
- Common pediatric surgical issues

These are outside the scope of this chapter, but contribute to the burden of global pediatric disease, and many have quite a different approach in a low-resourced setting than in a high-resource country.

Global Child Health Resources

WHO Global Burden of Disease Project
Available at: http://www.who.int/topics/global_burden_of_disease/en/
Lancet Global Burden of Disease Study 2010:
Available at: http://www.thelancet.com/themed/global-burden-of-disease
Lancet Child Survival Series – June 23, 2003. Volume 361:

1. Where and why are 10 million children dying every year?
2. How many child deaths can we prevent this year?
3. Reducing child mortality: Can public health deliver?
4. Applying an equity lens to child health and mortality: more of the same is not enough.
5. Knowledge into action for child survival.

Lancet *'Every Newborn' Series – May 20, 2014. Vol 384*

1. Who has been caring for baby?
2. Every newborn: Progress, priorities and potential beyond survival
3. Can available interventions end preventable deaths in mothers, newborn babies, and still-births, at what cost?
4. Every newborn: Health system bottlenecks and strategies to accelerate scale-up in countries
5. From evidence to action to deliver a healthy start for the next generation

Other Pre-Departure Resources

■ *The Mass General Hospital for Children Handbook of Pediatric Global Health* (2014)
  – Helpful resource for common medical conditions/topics

■ *Canadian Pediatric Society – Global Child & Youth Health Section*
  • A repository of links relevant to child Global Health
    – Available at: http://www.cps.ca/english/membership/Sections/GCYH/Links.htm

References

American Academy of Pediatrics (AAP). 2010. Helping Babies Breathe. Available at: http://www.helping babiesbreathe.org (accessed Oct 15, 2016).

American Heart Association. 2016. *Pediatric Advanced Life Support Provider Manual.* Dallas, TX: American Heart Association.

Bhutta, ZA, JK Das, N Walker et al. 2013. Interventions to address deaths from childhood pneumonia and diarrhea equitably: What works and at what cost? *Lancet.* 381: 1417–1429. doi:org/10.1016/S0140-6736(13)60648-0.

Black, RS, LH Allen, ZA Bhutta et al. 2008. Maternal and child undernutrition. *Lancet.* 371: 243–260. doi:10.1016/S0140- 6736(07)61690-0.

Blencowe, H, S Cousens, MZ Oestergaard et al. 2012. National, regional, and worldwide estimates of preterm birth rates in the year 2010 with time trends since 1990 for selected countries: A systematic analysis and implications. Lancet. 379: 2162–2172. doi:10.1016/S0140-6736(12)60820-4.

Conde-Agudelo, A, JM Belizan, J Dian-Rossello. 2011. Kangaroo mother care to reduce morbidity and mortality in low birthweight infants. *Cochrane Database of Syst Rev.* (3): CD002271. doi:10.1002/14651858 .CD002771.pub2.

Galeao Brandt K, MM de Castro Antunes, and GAP da Silva. 2015. Acute diarrhea: Evidence-based management. *J Pediatr.* 91 (6 Suppl 1): S36–S43.

Johansen REB, NJ Diop, G Laverack, and E Leye. 2013. What works and what does not: A discussion of popular approaches for the abandonment of female genital mutilation. *Obs Gyne Int.* 2013. doi:dx.doi .org/10.1155/2013/348248.

Katz, J, AC Lee, N Kozuki et al. 2013. Born too small or too soon: A pooled analysis of mortality risk among preterm and small-for-gestational-age infants in low- and middle-income countries. *Lancet.* 382 (9890): 417–425. doi:10.1016/S0140-6736(13)60993-9.

Maitland, K, S Kiguli, RO Opoka et al. 2011. Mortality after fluid bolus in African children with severe infection. *NEJM.* 364(26): 2483–2495.

Mayo-Wilson, E, JA Junior, A Imdad et al. 2014. Zinc supplementation for preventing mortality, morbidity, and growth failure in children aged 6 months to 12 years of age. *Cochrane Database of Syst Rev.* (4): CD009384. doi:10.1002/14651858.CD009384.pub2.

Mihanna, HM, J Moledina, and J Travis. 2008. Refeeding syndrome: What it is, and how to prevent and treat it. *BMJ.* 336: 1495–1498.

Patton, GC, SM Sawyer, JS Santelli et al. 2016. Our future: A Lancet Commission on Adolescent Health and Wellbeing. *Lancet.* 387: 2423–2478.

Pernica, JM, AP Steenhoff, H Welch et al. 2015. Correlation of clinical outcomes with multiplex molecular testing of stool for children admitted to hospital with gastroenteritis in Botswana. *J Pediatric Infect Dis Soc.* 1–7. doi:10.1093/jpids/piv028.

RTS,S Clinical Trials Partnership. 2015. Efficacy and safety of RTS,S/AS01 malaria vaccine with or without a booster dose in infants and children in Africa: Final results of a phase 3, individually randomized, controlled trial. *Lancet.* 386: 31–45.

Sawyer, SM. RA Afifi, LH Bearinger et al. 2012. Adolescence: A foundation for future health. *Lancet.* 379: 1630–1640.

Scott, JAG, JA Berkley, I Mwangi et al. 2011. Relation between falciparum malaria and bacteraemia in Kenyan children: A population-based, case control study and a longitudinal study. *Lancet.* 378: 1316–1323. doi:10.1016/S0140- 6736(11)60888-X.

United Nations Inter-Agency Group for Child Mortality Estimation (UN IGME). 2015. Levels and Trends in Child Mortality. Available at: http://www.childmortality.org/files_v20/download/IGME%20 report%202015%20child%20mortality%20final.pdf. (accessed Oct 15, 2016)

UNICEF. 2015a. State of the World's Children 2015: Reimagine the Future–Innovation for Every Child. Available at: http://sowc2015.unicef.org/. (accessed Oct 15, 2016)

UNICEF, World Health Organization, World Bank, and the Population Division of UNDESA. 2015b. *Level and Trends in Child Mortality Report 2015.* New York, NY: UNICEF.

Vogel, J, ACC Lee, and J Souza. 2014. Maternal morbidity and preterm birth in 22 low- and middle-income countries: A secondary analysis of the WHO Global Survey dataset. *BMC Pregnancy Childbirth.* 14: 56. doi:10.1186/1471-2393-14-56.

Walker, LF, I Rudan, L Liu et al. 2013. Global burden of childhood pneumonia and diarrhoea. *Lancet.* 381: 1405–1416. doi:10.1016/S0140-6736(13)60222-6.

World Health Organization (WHO). 2005a. *Handbook: Integrated Management of Childhood Illness.* Geneva, Switzerland: WHO Press.

World Health Organization (WHO). 2005b. *Pocketbook of Hospital Care for Children: Guidelines for the management of common illnesses with limited resources.* Geneva, Switzerland: WHO Press.

World Health Organization (WHO). 2011. Partnership for Maternal, Newborn and Child Health. Millennium Development Goal (MDG) 4. Available at: http://www.who.int/pmnch/media/press_materials/fs?fs _newborndeath_illness/en (accessed Oct 15, 2016).

World Health Organization (WHO). 2013a. Diarrhoeal Disease: Fact Sheet No. 330. April 2013. Available at: http://www.who.int/mediacentre/factsheets/fs330/en/ (accessed Oct 15, 2016).

World Health Organization (WHO). 2013b. Guideline: Updates on the Management of Severe Acute Malnutrition in Infants and Children. World Health Organization. Available at: http://apps.who.int /iris/bitstream/10665/95584/1/9789241506328_eng.pdf (accessed Oct 15, 2016).

World Health Organization (WHO). 2013c. WHO Methods and Data Sources for Global Burden of Disease Estimates 2000–2011. World Health Organization. Available at: http://www.who.int/healthinfo/ statistics/GlobalDALYmethods_2000_2011.pdf?ua=1 (accessed Oct 15, 2016).

World Health Organization (WHO) 2015. *Guidelines for the Treatment of Malaria* (3rd edition). World Health Organization. Available at: http://www.who.int/malaria/publications/atoz/ 9789241549127/en/ (accessed Oct 15, 2016).

World Health Organization (WHO) 2016a. Malaria in Children Under 5. Available at: http://www.who.int /malaria/areas/high_risk_groups/children/en/ (accessed Oct 15, 2016).

World Health Organization (WHO) 2016b. Female Genital Mutilation. Available at: http://www .who.int/ mediacentre/factsheets/fs241/en (accessed Oct 15, 2016).

You, D, L. Hug, S. Ejdemyr et al. 2015. Global, regional, and national levels and trends in under-5 mortality between 1990 and 2015, with scenario-based projections to 2030: A systematic analysis by the UN Inter-Agency Group for Child Mortality Estimation. *Lancet.* 386(10010): 2275–2286. http://dx.doi .org/10.1016/S0140-6736(15)00120-8.

Chapter 15

Obstetrics and Gynecology

Rachel Spitzer and Paul Thistle

Contents

The discipline of Obstetrics and Gynecology (OB-GYN) is unique in that it encompasses all aspects of women's health, including the medical and surgical management of the female patient. It is very much about families, parents and their infants. The global indicators of the health of women and their newborns, as exemplified in the Millennium Development Goals (MDGs) (WHO, 2015b) has been at the forefront in the assessment of quality of health and standard of living, especially in low-resource countries.

While many encounters in our field are pleasant with healthy outcomes, some of the emotionally challenging patient scenarios are among the most difficult and memorable tragedies we can witness in medicine. These are the deaths and disabilities of newborns and reproductive-aged women at the peak of their economically productive lives.

Burden of Illness

Despite the improvement in maternal and perinatal mortality in the past quarter century, great disparity still exists between nations. In Niger, for example, a woman has a one in seven risk of dying due to complications of pregnancy and childbirth during her reproductive years. By contrast, in Sweden, the lifetime risk of dying from these causes is much lower at 1/17,400 (Chan, Obaid, Phumaphi, and Veneman, 2008). Worldwide, 830 women die every day in pregnancy, delivery and postpartum; 99% of these deaths are in resource-limited settings. Leading causes of mortality include hemorrhage, infection, hypertensive diseases of pregnancy, complications of delivery and unsafe abortions (WHO, 2015a). In addition, more than 60% of newborn deaths occur in just 10 developing countries in Africa and Asia. Puerperal sepsis, obstructed labour, post-partum hemorrhage and neonatal sepsis remain significant causes of death and disability, rarely witnessed in a medical school teaching hospital of a developed country.

Women with gynecological conditions such as pelvic inflammatory disease and malignancy often present late in their clinical course, and their treatment options are limited in resource poor settings. For example, cervical cancer is the number one malignancy of women in many sub-Saharan African countries; 84% of cervical cancer cases occur in resource-limited countries, and 85% of deaths from this disease which is mostly preventable in developed nations (WHO, 2016). Many of these healthcare settings do not have equitable access to intensive care and oncologic services. Obstetric fistula is another condition rarely experienced in resource-rich settings but prevalent in the poorest parts of the world (Tunçalp et al., 2015). It should be noted that in the past 25 years, with the push from the WHO MDGs from 1990 to 2015 and now the transition to the Sustainable Development Goals (SDGs) to address the most significant health conditions and prerequisites around the globe, significant progress has been made in reducing the burden of maternal and neonatal mortality. As with so many conditions, the least change has been made in the poorest of settings (Wang et al. 2015).

As with other international electives, appropriate preparation of trainees in OB-GYN includes pre-departure training. A period of orientation and acclimatization on-site, and debriefing and reflection after return is critical. We highly encourage those interested in women's health to pursue opportunities to experience the excitement and challenge of OB-GYN in a variety of healthcare settings and some of you may choose a career in international settings as we have. We hope that what follows will provide useful insight to doing so, in as prepared and realistic a way as possible such that our experiences can help future trainees to limit any negative experiences and pitfalls. '*You must learn from the mistakes of others. You cannot possibly live long enough to make them all yourself*' (Sam Levinson).

Pre-Departure Preparation

Preparation to travel abroad is covered extensively elsewhere in this text but merits some specific comment in the context of OB-GYN. As the field is a surgical one, health and safety preparations must include consideration of surgical safety and post-exposure prophylaxis. Likewise, it is crucial for trainees to understand and prepare for the ethics of practice abroad by intending to practice within the scope of their existing knowledge and level of experience. This involves not only knowing your limitations, but also being cognizant to avoid inadvertent exposures to injury and infection more likely in someone insufficiently trained for independent surgical practice. Especially in low-resource settings, and in emergency relief situations, there are many ethical dilemmas, such as overstretched boundaries. There is the challenge and the consequence of deciding whether to take action with insufficient training versus not acting when there appears to be no alternative, such as the delivery of a breech baby when not trained to do so, or the delivery of an unanticipated second twin.

As a surgical specialty, the OB-GYN packing list should also include all personal protective surgical equipment. A trainee should inquire in advance if scrubs, gloves (sterile and unsterile), eye splash protection, surgical gowns and surgical shoes are easily available, and endeavour to bring supplies if necessary. Post-exposure prophylaxis for HIV is an important, and possibly expensive, decision. Do you bring your own, or rely on the host institution's program? In the event of needle-stick injuries, many local health authorities now have WHO-guided recommendations and anti-retrovirals to prevent HIV transmission to their own healthcare workers. However, if your elective is in a remote area, the drugs and the advice may not be immediately available.

Personal small containers of alcohol handwash often go a long way in settings where clean running water and soap might be scarce. Bring a good battery-powered LCD flashlight, a pocket Doppler and a finger pulse oximeter for that obstetric emergency. They will be lifesavers in crowded dimly lit obstetrical wards with aged equipment and few working electrical outlets. It is not romantic to perform a caesarean section by candlelight. The LCD headlamp is better! If you have basic training, a portable battery-powered laptop ultrasound is a modern miracle worker, allowing instant diagnosis of that placenta previa. It will be your travelling companion if you are a frequent volunteer overseas, or otherwise a fundraising goal as a gift to your host institution. You can leave it behind.

Do not overestimate the stated objectives of your elective or volunteer work and your intended contribution to women's health. You will learn from your national coworkers as much as you will give, and more. Do not think you will be saving the world; rather focus on saving the world of one mother. Think big, act small.

Aim for Straight *A*'s: Ability, Availability and Affability

The first A you will need is Ability. This will vary with your level of training and experience. Don't be fooled by the mild constellation of symptoms of your OB-GYN patient. A young woman can sit in an outpatient queue all day with a ruptured ectopic and two litres of hemoperitoneum. Her chief complaint as conveyed to the screening nurse is mild abdominal pain and dizziness. She was taught by her aunty that all expectant mothers experience such symptoms! This is where point of care ultrasound is a life saver, if you have basic training.

In many resource-limited settings, trainees are likely to encounter clinical scenarios in OB-GYN which are rare in North America. They can be extremely distressing even to the most seasoned practitioner of global OB-GYN. Examples include young women with advanced gynecologic malignancies, ruptured uteri and abdominal pregnancies, as well as neonates dying at gestational ages which are viable in our home setting. We are unique in OB-GYN in managing the challenges of a dyad of patients at many times – mother and baby – and balancing the needs of both. Neonatologists are in short supply. You are it! Sharpen your neonatal resuscitation in advance of your travel; be up to date on your NRP course; don't forget to put the pediatric diaphragm on your stethoscope before departure!

Your responsibility for two patients, mother and baby, potentially doubles the tragedy in the case of bad outcomes. Emotional preparedness is critical. 'Know yourself'. Trainees should be prepared to have some familiar coping mechanisms and comforts that they can practice abroad: exercise, planning to journal or blog (within appropriate confines of confidentiality), or having other outlets for relaxation such as books or videos at hand. Having an immediate supervisor or colleague on site with whom you can debrief is invaluable. That being said, expect to shed some tears within the first week of your elective.

However, just as important as Ability in OB-GYN is Availability – just being there for the mother and her relatives. Conditions change quickly and unpredictably. Ox-drawn carts ferrying the sick arrive at midnight. Ask to do your share of call. Let the national staff take the lead where possible. You may be working with national medical trainees on their core rotation, who are expected to grasp emergency obstetric skills prior to being attached to rural outposts where they may be the only physician or midwife. You will often be under resourced and understaffed, but in an emergency, you can do what you can with what you have where you are, working alongside your national colleagues. But you have to be there. OB-GYN is 24-hour specialty everywhere in the world!

Equally as important as Ability and Availability is Affability! This means being a team player among your national colleagues. It requires a sensitivity to the cultural attitudes and practices in the community. It was said in a recent health conference in Zimbabwe, that 'if you are poor, no one talks to you'. This might be true for an indigent rural obstetrical patient in the labor ward or the nurse aide responsible for her care. Let's make an effort to talk, and not to talk down. You cannot communicate enough. If you're not fluent in the local language, remember that body language speaks volumes.

Language and Culture

Language preparation (see Chapter 11) in the relevant foreign language is important in OB-GYN. A few words in the national language can break down barriers, even if your pronunciation produces smiles and laughter. We deal with female patients exclusively who may often be less educated than their male counterparts; in many international settings, women are far less likely to be educated in English or another European language introduced pre-independence. Knowledge of the local language will therefore help with patient interactions, and reduce the need for a local translator who may have other clinical duties to attend to.

'Getting along' requires the understanding and acceptance of existing healthcare culture even when you might not agree with everything you see. In many countries, midwives rule the roost. Let the physicians and students beware. They will have different training, experience and philosophy towards patient care. Similarly, if volunteers are male, they will need to appreciate the intimate professional relationship of the OB-GYN patient examination and respect a women's individual decision or community views on how they can be involved in patient care.

You might be the most gentle, most kind, most able volunteer to step into a labor and delivery ward on an international health elective, on call 24 hours a day – but beware, the patient may still not particularly be fond of you. The woman and the national staff may have had bad experiences with overseas volunteers in the past that left lasting negative impressions. You and/or the volunteers and students before you might have been afflicted with what we call the 'superior culture syndrome'. Superior culture syndrome flares up consciously or otherwise, when volunteers and students sense an imperative to impart and impose medical knowledge and cultural values upon their hosts and patients simply because they come from a more affluent society with a higher standard of healthcare. They do not see the silent protest of their wise, experienced and beleaguered national healthcare colleagues who prefer not to create a disturbance. Even the findings of the Cochrane data (www.cochranelibrary.com) base have to be placed in both a clinical and socioeconomic context. Some of our older mentors have insisted that OB-GYN is an art not science. In the middle of the night in rural Africa, you may have to very creative.

Ethical and Legal Concerns

Cultural understanding and preparation in OB-GYN must also include consideration of varied international laws in the area of reproductive health, and how they apply in the specific setting. There are many ethically challenging situations in OB-GYN. The law and/or commonly held beliefs around women's rights and opportunities and practices such as abortion, independent access to contraception or consent for sexual activity may differ significantly from that of your home country. For example, in Zimbabwe, the male partner makes the final decision in the use of contraception, especially permanent methods, despite the health risk and dangers associated with a future pregnancy.

Likewise, many women may present having had female genital mutilation (FGM); while internationally decried, we would never wish to make women, who have experienced this practice, feel shameful about their bodies. Practicing within these different confines may provide significant frustration for the trainee but it needs to be clearly understood that a single (or even repeat) visit abroad is not the time or place to challenge national laws or perceptions! In some circumstances, to do so could create awkwardness, problems, or even danger for the local practitioners who stay behind after the trainee departs. Therefore, at least at the time of the elective, these differing regulations need to be politely respected and taken as part of the broad cultural experience.

Coming Home

It is not the intention of this chapter to condone infractions of women's rights, merely to suggest what constitutes safe professional practice at the time of the elective or volunteer stay. Individuals can become involved from home in campaigns and other opportunities for meaningful change in international practices and regulations should they so desire; it is these sorts of experiences found in overseas elective and volunteer work that form the basis of interesting reflection and discussion upon returning home, or with their supervisor while still abroad. A thorough debriefing and opportunities to express oneself in avenues such as personal writing, or with a mentor experienced in international health, will help foster understanding of the diverse realities in our world.

References

Chan, Margaret, Thoraya Obaid, Phumaphi Joy, and Veneman Ann M. 2008. Maternal, newborn, child and adolescent health: Cover our mothers and babies. World Health Organization (WHO). http://www .who.int/maternal_child_adolescent/news_events/events/2008/mdg5/article/en/

Tunçalp, Ozge, Tripathi, Vandana, Landry, Evelyn, Stantonc, Cynthia K, and Ahmed, Saifuddin. 2015. Measuring the incidence and prevalence of obstetric fistula: Approaches, needs and recommendations. Bulletin of the World Health Organization (WHO). http://www.who.int/bulletin/volumes/93/1/14-141473/en/

Wang, Haldong et al. (GBD Child Mortality Collaborators). 2016. Global, regional, national, and selected subnational levels of stillbirths, neonatal, infant, and under-5 mortality, 1980–2015: A systematic analysis for the Global Burden of Disease Study 2015. *The Lancet* 388 (10053):1725–1774.

World Health Organization (WHO). 2015a. Media Centre: Fact sheet N°348. Maternal mortality. http:// www.who.int/mediacentre/factsheets/fs348/en/

World Health Organization (WHO). 2015b. Millennium Development Goal 5 2015. Improve Maternal Health. www.who.int/topics/millennium_development_goals/maternal_health/en/

World Health Organization (WHO). 2016. Media Centre: Fact Sheet No. 380 Human papillomavirus (HPV) and Cervical Cancer. http://www.who.int/mediacentre/factsheets/fs380/en/

Chapter 16

Midwifery: 'With Women' across the Globe

Karen Hays

Contents

Since the re-emergence of U.S. midwifery education in the late twentieth century, midwife trainees have participated in international experiences to enhance their education (Hays, 2001; Latta et al., 2011; Levi, 2009; NARM, 2016). These trips can last a few weeks or several months, and might focus on clinical, public health and/or community settings. The reasons for seeking an international experience are varied, but students are typically inspired by three intertwining motivations.

1. *To serve humankind by helping others* (Delorme, 2012; Koopman, 2008; Lasker, 2016; Latta et al., 2011; Thiessen, 2012)
2. *To explore pregnancy, birth, motherhood and healthcare from a cross-cultural perspective* (Dowell and Merrylees, 2009; Hays, 2001; Latta et al., 2011; Levi, 2009)
3. *To provide access to a clinical setting where large numbers of patients*: In this case pregnant women – seek care, in order to expand learning experiences and skills through 'high-volume' exposure (Hays, 2001; Martin, 2014; Nestel, 2006; White and Cauley, 2006)

Although the first and second motivations listed are common and may be more emotionally driven, the third motivation is usually central for most midwifery students and will therefore be the focus of the following discussion.

You may believe that a clinical rotation in a busy maternity ward could be exciting, interesting and accelerate your learning. However, it is important to balance the focus on yourself with what you are able to contribute. In order for your experience to prioritize the needs of the patients and the host community, you must be thoughtful in your preparation and be willing to consider what kind of contribution you can realistically make (Delorme, 2012; Hays, 2001; Martin, 2014; Nestel, 2006; Schytt and Waldenstrom, 2013).

Preparing to Go

Making arrangements to participate in a midwifery global health elective is similar to other health professional trainees (Latta et al., 2011; Lasker, 2016). These activities include the following:

- Choosing (or being assigned to) a location and then learning about the place and its people
- Identifying learning objectives, completing school paperwork and planning travel details
- Demonstrating that your clinical judgment, skills and emotional maturity are appropriate for an international placement

Each midwifery school will have a different approach to student preparation. Unfortunately, even rotations that are part of well-established credit-bearing courses may sometimes have minimal preparation. Therefore, you should inquire *early* in the planning process about what the school is responsible for and what you are expected to do. Note if the school's policies and guidelines for global health preparation programs incorporates feedback, expectations and advice from members of the host community – healthcare providers, patients and others. If possible, talk to midwifery students who have gone before you and ask them what they wished they would have known before departing.

One indicator of a thorough international elective preparation program is a requirement for students to think about their motivations and positionality (Nestel, 2006, 69–83; Lasker, 2016, 92–97; Martin, 2014, 48). This means that the school recognizes that international clinical rotations can be ethically challenging and potentially harmful. One issue is that students from relatively rich countries travel to volunteer in busy maternity wards, often in charity or government hospitals, where the patients and healthcare workers are often from less privileged backgrounds. Discussions about 'voluntourism' are currently taking place within various health professions, including midwifery. Familiarize yourself with the literature in this area to appreciate some of the ethical debates and explore your own motivations for participating in an international clinical rotation. It is important to reflect on how your gender, race/ethnicity, privilege, spiritual beliefs and other factors may influence your perceptions and experiences, as well as how your presence might impact the host community and the individuals with whom you will come into contact.

Preparing to Provide Midwifery Care in an International Setting

If you intend to be active in a labor and delivery ward during your international rotation, you should have frank conversations with experienced midwives and other knowledgeable clinicians about potential realities you are likely to encounter, including how to cope with difficult situations. Discussions about on-site supervision, resource limitations that may lead to poor medical outcomes, and the status of women should be covered. The scope of your involvement and your ability to provide healthcare that benefits the patients must be clarified as much as possible before departure.

Supervision

Midwifery students deserve and require supportive, on-site mentorship and supervision in any clinical setting. In the past, midwifery trainees would frequently arrive in another country, after minimal arrangements, to volunteer in a maternity hospital for several weeks in exchange for some distant support from a U.S.-based training school (i.e. donations of money, equipment or supplies). The burdens placed on local staff to supervise an unknown visiting trainee, the lack of on-site support for students when poor patient outcomes or interpersonal conflicts occur, and an unfortunate track record of visiting students behaving in ways that are culturally incongruent with the norms of the host community have led to the conclusion that U.S. educational institutions must take more responsibility for their students while onsite (Delorme, 2012; Martin, 2014).

Therefore, you should ensure that an experienced faculty member from the home institution or a well-trained and institutionally supported local preceptor from the host community is present whenever you are in the clinic or hospital. This supervisor should be prepared to both mentor and evaluate you. The supervisor should speak the language used in the healthcare institution; have legal authority to provide nursing, midwifery or medical care in the country; and have a trusting, working relationship with key personnel in the maternity ward. You may also require authoritative assistance with diplomatic negotiations regarding issues such as ensuring that you do not 'compete' with local midwifery students on the ward, deciding which types of hands-on clinical care is appropriate for and expected from you, and if you will be invited to observe or participate in other types of learning opportunities (e.g. the operating room, high-risk newborn unit, morbidity and mortality reviews, midwifery school classes or community outreach mobile clinics).

Resource Limitations

Healthcare institutions in low- or middle-income countries where most midwifery trainees are placed present challenges regarding the quality of care students will witness and in which they will participate. If you are accustomed to healthcare settings where supplies are abundant and where trained personnel necessary for managing medical emergencies quickly appear, you might find yourself shocked, confused and frustrated in an environment where the opposite is the norm. When discussing such realities during preparation activities, you may suspect that your teachers are merely pointing out the obvious. But, until you experience it for yourself, it is impossible to predict how these conditions will make you feel, especially if the skill set you brought from your home setting did not prepare you to function in a low-resource environment. One suggestion is while still at home and with preceptor approval, you can strengthen as many midwifery skills as possible that require 'hand skills' instead of machines (e.g. using Naegele's rule to calculate a due date, a manual cuff to take a blood pressure and a fetoscope to hear the fetal heart). Also before departure, you should ask experienced faculty and preceptors to lead you through difficult case studies to help prepare you for managing maternal and newborn complications with limited technology, including strategies for coping with sad outcomes that can trigger strong emotions.

Status of Women

Midwifery is a profession that focuses on caring for women. Therefore, noticing how the status of women and gender politics play out differently from your own familiar cultural milieu can be confusing and sometimes distressing. You will need to practice humility and sensitivity so as to not be disruptive and overly self-focused in an environment where the complexities of human interaction are not easily (or ever) understood by an outsider. This might be most difficult if you are judging that the treatment of the patient is poor or unfair. Therefore, during preparation activities, several scenarios should be explored that highlight issues such as when female patients cannot give their own informed consent for medical care, the treatment of underprivileged or ethnic minority women that may differ from care given to wealthier women from the dominant culture, and the use of what you might consider outdated obstetrical practices (e.g. enemas, episiotomies and rules forbidding birth companions). The teaching scenarios should cover situations that may be the norm in the country and culture, but must minimize (ideally, eliminate) stereotyping, prejudicial assumptions and negative judgments. This type of pre-departure activity would optimally be conducted with assistance from a knowledgeable culture broker (NCCC, 2004) – a person from that country who can represent the people and culture that promotes dignity, respects traditions and can shed light on current cultural and institutional healthcare practices and the complexities of historical phenomena (e.g. colonialism, racism, intergenerational trauma and religious influences).

Student Involvement and Benefits/Risks to Patients

Midwifery trainees, due to the nature of the profession, encounter women during times of personal vulnerability associated with the intensity and unpredictability of labor and birth, as well as the sudden public exposure of what are normally private body parts. Thoughtful anticipatory guidance should prompt you to reflect on how you might impact the patient's experience during such a memorable time in her life. Three important areas to consider are consent for care by you (a foreigner and a student), your language abilities and your clinical expertise.

First, foreign students should not expect that they will be accepted by the patients they have come to serve. Women everywhere have preferences, although not always choices, regarding who takes care of them in medical settings. Maternity patients should be given the option of accepting or declining care from you, and their reasons for declining (e.g. they prefer a more experienced provider, are uncomfortable with the student's gender or are fearful of someone who appears so different) should not be questioned or minimized.

Second, protocols should be in place so that students who cannot communicate due to language barriers are never left alone with a woman in active labor or who has recently delivered. Although much communication can take place non-verbally in the labor room, it is recommended that, before or immediately upon arrival, you should memorize 10 initial, essential phrases in the patient's local language(s): 'hello', 'please', 'thank-you', 'okay', 'breathe', 'push', 'good', 'boy', 'girl' and 'I'm sorry'. Although these few words are not a replacement for the presence of a fluent interpreter, speaking in the local language can help develop rapport and demonstrate your interest in building cross-cultural bridges.

Finally, students who are medically unskilled or personally overwhelmed may discover that their presence is neither helpful to the staff nor therapeutic for the patients. Before departure, you should think about potential clinical circumstances in which you might be in over your head and thus not adding value to the situation. You should know what your options are so that, first and foremost, the patient can get her needs met, but also so that the local staff are not unnecessarily burdened by your needs and you are protected from accusations of malpractice. As with all health professional training, midwifery trainees are expected to attempt sequentially more difficult tasks to build their clinical skills, but this should *never* be at the expense of the patient receiving the highest quality of care possible (Raisler et al., 2003). This brings the conversation back to the requirement for supportive supervision at all times while you are caring for patients.

Post-Trip Issues

As all students who return from a global health elective, midwifery students will need guidance through the potential reverse 'culture shock' and to make sense of their experiences. You might wonder how to integrate your new knowledge and skills into your practice back home (more on in the next paragraph), and you may struggle with ethical distress when you recall the experience. In the surveys by Hays (2001) and Latta et al. (2011), several midwifery students expressed uneasiness with their memories of the resource limitations, quality of care and treatment of women. However, this can also provide insight into global healthcare, privilege in higher-resourced countries and potential activism to increase awareness of these issues and decrease global health disparities. As with preparation activities, you should look for indicators of a well-thought-out institutional program for re-entry: structured meetings with objectives and evaluations, plus continuing monitoring and support by school faculty and, if needed, by professional counselors (Delorme, 2012; Elit et al., 2011; Green et al., 2008; Latta et al., 2011; Martin, 2014).

One important area of professional integration and development that midwifery students should explore with faculty and preceptors back home is how to reground oneself in the professional and legal scope of midwifery practice in the United States. Each state has its own regulations, and you should not graduate from midwifery school under a false impression that you can offer clinical care that follows the standards of practice in the country where you completed an international elective. For example, if you attended twin deliveries overseas you may believe that you can add that service to your professional practice upon graduation. But attending twin deliveries might be outside the legal scope of practice in your home jurisdiction. Even if midwifery management of twin births is standard local practice, you still need mentorship for how to provide appropriate care of multiple pregnancies in your home community.

Time must also be reserved after the trip in which opportunities to (a) critically evaluate the long-term sustainability of the international partnership, (b) craft tactful recommendations for improvement and (c) create resources that could be shared with future students interested in the site. In addition, pondering and exploring the bigger issues of equity, reciprocity, privilege, oppression and racism are fundamental to analyses of cross-border and cross-cultural encounters. Although such discussions can be difficult and no easy answers exist, this is a valuable opportunity to deepen your understanding of the power and privilege, and therefore responsibility, that comes with access to higher education, joining a professional discipline and having the resources required to explore the world. It is often wondered whether the money spent on the trip might have been put to use in ways that could have otherwise benefited the mothers and babies, or the local midwives, in the host community.

References

Delorme, Lisa. 2012. *Proposed Guidelines for a Global Service-Learning Program for the Department of Midwifery at Bastyr University.* Kenmore, WA: Bastyr University Library.

Dowell, Jon, and Neil Merrylees. 2009. Electives: Isn't it time for a change? *Medical Education* 43 (2): 121–26.

Elit, Laurie, Matthew Hunt, Lynda Redwood-Campbell, Jennifer Ranford, Naomi Adelson, and Lisa Schwartz. 2011. Ethical issues encountered by Medical Students during International Health Electives. *Medical Education* 45: 704–11. 10.1111/j.1365-2923.2011.03936.x

Green, Barbara F., Inez Johansen, Megan Rosser, Cassam Tengnah, and Jeremy Segrott. 2008. Studying abroad: A multiple case study of nursing students' international experiences. *Nurse Education Today* 28 (8): 981–92. 10.1016/j.nedt.2008.06.003

Hays, Karen E. 2001. *Seattle Midwifery School Survey of Graduates Regarding Foreign Training Sites*. Seattle, WA: Seattle Midwifery School (unpublished manuscript).

Koopman, Sara. 2008. Imperialism within: Can the master's tools bring down empire? *ACME: An International E-Journal for Critical Geographies* 7 (2), 283–307.

Lasker, Judith. 2016. *Hoping to Help: The Promises and Pitfalls of Global Health Volunteering*. Ithaca, NY: Cornell University Press.

Latta, Summer, Mary Ann Faucher, Sarah Brown, and Martha Bradshaw. 2011. International clinical experience for midwifery students. *Journal of Midwifery and Women's Health* 56 (4): 382–87. 10.1111/j.1542-2011.2011.00035.x

Levi, Amy. 2009. The ethics of nursing student international clinical experiences. *Journal of Obstetric, Gynecologic and Neonatal Nursing* 38 (1): 94–9. 10.1111/j.1552-6909.2008.00314.x

Martin, Merka G. 2014. *International Health Electives: Preparation, Participation, and Assimilation. A Workshop for Student Midwives*. Kenmore, WA: Bastyr University Library.

National Center for Cultural Competence (NCCC). 2004. *Bridging the Cultural Divide in Health Care Settings: The Essential Role of Culture Broker Programs*. Georgetown, VA: Georgetown University.

North American Registry of Midwives (NARM). 2016. *Revised Policies Concerning Training of CPMs in Out-of-Country Clinical Sites*. http://narm.org/news/revised-policies-ooc/

Nestel, Sheryl. 2006. *Obstructed Labor: Race and Gender in the Re-Emergence of Midwifery*. Vancouver, BC: University of British Columbia (UBC) Press.

Raisler, Jeanne, Michelle O'Grady, and Jody Lori. 2003. Clinical teaching and learning in midwifery and women's health. *Journal of Midwifery and Women's Health* 48 (6): 398–406.

Schytt, Erica, and Waldenstrom, Ulla. 2013. How well does midwifery education prepare for clinical practice? Exploring the views of Swedish students, midwives, and obstetricians. *Midwifery* 29 (2): 102–9. doi: 10.1012/j.midw.2011.11.012

Thiessen, Rebecca. 2012. Motivations for learn/volunteer abroad programs: Research with Canadian youth. *Journal of Global Citizenship and Equity Education* 2 (1). http://journals.sfu.ca/jgcee/index.php/jgcee/article/view/57/43

White, Mary T., and Katherine L. Cauley, 2006. A caution against medical student tourism. *Virtual Mentor* 8 (12): 851–54.

Chapter 17

Nursing during Global Health Experiences

Lorena Bonilla and Carolyn Beukeboom

Contents

Introduction

The *International Council of Nurses Code of Ethics for Nurses* (ICN, 2012) states that nurses have four fundamental responsibilities that include promoting health, preventing illness, restoring health and alleviating suffering. Nursing, as a human caring science, holds the social responsibility of addressing issues that affect the health of the people it serves on a local, national and international level. Nurses provide a valuable human resource for achieving the United Nations Sustainable Development Goals that include eradicating extreme poverty and hunger; achieving universal primary education; promoting gender equality and empowering women; reducing child mortality; improving maternal health; combating human immunodeficiency virus/acquired immune deficiency syndrome (HIV/AIDS), malaria and other diseases; ensuring environmental sustainability and developing a global partnership for development (United Nations, 2016).

Nurses and nursing students may care for people in various international settings including community outreach, health promotion and education, and acute care hospital placements. Global health experiences include humanitarian emergency crisis responses, public health and research opportunities, as well as short and long-term community development projects. The ability of nurses and nursing students to participate in such activities provides them with an opportunity to learn about cultural diversity, poverty and working with limited resources. International nursing work emphasizes the importance of strength-based care that focuses on human resilience while finding the right balance between individual strengths, problems and deficits. Strength-based nursing care focuses on empowering people by working with individuals, families and communities to find the necessary tools to maintain and improve their health and quality of life (Gottlieb, 2013). This chapter addresses key issues that affect nursing practice during international placements including specific considerations for students and nurses, ethical distress, interprofessional collaboration and communication, as well as healing within different cultures. The term 'nurses' in this chapter refers to nurse practitioners, registered nurses and registered practical nurses in their respective roles, as well as the students in each of these roles who may be involved in international experiences.

Planning and Organizing International Placements

A review of the literature suggests various issues to consider in general for anyone involved in planning ethical and sustainable global health experiences. These include the goals and purpose of the trip, length, available resources, weather, transportation, food, lodging, taxes and fees, administrative and financial issues, communication and relationships with the communities that will receive care, as well as the determination of needed medical supplies (Daniels and Servonsky, 2005; Solheim and Edwards, 2007). Other important concerns are the safety of the participants, recruitment criteria of volunteers, and the appropriate training and debriefing before, during and after the international placement.

The majority of available literature regarding short-term placements focuses on the importance of planning and organization, as well as the need to provide students and nurses with international experiences given the benefits of volunteering internationally (DeCamp, 2014; Memmott et al., 2010; Solheim and Edwards, 2007). Practical considerations for nursing faculty planning and organizing such placements for nursing students include an appropriate fit within the curriculum, the selection of an appropriate model to deliver the experience, and the finances required to implement the experience. The recruitment of appropriate faculty, establishment of relationships with the international placement site, selection of students, development of curriculum and evaluation of the international placements are also key elements in the process of organizing and developing international placements for nursing students (Memmott et al., 2010).

The planning and organization phase of international placements must consider and explore sustainability, ethical issues, community development and capacity building following fundamental global health responsibilities based on the principles of social justice and human rights. To ensure meeting people's needs in a safe, ethical, culturally relevant and competent manner, the effectiveness and limitations of the nursing care provided must be evaluated from the communities' perspective. A review of the literature suggests that only a few studies actually explore communities' perceptions of the care received during global health experiences (DeCamp et al., 2014). Consequently, there is a need for research that gives voice to communities that receive healthcare during global health experiences. It is also necessary that nurses and healthcare professionals in general, take the time to assess and evaluate people's needs before they provide care.

Considerations for Nurses and Nursing Students

There are many opportunities to work with a wide range of organizations during humanitarian emergency crisis responses, short and long-term placements, as well as community development projects. A careful consideration of the purpose and goals of particular organizations and available opportunities is very important prior to participating in any international placement. It is essential to have an understanding of the vision and purpose of the organization, as well as its before role within the community, and the established relationships with the people that will receive care. All of these factors will promote sustainability, and assist with the follow-up and evaluation of the care provided. The type of nursing role and function that the nursing student or nurse would like to perform and is competent to perform must be carefully considered. Depending on the organization of the international placements, nursing students may have an observational educational type role. Possible nursing roles include direct patient care, supervisory positions, mentorships, research, education, administration and intra/interprofessional collaboration and teaching.

International placements can renew a nurse's respect for teamwork, holistic practice, the importance of clinical assessments in the absence of technology, as well as the dedication to improving the health of people everywhere. Other critical issues to consider before volunteering include the language spoken in the country of destination, political instability, vaccinations and health insurance, as well as the need of a nursing license to practice internationally. Nurses must be aware of the limits of their scope of practice, professional and legal issues that can affect their ability to provide safe, ethical and competent care during their international placements, as well as the type of nursing role required that might include teaching, supervising and hands-on care (Memmott et al., 2010). Organizations have different set of rules, policies and regulations regarding nursing practice. Nurses and student nurses must clarify the available support, mentorship and their expected legal and professional accountability during an international placement. The institutional, international and professional policies governing international placements, whether volunteering or completing a required learning experience, must be clarified prior to becoming involved. Refer to Chapter 7 for further information regarding the preparation needed to go abroad.

Reflection and critical thinking about nursing practice and the care provided are essential during international placements. Students, nurses and faculty must be knowledgeable about appropriate ethical frameworks, relevant best practice guidelines, and their scope of practice during international placements. Learning about cultural diversity and respect for other ways of life must begin with the awareness of personal and professional differences that affect the nurse's ability to provide culturally safe, competent and relevant nursing care anywhere in the world. For this reason, it is critical that nursing students and nurses receive the appropriate preparation before they participate in an international placement.

Ethical Distress

Ethical distress during international placements occurs for various reasons (DeCamp, 2014); therefore, nurses and nursing students will benefit from guidelines that can assist to problem-solve situations given the challenging circumstances they may encounter. Appropriate preparation and training before departure can help students and nurses prepare for the possible practical and ethical challenges they can encounter. This preparation should include learning about the country, culture, language and health-related values, beliefs and behaviours. The application of available ethical frameworks, professional and legal guidelines to challenging situations that may be encountered abroad can help to prepare for difficult clinical decision making. The more information people can receive about their placement, guidelines regarding safe and competent nursing care, as well as different ways of life, the easier it will be for them to adapt their practice and evaluate the context of the placement in a holistic, caring and ethical manner.

Cultural conflicts, lack of resources, and competency with certain clinical skills can lead to experiencing challenging ethical situations. For example, nurses can experience ethical distress when they have to ignore their female patients' wishes in patriarchal societies where women are not allowed to make decisions regarding their care. In certain countries, women must obtain permission from their spouse, or a significant male in their life, to be able to receive medical treatment. The life of a woman, and her baby, who is not allowed to receive a C-section will be put in danger because of religious and cultural beliefs. It is therefore important for everyone in the medical team to discuss patient situations and consider the safest, most ethically competent way to proceed, which would incorporate different stakeholders' needs, as well as the context of the situation. Nurses play an important role in facilitating an open and honest communication with all the team members that include the local healthcare practitioners who understand the language and cultural context better. Given the lack of resources, a medical team may be required to decide whether to continue with life-saving treatment in the absence of appropriate equipment needed for further treatment. Although the right or least wrong decision may not be clear in certain situations, the appropriate discussion and debriefing about the situation with the health care team members, including the local and international team, are essential.

During international placements, nurses and nursing students may be asked to complete tasks they are not qualified to do in their home countries such as starting intravenouses (IVs), taking blood samples and delivering babies, which can lead to practical and ethical dilemmas that cause ethical distress. Some might say that 'there is no one else who can do it, so you may as well just do it'. Regardless of the location and context for nursing practice, students and nurses must adhere to their homeland's scope of practice and become aware of legal, ethical and practical guidelines that affect their nursing care within the international context (ICN, 2012). In such situations, appropriate responses may include: 'I have not been trained to do that skill', 'I don't feel comfortable performing that skill' or 'I would be happy to watch and help you, but I am not trained to perform that skill'. For nursing students, the basic preparation before an international placement must include a review of fundamental skills such as head to toe assessments and taking vital signs without relying on the use of technology that may not be available in developing countries. It is very important that students and nurses feel as confident as possible with their skills, as well as communicating with people that may not speak their language. Students always require the supervision of faculty or nurse preceptors that possess the necessary preparation to mentor, guide and assist them to problem-solve within the context of an international placement. Nursing faculty and preceptors must discuss and clarify their scope of practice, as well as the students', with the placement agency to ensure the safety of patients, students, and the health care team, as well as promote and support safe, ethical and competent nursing practice

Personal and professional values and beliefs may be compromised during placements for a variety of reasons. It is therefore necessary for nurses and nursing students to develop an ability to assess and understand situations in a holistic, culturally sensitive and ethical manner. Given the lack of resources and context of international placements, the application of various ethical frameworks, standards of practice, and legal guidelines to different situations can ensure the delivery of safe, culturally competent and ethical nursing care.

Interprofessional Collaboration

In many developing countries, culture, available resources, hierarchy and education issues in the medical system play an important role in the delivery of healthcare services. Depending on the country, healthcare providers may include health promoters, community health workers, midwives, nurses, clinical officers, surgeons and physicians. Nursing education, accountability and the scope of practice of nurses and nursing students vary in different countries and within different settings. In some places in rural Africa, there is no formal nursing education, and therefore many nurses are trained by international non-governmental organizations (NGOs) working in the area. Clinical officers, a role utilized in many African countries, usually have a 3-year education and similar scope of practice as physicians (Mullan and Frehywot, 2007). Physicians are well respected and treated accordingly, while nurses occupy a subservient role to the physicians who are well respected. Nurses do not possess the professional autonomy of nurses in developed nations (McKay and Narasimhan, 2012). Regardless of the context and location, it is critical that students and nurses participating in international placements value and respect the skills, knowledge and expertise of the local staff, particularly the nurses and nursing students. The local health care team can educate foreign students and professional healthcare workers about diseases and other conditions unknown in developed countries, as well as guide the implementation of culturally sensitive and ethically appropriate care. Local staff nurses and nursing students usually work as interpreters and facilitate the implementation of care to people in their native language.

Communication and Healing within Different Cultures

Students and nurses must practice and provide nursing care according to fundamental nursing values and beliefs (ICN, 2012). Regardless of location and context, the ability to establish therapeutic nurse–client relationships based on mutual respect and trust is essential when working with individuals, families and communities in order to empower them, assess their needs holistically and facilitate the achievement and maintenance of health, wellness and quality of life (Gottlieb, 2013; ICN, 2012). International placements provide an opportunity for students and nurses to deliver safe, ethical and competent care while improving their communication and assessment skills without the use of technology and various equipment. Fundamental nursing assessment competencies include the auscultation of lungs without access to X-rays, assessment of poor blood circulation of the extremities without oxygen saturation monitors, and assessment of anemia without blood testing. Working in other countries with different ways of life and language require that nurses rely on interpreters, which presents different challenges when providing nursing care. Barriers to verbal communication with patients provide an appreciation for effective and therapeutic non-verbal communication such as hand gestures, facial expressions, touch and the use of eye contact that vary in meaning and appropriateness depending on the cultural setting.

Variation within cultural settings opens one's eyes to the practice of Western medicine and the acceptance of complementary and alternative healing including the use of plants, herbs and rituals. Many people in developing countries cannot afford and do not have access to Western medicine; therefore, they have to rely on herbal teas, shamans, ritualistic curing practices and bone healers to provide most of their health care. Foreign practitioners must be aware and become knowledgeable about alternative practices that do not to cause harm to the patient.

All healthcare-related cultural practices require sensitive and open communication between the health care professionals and the people receiving care. It is therefore critical for foreign healthcare professionals to be open minded while carefully considering and discussing with people the safety of alternative methods of treatment, as well as their impact on health, wellness and prevention of illness. In one country in South America, a child experiencing seizures came to the hospital with the parents. The medical staff started to give medication in an attempt to stop the seizure, while the parents wanted to perform a healing ritual over the child's body. Once the medical team realized the ritual would cause no harm to the child, they allowed it to take place while providing the necessary medication to stop the seizure. The team and the parents were equally pleased with the outcome of their collaboration after the seizures stopped. In another situation, local health workers from rural communities discussed with farmers how to treat machete cuts obtained while working in the field, far away from any medical resources and without adequate water for cleaning the wound. The health workers proposed urine as a sterile product to use for cleaning machete wounds. Although not scientifically proven, many natural healing organizations promote using urine as an effective treatment. Along with an open mind and acceptance of different cultural norms, the health care professional must be aware of harmful practices such as putting mud on the umbilical cord of a newborn baby, which can lead to tetanus infection and ultimately death of the child. In each of these scenarios, nurses can support and encourage the necessary dialogue between patients, families and communities to explore the benefits and/or harms related to established cultural practices. Nurses and nursing students provide direct patient care and therefore the development of trusting and respectful relationships between the patient and other healthcare providers is essential to broker cultural differences.

Conclusion

According to ICN (2012), nurses have a social and moral obligation to help people maintain and regain health, wellness and quality of life regardless of the location where nursing care takes place. Advocacy, social justice, human rights and policy changes are key elements in the delivery of safe, ethical, accountable and competent nursing care. International nursing practice must demonstrate respect and understanding of cultural diversity following nursing and transcultural nursing theories. Reflection and critical thinking about ethics, standards of practice and legal issues that guide nursing care are essential. Nurses must critically consider the benefits versus possible harm caused by their practice, responsible use of resources, scope of practice, and the need for policy change in international settings. In developed countries, nurses recognize the importance of assessing and understanding people's needs, building capacity and remaining open to diversity, as well as avoiding paternalistic attitudes and deficit-thinking approaches to health care. International nursing practice must follow standards congruent with intercultural nursing theories to avoid perpetuating marginalization and paternalistic attitudes and behaviours that will not assist people to meet their needs and improve their quality of life. Given the findings in the literature (DeCamp et al., 2014; Memmott, et al., 2010; United Nations, 2000), the implications for global health and nursing curricula, nursing leaders must develop appropriate frameworks for practice while educating nurses and nursing students about safe, ethical, competent and culturally relevant nursing care during international placements.

References

Daniels, L., and Servonsky, J. (2005). Guide for a successful international mission. *Journal of Multicultural Nursing and Health*, Vol. 11, No. 3, 57–61.

DeCamp, M., Enumah, S., O'Neill, D., and Sugarman, J. (2014). Perceptions of a short-term medical programme in the Dominican Republic: Voices of care recipients. *Global Public Health*, Vol. 9, No. 4, 411–425.

Gottlieb, L. N. (2013). *Strengths-Based Nursing Care: Health and Healing for Person and Family*. New York, NY: Springer.

International Council of Nurses (2012). *The ICN Code of Ethics for Nurses*. Geneva, Switzerland: ICN.

McKay, K.A., and Narasimhan, S. (2012). Bridging the gap between doctors and nurses. *Journal of Nursing Education and Practice*, Vol. 2, No. 4, 52–55.

Memmott, R. J., Coverston, C. R., Heise, B. A., Williams, M., Maughan, E. D., Kohl, J., and Palmer, S. (2010). Practical considerations in establishing sustainable international nursing experiences. *Nursing Education Perspectives*, Vol. 31, No. 5, 298–302.

Mullan, F. and Frehywot, S. (2007). Non-physician clinicians in 47 sub-Saharan African countries. *Lancet* Vol. 370, No. 9605, 2158–2163. Retrieved from http://www.thelancet.com/pdfs/journals/lancet/PIIS0140 -6736(07)60785-5.pdf.

Solheim, J., and Edwards, P. (2007). Planning a successful mission trip: The ins and outs. *Journal of Emergency Nursing*, Vol. 33, No. 4, 382–387.

United Nations (UN). (2000). *United Nations Millennium Declaration*. Retrieved from http://www.un.org/en /ga/search/view_doc.asp?symbol=A/RES/55/

United Nations (UN). (2016). Sustainable Development Goals: 17 Goals to Transform Our World. Retrieved from http://www.un.org/sustainabledevelopment/sustainable-development-goals/

Chapter 18

Disability and Rehabilitative Experiences

Stephanie A. Nixon and Debra Cameron

Contents

Introduction to Rehabilitation in Low- or Middle-Income Countries

International electives in rehabilitation are typically undertaken by students in the fields of physical therapy (PT), occupational therapy (OT) and speech-language pathology (SLP). It is also possible for medical, nursing and other students (including those trained as aides – for example, physiotherapy aides) to undertake rehabilitation-focused electives; however, the majority are students in the rehabilitation professions. 'Rehabilitation' tends to focus on ability and disability, movement, function, inclusion, social participation and meaningful occupation. As such, rehabilitation providers are involved not only in activities directly linked to health but also to wider social change that promotes engagement and inclusion. Underpinning these issues is a human rights-based approach as articulated in the United Nations Convention on the Rights of Persons with Disabilities (CRPD), which was adopted in 2006 (UN, 2006). The CRPD is supported by the World Report on Disability, published by the World Health Organization and World Bank (2010). The CRDP and the World Report on Disability are part of the wider response to the enormous burden of disability worldwide. More than one billion people live with some form of disability, with the majority residing in low- or middle-income countries (LMIC). Global data on unmet rehabilitation needs do not exist but estimates suggest significant gaps, especially in resource-poor settings (World Health Organization and World Bank, 2010, p. 201). The following two frameworks help characterize the scope of rehabilitation in low- and middle-income settings.

International Classification of Functioning, Disability and Health: First, the World Health Organization's (WHO) International Classification of Functioning, Disability and Health (ICF) is a widely accepted approach for understanding rehabilitation in both resource-rich and resource-constrained settings (World Health Organization, 2001). The ICF describes facets of human functioning affected by a health condition. In contrast to a biomedical approach, the ICF focuses on the impact of health conditions at three levels: body functions and structures, *activity* and *participation*. The ICF also understands environmental and personal contextual factors as shaping experiences at these three levels. As such, the ICF understands disability as created when individual impairments intersect with limiting environmental conditions. The ICF has been widely used to investigate many diseases and disabilities. *The ICF is not linear or sequential.* As such, there is no requirement for health-related experiences to be understood in terms of impairments leading unidirectionally to activity limitations and participation restrictions, which allows for a more dynamic and realistic understanding of lived experiences. Finally, *the ICF takes a positive, assets-based stance focusing on capacities as opposed to problems.* The ICF takes abilities and strengths as its starting point as opposed to challenges. This approach enables examination of not only problems but also the creative means by which people demonstrate resilience in the face of adversity.

Community-based rehabilitation: The other dominant framework is 'community-based rehabilitation' (CBR). This model is not just about *where* rehabilitation is delivered (i.e. in a community); it is a comprehensive, multisectoral approach to improving the equalization of opportunities and social inclusion of people with disabilities while combatting the perpetual cycle of poverty and disability. CBR privileges local expertise and resources and focuses on empowerment across a range of life-related concerns. CBR as a model was initiated by the WHO following the Declaration of Alma-Ata in 1978 in an effort to enhance the quality of life for people with disabilities and their families, meet their basic needs and ensure their inclusion and participation. The CBR approach is dominant in resource-poor settings, but stands to benefit high-income communities as well.

Educational Requirements

The clinical practice component of the curricula of rehabilitation training programs typically includes multiple on-site clinical education electives. Students in rehabilitation programs in North America may have the opportunity to participate in one or more of the clinical electives in resource-poor settings. Requirements are specific to each discipline and each jurisdiction and may vary according to the length of the electives (e.g. 3–12 weeks), the requirements for supervision (e.g. on-site vs. virtual supervision) and clinical experience required (e.g. an SLP program may require clinical education experience in highly specified clinical domains). Logistical arrangements for placements can be complicated by university requirements for legal contracts and various forms of insurance (malpractice, work place safety) that facilities in LMIC countries may find difficult to provide.

Clinical Settings

Access to rehabilitation is extremely limited in many LMIC settings. Public funding is rarely available and services are supported by a diversity of international and local players, including for-profit clinics, non-governmental organizations (NGOs) and churches. As such, students may experience models of rehabilitation delivery that differ from North America. Hospital-based care remains common. However, rehabilitation in the community is often provided by community rehabilitation workers, who have local expertise but little formal credentialing, under the supervision of a licensed therapist. As such, it is not uncommon for rehabilitation professionals to see clients only once or twice in a year or sometimes, only once ever. Rehabilitation can also be provided in short-term, intensive 'treatment weeks', whereby families and their children with disabilities live for a week in a clinical setting to receive hands-on education to support families in carrying out rehabilitation when they return home. These programs also allow families to give and receive mutual support from other each other. Box 18.1 outlines a range of considerations for students undertaking rehabilitation electives.

Patient Populations

Patients in rehabilitation electives are typically adults and children who experience forms of disablement resulting from health conditions or injuries. Following the language of the ICF, patients typically experience impairments in body structure or function, activity limitations and/or participation restrictions that can be addressed by rehabilitation. The health conditions causing these forms of disability are diverse and include both conditions that are common in high-income settings as well as infectious diseases like human immunodeficiency virus (HIV), polio, malaria and tuberculosis (TB) that are more prevalent in resource-limited communities. Students may also provide rehabilitation to adults and children whose challenges result from lack of medical care, including untreated hydrocephalus and a higher prevalence of cerebral palsy. In all cases, the determinants of health play a pivotal role in shaping both the patient's experience and the rehabilitation provider's approach.

Nature of Rehabilitation Interaction

The practice of rehabilitation in North America typically focuses on approaches that are collaborative and interprofessional. The therapeutic interaction often involves trust developed over time and a commitment to patient-centred care. Empowerment is often a goal to enable patients to manage their own rehabilitation in partnership with the therapist. These common rehabilitation approaches may be present in low-resource settings, but they may also be challenging by contextual constraints. For instance, the medical model and authority of physicians over other healthcare providers predominates in many settings, which can challenge the rehabilitation focus on social participation and inclusion. Furthermore, rehabilitation providers may be expected to practice under the supervision of physicians in some settings, limiting clinical problem-solving and autonomy. The approach to patient advocacy and empowerment may also need to shift in different sociocultural contexts. For instance, whereas government policy makers may be a target for change in some settings, this approach may be less effective in other environments without public funding for rehabilitation.

BOX 18.1   CONSIDERATIONS FOR STUDENTS UNDERTAKING REHABILITATION ELECTIVES

Before the elective:

■ You should find out the following about the destination country:
   - Current information on disability prevalence and rehabilitation services: Sources may include the World Report on Disability and country profiles on the websites of the global health professions associations (e.g. World Confederation of Physical Therapy).
   - Detailed information on impairments that are common for that region that may not be seen in one's home environment: for example, injuries that may be less familiar (such as snakebite, machete injuries) or impairments resulting from lack of medical services.
   - Beliefs about disability: There is a diversity of beliefs about the causes and implications of disability in *all* settings, and it is useful to learn about some of the common disability understandings in the destination area ahead of the elective to be more sensitized to one's assumptions and the implications for rehabilitation practice.
   - Language spoken by therapists and other workers: If not one's own language, students should prepare by learning some key phrases related to etiquette and to rehabilitation.
■ You should find out about the elective facility, including the following:
   - Typical patients and common impairments that are treated
   - Type of intervention approaches commonly used
   - Models of service delivery: CBR, intensive weeks, consultation and direct treatment
   - Resources available: For example, number of therapists and other workers, equipment, assessment tools
   - Needs of the facility: What students could bring to meet identified needs of the facility (e.g. rehabilitation equipment, assessments or educational materials)

During the elective:

■ You should always work within your scope of practice:
   - Generally speaking, if a student cannot undertake a particular practice in her or his home country, then it should not be done elsewhere.
■ You should recognize that local rehabilitation providers are experts in service delivery in their context:
   - You should attempt to learn what you can from these local experts.
   - You should support the position of local therapists as the expert even if (and especially if) you are treated as more knowledgeable.
■ You should consider resources that are available when suggesting new approaches or equipment:
   - For example, availability of parts, batteries, expertise to repair, expertise to instruct on use.
■ You should focus on sustainability of your interventions:
   - When providing care, consider from the start how this course of treatment can be continued beyond the student's departure.

Differing Perceptions of Disability

While many contextual differences can shape internship experiences, understanding of *disability* is central to rehabilitation. Differing perceptions of disability are also common in North America, yet they may be even more clear in resource-poor settings. Roush and Sharby (2011) offer a framework for thinking about disability as follows: the medical model, the social model and the moral model. At the core of this approach and others is recognition of disability as a social construct or set of ideas that are seen as a norm. Students need to develop their capacity for critical analysis to be able to recognize the assumptions that underpin these various understandings of disability, since they will impact expectations about rehabilitation. For instance, one may consider the view of disability as (1) a physical problem to be fixed (the medical model); (2) a problem imposed on people with differing abilities by the environment, policies or attitudes (the social model) or (3) a blessing or curse (the moral model).

Stigma and discrimination are part of each of these approaches and can itself be disabling. For instance, people with disabilities may be a source of shame for families and, thus, hidden away, which limits access to rehabilitation or requires the trust built into CBR in order to enable intervention within people's homes.

Another core concept is *ableism* or the assumption that being able-bodied is the normal and natural way to be in society (Goodley, 2014). This is the dominant approach in most settings and results in the production of norms, policies and buildings that meet the needs of able-bodied people first, with accessibility for people of differing abilities viewed as exceptions. Ableism is so entrenched in society as to be almost invisible – yet, it remains one of the most disabling forces limiting the opportunities of disabled people and is a core focus for rehabilitation.

Ethical Challenges

Global health principles related to humility and critical thinking (Canadian Coalition for Global Health Research, 2015) are particularly important in rehabilitation electives because of the different positions of rehabilitation and disability within diverse healthcare systems. Students may experience moral distress as a result of differing approaches to discipline with children (Nixon et al., 2015) or challenges related to the lack of evidence for certain interventions. For instance, there may be a preference for massage for children with cerebral palsy, which is not evidence based but seen as closer to traditional practices and therefore more accepted and expected in a local setting. Students should also be prepared to recognize and mitigate ethical challenges related to power differentials whereby Global North (and especially white) students' perspectives are valued over and above local therapists with more experience. A further challenge relates to working in settings of extreme resource limitation whereby resourcefulness and ingenuity become crucial skills (Cassady et al., 2014). Commitment to sustainability is crucial, such that students' actions can continue to be carried out by others when they leave. This commitment leads to suggestions of equipment or other adaptations that use locally sourced materials. Finally, given the scarcity of rehabilitation professionals, students and their home universities must recognize the cost to local sites in terms of time lost when local providers use any of their limited availability to provide supervision and teaching to students. This is one of many costs borne by local hosts and their sites that often go unrecognized and unreimbursed in the context of international internships.

Types of Elective Experiences: A Few Examples

■ **CBR experiences:** While rehabilitation professionals assess and provide treatment plans, most direct service within CBR is delivered by community workers with local neighbourhood-level trust and expertise who travel to family homes to provide individual treatment. For example, CBR electives have been occurring at a NGO in Moshi and Dar es Salaam, Tanzania for over 10 years with OT, PT and SLP students travelling from several universities in North America. The elective includes week long intensive educational programs with rehabilitation professionals and students where the families of pediatric patients live together at the clinic. This approach helps meet the needs of families who struggle to find available services and/or who travel long distances to seek therapy.

■ **Remote and rural experiences:** International electives can offer particular challenges where rehabilitation services and resources are extremely scarce. A community-based organization in a very rural part of Kenya has been offering clinical internships to students from several Canadian universities for over 10 years. In this elective, the visiting students live with a local family and learn about providing rehabilitation services to remote communities. Clinics are held in surrounding rural towns and villages where clinical supervision is provided by locally trained therapists. For OT students, one of the challenges has been promoting a participation-based approach to therapy with clients who are used to more passive interventions, such as physical handling or massage since massage is perceived by some to be similar to more traditional healing methods. Access to learning about an evidence-based approach to clinical decision making can be challenging for practitioners in remote areas given limited Internet access. As such, the director of this clinic encourages students to provide workshops on evidence-based practice and the site also participates in collaborative research on HIV and rehabilitation as part of their broader international relationship.

■ **Experiences where there are few locally educated rehabilitation professionals:** Building on a 15-year OT relationship, one program in Trinidad and Tobago has recently added SLP and PT students despite the scarcity of locally trained rehabilitation professionals. As such, supervision for rehabilitation students has been provided primarily through Canadian therapists who travel to provide on-site supervision for part of the elective and provide remote, virtual supervision for the rest of the time. Students have been offered broader opportunities within the country, including presentations at local conferences, advocating for OT during displays at local malls, profiling the professions at local high schools and providing input into the first publicly funded interdisciplinary assessment and treatment clinic in the country. This elective is also unique because it offers interprofessional internships whereby students from different disciplines train together. This interprofessional approach offers opportunities for collaborative assessments and enhances implementation of recommendations from all three professions when, for example, OT students overlap with SLP students at one point, and with PT students at another time in the year.

■ **Electives with students from multiple universities:** At one NGO in India, OT, PT and SLP student electives are coordinated by Canadians. At least four different Canadian schools send their rehabilitation students. By involving a number of schools whose placements occur throughout the year, more sustainable services have been provided to children with disabilities at this clinical centre. Interprofessional opportunities to learn from each other and to share supervision are facilitated.

References

Canadian Coalition for Global Health Research. 2015. CCGHR principles for global health research. http://www.ccghr.ca/resources/principles-global-health-research/

Cassady, Christina, Mehru Rehana, Chan, Nga Man Carmen, Engelhardt, Julie, Fraser, Michelle, and Stephanie A. Nixon. 2014. Physiotherapy beyond our borders: Investigating ideal competencies for Canadian physiotherapists working in resource-poor countries. *Physiotherapy Canada* 66(1):15–23.

Goodley, Dan. 2014. *Disability Studies: Theorising Disablism and Ableism*. London: Routledge.

Nixon, Stephanie A., Lynn Cockburn, Ruth Acheinegeh, Kim Bradley, Debra Cameron, Peter N. Mue, Nyingcho Samuel, and Barbara E. Gibson. 2015. Using postcolonial perspectives to consider rehabilitation with children with disabilities: The Bamenda-Toronto dialogue. *Disability and the Global South* 2(2):570–589. https://disabilityglobalsouth.files.wordpress.com/2012/06/dgs-02-02-01.pdf

Roush, Susan E., and Nancy Sharby. 2011. Disability reconsidered: The paradox of physical therapy. *Physical Therapy* 91(12):1715–1727. doi:10.2522/ptj.20100389

United Nations. 2006. Convention on the Rights of Persons with Disabilities. http://www.un.org/disabilities/convention/conventionfull.shtml

World Health Organization and World Bank. 2010. World Report on Disability. http://www.who.int/disabilities/world_report/2011/en/ (accessed: March 2, 2017).

World Health Organization. 2001. *International Classification of Functioning, Disability and Health (ICF)*. Geneva: World Health Organization.

Chapter 19

Developing and Preparing Appropriate Social Work Placements

Lesley Cooper

Contents

Introduction

Going abroad can be both exciting and daunting. Students find it exciting because they can practice learning in non-traditional agencies but are cautious as they are leaving a comfortable environment to one where there is no certainty and often no social and family contacts. This chapter focuses on the potential challenges faced by students as they prepare for, undertake and conclude their international programs.

As a social work student, you may be motivated to go abroad for placement for a variety of reasons, including interest in learning about another culture, interest in how services are delivered and the challenges in working with people and agencies where languages and practices are different from your own. Such experiences may be part of your practicum, short-term study abroad programs, volunteer experience or a component of an academic subject on international social work.

You might be placed with a non-governmental organization (NGO) with long-standing connections between your sending university staff and the host organization. Such connections are frequently reciprocal with specific responsibilities to the host organization and your home institution. This relationship provides the context for practice. Your learning is not only influenced by the partnership arrangements but also grounded in core educational and culturally explicit principles. In a similar way to other professions, learning abroad should be subject to critical examination, influencing selection of experiences and the preparation of students.

How Is Social Work Practiced around the World?

Good health is influenced by a range of social determinants including income and its distribution, levels of education, education and development of children, levels of unemployment, food security, housing, and the extent of inclusion and exclusion in community life. Social workers have a commitment to ensure that people are treated equitably and that factors influencing poor health outcomes are ameliorated for individuals, families and communities with specific change strategies.

Social workers use a variety of social development activities. Social development is a purposeful process of planned change intended to bring about social improvements in a community (Midgley 2003). Planned change means working with many stakeholders that include large NGOs, governments, other professions and local communities. Social workers focus on raising living standards, increasing access to health services and addressing the needs of vulnerable women, children, and other groups oppressed by their social and political circumstances. Participatory approaches based on mutuality and community involvement are core to their work.

The range of social work methods and target groups vary among nations and from one NGO to another. Social workers in the Global North are educated to use diverse practice methods incorporating working with individuals and families, research, community organization and social development, group work and social policy. At the undergraduate level, students may have basic skills in all these areas but there will be a higher degree of specialization at postgraduate level. Students cannot assume that the clinical practices common in the Global North are available in the Global South. In many international placements, there is a greater emphasis on community work and program development. Recognizing the challenges posed by language difficulties, social workers will aim to enhance the participation of the community in improving health outcomes, work actively to form coalitions to address injustices and organize to improve services.

In many Western nations, working with individuals and families is the dominant practice method with many social workers employed in hospitals, specialist units (mental health or working with children) and community health centres. The specific focus of the practice depends on the policy and presenting health and social problems. Working with individuals and families is often referred to as casework, counselling and less frequently therapy. These individual-oriented methods may not be as strongly evident in developing countries where community work and social development methods prevail. These latter methods work at the population level to engage groups and community to work collaboratively for the common good.

Range of Placements

There is very little detailed information about the range and nature of international placements as each university has particular preferences and individualized arrangements. In her international

collaborative study, Cleak et al. (2016) examined the placement practices of two universities: Queen's University, Belfast and Latrobe University, Australia. She found that students worked in a wide variety of international placements but children and families, displaced children in orphanages, and the education of disabled children and young people with intellectual disabilities were dominant areas. Students were also linked with mobile health vans, human immunodeficiency virus infection/acquired immune deficiency syndrome (HIV/AIDS), immigrants and refugees, human trafficking and community-based living. These finding may not necessarily be representative. Cleak et al. (2016) also found that community development, aid work, research and evaluation and social policy were common. She also indicated that some students did one-on-one work, but the specific context was not elaborated. It is assumed that this was because some students went from a European nation (Northern Ireland) to another developed country where English was the common language.

There are many impediments to working with individuals and families in international settings. The extent to which students undertake one-on-one activities will depend on their language skills, length of placement, level of experience, appropriateness of one-on-one work in the social context and NGO activities. In high-income countries (HIC), social work practice uses a deliberate and directed conversation as the basic practice tool. If students are not fluent with the local language and dialect and do not understand local cultural practices then direct practice may not be possible and certainly not effective. The placement length is another decisive factor. In 2 weeks, observation and sharing of information about services may be all that is possible. Greater collaborative opportunities exist over a semester of 13–14 weeks, but this does not necessarily include working with individuals in a therapeutic capacity. Some practitioners question whether students with no experience in individual work should learn their casework practice in international settings with possibly limited guided learning. This is ethically questionable and may be harmful to individuals. Other academics argue that our Western approaches to social work practice may legitimate such practices in cultures, which have their particular indigenous and cultural ways of working (Cornelius and Greif 2005). Whatever the practical and ethical challenges posed, students and their academic teachers are committed to social justice and an equitable society.

Questioning International Experiences

What students do in offshore learning experiences is influenced by the values and experiences of their teaching staff. International experiences are not necessarily viewed positively in the academic community. Scholars question whether international placements are perpetuating professional imperialism. Razack (2009) raises the issue of superior positioning by Western universities. She uses colonization as her starting point outlining the way in which European countries conquered and exploited people and resources. As a result, indigenous people were subjugated, left without capacity to accumulate capital and made to feel inferior to white settlers. Racism at home and abroad is one manifestation of imperialism and is addressed as a significant aspect of social work education.

It behoves us to examine the social work curriculum as a whole and prepare students to recognize that social work education goes beyond local contextualized practice to one where social workers are prepared for international practice with abilities to *work with* diverse groups at home and internationally. *Working with people is very different to the position of doing for or working on behalf of others.* The curriculum as taught requires thoughtful examination, in particular considering the exclusiveness of the Western intellectual paradigm as manifested in social work, with its strong clinical traditions and hegemonic constructions (Parker et al. 2015). Examination of curriculum also means considering ideas embedded in human social development and the delivery of human services. Neo-liberal strategies for the solution of social problems also need careful examination along with ethical frameworks emphasizing individuality and self-determination. If these are the critical debates about curriculum and preparation, students will arrive in their international placements understanding the way power and privilege are contained with norms and values and exercised in social work practice.

Preparation for Programs

Many universities address global social work practice as a standard requirement in both graduate and undergraduate curricula. Social workers would be expected to take a human rights perspective and address global issues at the macro policy level, program level and individual perspective. Intellectual understanding of global issues in the classroom is very different to a practical understanding of work and use of self in international settings. It requires very specific student (and worker) preparation.

Universities in the West take preparation for student learning in other nations seriously and are guided by key principles. Learning occurs when students become aware of global inequalities, poverty and social problems; have personal space and support to confront and reflect on the personal contradictions and dilemmas posed by this awareness and develop new ways of thinking and acting. Five principles supporting student learning have been developed for effective administration of international placements.

These principles are *role taking, support, reflection, intensity* and *reciprocity* (Lough 2009). Role taking refers to situations where students have real social work responsibilities and activities, which simultaneously allow for application of critical thinking. Activities are made more complex when students are required to consider not only their particular activities or interventions, but also the cultural assumptions behind the actions. This is easier if the participant's language is English and complicated when students are required to work in the native language as they miss the real meanings and nuanced way language is used.

Support is the next key principle referring to good preparation, regular supervision and consistent contact between the university and host agency. Reflection in and on practice is core to learning and critical in developing nuanced cultural understandings. Approaches include use of journals, logs, blogs and peer-to-peer discussion. Supervision on-site or via Skype allows for a deliberate reflective process on a regular basis noting that lifelong reflection is part of being professional.

The fourth principle, intensity, addresses the length of the placement and regular attendance thus supporting personal development. Three months is considered the norm for social work placements, although the length of the placement is often compromised by factors such as visa restrictions, religious and cultural celebrations and the length of semester breaks.

A reciprocal relationship between host organization, service agency and community is a fundamental principle of good practice. Successful student placements are built on sustained and nurtured relationships between organizations. The principle of reciprocity is buttressed by respectful equal relationships, consideration of the needs of the host agency and the needs of students so that all may benefit. Reciprocity should not be perceived as a one-off relationship, but one that continues over time and involves not only placement of students but visits by and involvement of faculty and service providers. In many local placements, the university provides privileges for those agencies working directly with students and recognition for personnel actively with students. This includes recognition of agencies for their work with students, providing adjunct professorial status, showcasing the work of agencies and providing staff training and development (Cooper et al. 2010). We are all challenged to consider the best way to recognize the contribution of international agencies to students. These principles are critical in the preparation for international placements.

In any program, faculty are key leaders as their involvement and commitment aid high-level learning outcomes within and across subjects. These learning outcomes include high-level analytical skills; capacity to translate knowledge across domains of practice; evaluation of policy, processes and practice and application of skills from a Western academic and practice orientation to the practices found in other nation states. In addition, faculty can play a role at a personal level in responding to student anxieties, discussing practical matters and deliberating about future careers.

Preparation for Students

Preparation of students prior to departure is paramount. Some authors focus on the pedagogical preparation (Nuttman-Shwartz and Ranz 2017), and some prefer to begin with an intellectual understanding of globalization, internationalism and colonialism while not neglecting the practical (Nuttman-Shwartz and Berger 2012; Razack 2009). One common approach is dividing the preparation into phases that include a specific preparation phase, a stay abroad phase and returning home phase. Of all these phases, the preparation receives most attention in the home institution.

Cognitive and affective preparation is essential. The cognitive includes formal learning in the classroom prior to departure taking account of the knowledge and critical reflective practice skills necessary for informed and thoughtful social work. Nuttman-Shwartz and Ranz (2017) advocate learning about the historical context and power relationships within and between nations, including the economic and political reality of the host country.

All students are expected to learn about the host agency before arriving on placement. This enables thoughtful preparation, and conveys interest and excitement to the hosts. The discovery process may be challenging if the agency is small, does not have a website or the language is not English. Access to a university database, government or United Nations Reports, previous student reports on agencies, and personal or professional contacts are all valuable as part of preparation. Understanding complexities may be difficult when the environment is unfamiliar. Students can look for people with similar personal and professional interests beforehand and discuss the potential opportunities for social work so this task is made easier.

Cognitive and affective dimensions are enabled when students work in small working groups to obtain visas, find appropriate accommodation, purchase tickets or discuss cross-cultural matters. Contributions of those faculty and staff who have 'gone before' add enormous value to the learning.

On the other hand, the affective dimension is a necessity enabling students to reflect on their motivations for wanting to practice abroad, to anticipate challenging situations and to consider their response to these situations. Some potential affective issues for students in preparing for placements are their over-identification with the host country or one's own country; appreciating what it is like to have minority status in another country; feelings of superiority and a willingness to judge based on that superiority, shame or feeling inferior for being privileged or just fear about an unfamiliar environment (Nuttman-Shwartz and Berger 2012). Attending to the emotional dimensions prepares students to cope with the unanticipated events and incidents that inevitably arise (Nuttman-Shwartz and Berger 2012).

Management of Risk

Learning professional practice skills means that students are exposed to the same dangers and risks as other employees. However, many students in international locations work outside the safe and supported confines of agencies and the guidance of supervisors. This has been clearly illustrated in Chapter 1. Dangers are of greater concern when students are novices and placed in unfamiliar locations or when workplace standards are not specified and where risks are unknown. These risks are not confined to workplaces but also personal conduct after hours.

Administrators with responsibility for the well-being of students and professionals with a commitment to clients and communities are alert to the potential risks when students go offshore and stress the importance of orientation to external agencies. This includes open dialogue between host agencies and the university about such matters as student orientation, regular supervision to minimize errors and review after students return. If possible, it is important to consider the suitability of working environments for students and prepare students for likely risks and dangers in the workplace and in the location. It is important for students to understand risks, how best to manage these risks and the steps to take if an incident occurs.

Personal safety and health are discussed in Chapters 8 and 9. Emotional ups and downs occur in many placements irrespective of the location, as placement may be the first occasion when students decide whether social work is really the career for them. Emotional vulnerability and dealing with any feelings of helplessness, personal esteem, interpersonal relationships in the workplace and related to the actual placement may occur. From time to time, our national governments provide travel advisory information that includes informed advice to minimize risk and maximize personal safety. At such times, and in response to a threat, we are asked to exercise caution and consider the need to travel to particular areas or to not travel. Students and practicum programs are well advised to heed the university's direction on this matter. Care for students and faculty will be paramount.

Though language preparation is useful and sometimes essential, there are limitations. The value is found in a desire to understand and appreciate another culture and a willingness to cooperate with others. Nevertheless, it is challenging to use our professional concepts in a language and culture where the professional concepts are not known and where the student does not have full competence. Misunderstandings and communication problems inevitably arise. Students may be able to access and use interpreters and knowing the local protocols for working with them could be a useful aspect of student preparation. Generally speaking, all participants may need to employ sensitive improvisation in communicating across cultures.

During the Placement: The Learning Process

Many students in semester-long placements are formally assessed and grades recommended to their home institutions. As part of the learning process, students are expected to specify achievable contextualized learning goals that may include methods and learning about services in a cross-cultural environment. Students expect qualified supervisors with more than 2 years of practice experience and supervisory training as supervision is the core of learning practice. Despite this, the responsibility for learning remains with the student, their motivation to success and the opportunities to maximize learning.

Post Experience

Returning home brings a mixture of conflicting emotions. Regrets at leaving behind newly formed friendships and desire to reconnect with family and friends; a willingness to share cross-cultural experiences and new ways of working and ideas about future career opportunities. All parties need to review and evaluate these experiences (see Chapter 25). Students need to digest their specific experiences and share with others, especially students contemplating similar placements. This sharing can be done in small groups as part of de briefing, specially convened student conferences or presentation of posters.

Conclusion

Students with financial resources and commitment to cross-cultural learning have opportunities to experience social work practice in international settings. These international experiences differ markedly from the practice experiences in developed countries where work with individuals and families dominate. Placements are arranged with the understanding that there is a growing critical analysis of the value of exchanges, especially concerns about colonization and the implicit exercise of power. Their value is enhanced with a thorough preparation of students attending to the affective and cognitive domains and a supportive host institution valuing learning and reciprocity with their partner agency.

References

Cleak, H. Anand, J., and Das, C. (2016) Asking the critical questions: An evaluation of social work students' experiences in an international placement. *British Journal of Social Work*, 46:389–408.

Cooper, L., Orrell, J., and Bowden, M. (2010) *Work Integrated Learning: A Guide to Effective Practice* (London: Routledge).

Cornelius, L.J., and Greif, G.L. (2005) Schools of social work and the nature of their foreign collaborations. *International Social Work*, 48:823–833.

Lough, B.J. (2009) Principles of effective practice in international social work field placements. *Journal of Social Work Education*, 45:467–480.

Midgley, J. (2003) Social development: The intellectual heritage. *Journal of International Development*, 15:831–844.

Nuttman-Shwartz, O, and Berger, R. (2012) Field education in international social work: Where are we and where we should go. *International Social Work*, 55:225–243.

Nuttman-Schwartz, O., and Ranz, R. (2017) Human rights discourse: An experience of social work students from Israel and India. International Social Work, 60: 283–296.

Parker, J., Crabtree, S.A., Azman, A., and Carlo, D.P. (2015) Problematizing international placements as a site of intercultural learning. *European Journal of Social Work*, 18:383–396.

Razack, N. (2009) Decolonizing the pedagogy and practice of international social work. *International Social Work*, 52:9–21.

Chapter 20

Surgical Team Experiences

Maija Cheung, Michael Hall and Doruk Ozgediz

Contents

Recent years have seen an extraordinary surge of interest among students and residents in global surgery. Many trainees seek a clinical experience in a resource-poor area to learn more about the challenges of surgical care in these environments and also to make a contribution to teaching, research or service delivery programs. This interest is likely to increase even more as the surgical community becomes more involved in global health, a field traditionally with a focus on communicable diseases and large-scale public health programs. Recent work has highlighted the significant role of surgery in the public health of low- and middle-income countries (LMICs) with estimates of the treatment for surgical conditions encompassing approximately 30% of the global burden of disease (Meara et al., 2015; Mock et al., 2015; WHO, 2014). This chapter presents some practical information for trainees on a surgical elective in a resource-poor area.

Preparation: General Overview

Preparing for an international surgical experience can be simultaneously exhilarating and overwhelming. Several recent works provide an excellent resource for trainees beginning work in this area (Leow et al., 2012; Tarpley et al., 2007; Chu, 2010; Cunningham, 2013). Perhaps the most important place to start is to have an honest conversation with yourself about primary motivations for global engagement in surgery: Is it faith-based? Service-based? A desire to learn more about uncommon disease presentations? Or a desire for adventure (Philpott, 2010)? One may point out that there are substantial disparities in healthcare in our local environment, so why go so far away when local populations also require assistance? These are all important to consider personally, and many trainees may realize that similar sets of skills are required to care for vulnerable populations both at home and in resource-poor areas abroad.

Because global surgery electives vary so much in scope, location, cultural issues and surgical needs, one should consider some of these very broad topics to help narrow down the focus. The main goals of the elective, such as the purpose of the trip (surgical mission vs. academic exchange), the different populations that will be served (cultural differences, religious differences, pediatric and other special populations), the types of cases one will be observing/assisting/performing and the team make-up (individual vs. a group trip) define the trainee experience. In surgical missions, the emphasis is more on operative experience and an accompanied preceptor is ideal, whereas in an academic exchange, the goals may be more focused on research or education and can lend themselves to a more fluid and self-defined experience.

The team make-up can dictate many of the goals as well as determine what surgical needs can be adequately and appropriately addressed. Team composition can range from only licensed healthcare providers such as surgeons, anesthesiologists, nurses and residents and students to bio-medical engineers, sociologists or undergraduate students, all of whom bring very different skills, practical experiences and cultural views. The team composition can also range from members of academic departments from a single institution to collections of individuals only loosely affiliated by either intra-institutional partnerships, geography or the organization facilitating the trip. Meetings during the planning stages to discuss goals can be useful. Learning from past mistakes is equally, if not more, valuable in setting up a team for success. Speaking with colleagues who have had similar experiences and compiling an institutional database of helpful information in an electronic or paper form that can be passed around can provide a good starting place prior to the final planning stages. Group meetings are also important for logistical planning, as often large amounts of supplies need to be divided and carried between team members.

In a similar fashion, one must familiarize themselves with the host team. Supply of specialist surgeons is extremely limited in many of the low-income countries and some countries have an explicit policy supporting non-physicians to perform surgery, and most of the anesthesia also may be provided by nurse anesthetists (Chu et al., 2009). Despite a lack of specialist training, these clinicians often have a great deal of clinical experience and expertise and are an invaluable source of information for a visiting trainee.

Surgical needs and the scope of cases encountered will vary immensely depending on the variables discussed above. The scope of surgical work at most district or general hospitals includes mostly emergency surgery, including trauma care (generally a result of road traffic crashes) and obstetric emergencies. Common injuries include blunt chest/abdominal/head trauma and orthopedic injuries. Additionally, emergent general surgery cases such as intestinal obstructions, bowel perforations and incarcerated hernias are also common. Malignant solid tumors often present at advanced stages, and elective pathologies such as goiters can progress to cause substantial morbidity (WHO, 2003). Familiarizing yourself with the management of traumatic injuries such as laparotomy for trauma and simple urologic and gynecologic procedures such as the placement of suprapubic tubes, management of testicular torsion and cesarean sections, ectopic pregnancy, and dilation and curettage can be useful in preparing for these possibilities. The population demographics should also be considered since many low-resource countries have an extremely high percentage of their population under the age of 18, and therefore a high burden of disease specific to pediatric general surgery interventions.

In the United States, there are clearly established criteria for formal electives set by the American Board of Surgery and the Residency Review Committee (Charles et al., 2015). In Canada, despite numerous residency electives, the Royal College of Surgeons has no formal international elective requirements. A number of studies have demonstrated the unique value added by global health experiences in surgery when traditional competencies are considered (Henry et al., 2013; Ozgediz et al., 2008). Currently, a select group of residency programs offer accredited electives to their trainees and many residents in other programs seek similar experiences but may not have an established program.

There has been a call to organize these efforts, so a greater number of residents can benefit from these experiences and each residency program does not expend unnecessary administrative resources (Mitchell, 2011). The American College of Surgeons 'Operation Giving Back' program serves as a clearinghouse of opportunities and resources for surgeons and trainees for global engagement (Operation Giving Back, 2016). Some trainees seek more structured training such as a Master's in Public Health or other research degree to gain additional skills as a clinician-researcher for surgery in resource-poor areas. A number of recent resources can assist the student or trainee especially interested in the career development of an 'academic global surgeon' (Swaroop and Krishnamswami, 2015; Calland et al., 2012).

What to Bring on a Surgical Elective

For groups or those going on established electives, pre-deployment information packets can be extremely useful. These often include basic logistical information such as the itinerary, contact phone numbers, emergency phone numbers for team family members, maps, recent situation reports and a short document of medically related terms and frequently used expressions.

Often, you will be bringing items that will be left behind such as surgical supplies and educational resources for local providers. Electronic (PDF) copies of surgical textbooks or other information (trauma manuals, Advanced Cardiac Life Support [ACLS]/PALS algorithms) that can be shared with local students and providers can be very helpful. Much of what to bring on a surgical elective would not greatly vary with a medical or other elective (see Chapter 7). Following are a few specific items to consider:

1. Headlamp to use in the operating room (OR)
2. Eye protection
3. Surgical loupes
4. Your own scrubs, caps and masks and OR shoes
5. Hand sanitizer
6. Sterile surgical gloves for yourself, especially for small sizes
7. Swiss army knife/leatherman
8. Pulse oximeter

Health, Safety and Well-Being

As with other electives, the trainee and the organization involved should clarify the necessary registration documents for trainees, as well as the need (or not) for malpractice insurance. Centers for Disease Control and Prevention (CDC) recommendations for vaccinations and other advice should be heeded, such as malaria prophylaxis in the tropics. The organization/university should have evacuation insurance in place for you; otherwise, you must look into purchasing this for a short period. Especially for human immunodeficiency virus (HIV) endemic areas, you will need to ensure that post-exposure prophylaxis is available locally or bring it with you. Risk of needle-stick injury or sharps injury may be higher on surgical than other electives. Any needle-stick injury should be immediately reported to one's home surgical program in addition to the local hospital and preceptors.

You must adapt to local resources in the OR and follow general precautions for blood-borne pathogens, which can sometimes be difficult in an environment that may lack many basic safety and hygiene measures, such as running water and sanitizer; poor instruments in the theatre and limited gloves and supplies. Bringing some of your own protective equipment as mentioned above can help offset any limited supplies and ensure your own safety.

In addition, you must be prepared for outcomes that may not match the outcomes for certain diseases in the home institution, and you may encounter more mortality and disability than at your home environment. Healthcare may not be readily available, even for the hospitalized patient, if the system or hospital functions poorly. This may create emotional distress for trainees on electives, and key coping strategies are to rely on your team to discuss some of these issues as they arise and to build relationships with the local providers who cope with such challenges on a daily basis.

Preparation for Clinical Challenges and the Service Delivery Environment

The burden is on the visiting teams and programs to provide the optimal preparation for their trainees, to minimize any burden on host providers who may use valuable clinical time to orient new trainees. The program may designate a local preceptor and potentially compensate them or provide them an official title in turn for the education provided to their trainees or the program may provide alternative forms of reciprocity.

Even advanced trainees may be unfamiliar with the surgical options and operative approaches utilized in low-resource countries, especially in niche clinical scenarios such as disaster relief and war zone areas (Lorich, 2010). Multiple resources cover the types of conditions that might be encountered, both as a general surgeon, but also as a sub-specialist surgeon (plastics, orthopedics, pediatric surgery, trauma) (Semer, 2007; WHO, 2007; Carter, 2003; Gosselin et al., 2014; King et al., 1990; Ameh et al., 2011). These may also be useful electronic resources to share with your colleagues. In addition, trainees may benefit from hands-on courses such as the humanitarian surgery courses offered at annual national meetings or individual universities. Others will undergo more intensive surgical training as required by the humanitarian surgical organizations involved in conflict zones covering war surgery in greater depth (Giannou and Baldan, 2009). In general, there are certain clinical challenges to be aware of, and prepare for, prior to travel:

1. *Expect advanced presentations of common diseases in typical disease categories*: Surgical infections, oncology, obstetrics, trauma, and so on. Treating these in a resource-poor area can be extremely challenging. Local clinicians are often the 'experts' in most appropriate management in this context. See the section 'Case Selection'.

2. *Allow yourself to learn from barriers to care*: The 'three delays' model of obstetric care has been recently applied more broadly to surgical conditions and refers to the delay in the decision to seek care, the delay in reaching healthcare and the delay in receiving healthcare at the institution (WHO, 2011). All delays play a role in advanced presentation of disease. Every patient encounter has something to teach us about the types of interventions that can

improve access to care, and these clinical interactions may provide the seed for innovative solutions. For example, many patients with a deformity or growing mass may initially seek the care of a traditional healer prior to accessing a more formal health service, due to religious or cultural beliefs.

3. *Educate yourself about the disease entities that might be endemic to certain areas or regions*: For example, typhoid perforation is a particular scourge in the tropics, but rarely seen in high-income countries. The disease can present as a broad spectrum, and some advance preparation may help be prepared for surgical and medical options for treatment (Ameh and Abantanga, 2011).

4. *Also educate yourself about comorbidities that can affect workup and treatment*, such as high HIV–tuberculosis (TB) endemic areas, malaria in the tropics, undernutrition and parasitic infestations. For example, an early postoperative fever in a high-income setting may be from atelectasis or simply an inflammatory response, while in the tropics a blood smear may detect malaria in a malaria endemic region.

5. *Hone your physical exam skills*: Resource-poor areas force economy in diagnostic studies and lab work. Some of the more advanced diagnostics (i.e. computed tomography [CT] scan, magnetic resonance imaging [MRI]) may not be available, and if available, very costly to patients and families. Plain imaging (X-rays) and ultrasound may be more available, therefore some familiarity with these modalities can help. Decisions for and against surgery may need to be made based on more limited information.

6. *Recognize the role of families in patient care*: In most settings, nursing staff is extremely limited, and families provide all of the bedside care – clothing, feeding, mobilizing and even essential care in some places (giving medications, fluids, etc.). Education of families and empowering them in this role can make a tremendous difference. In addition, building a close relationship with the limited ward nurses is also critical. Trainees can often assist with nursing tasks, and this can help build camaraderie with the local healthcare team.

7. *Communication*: This can be a challenge if the patients and families do not share the first language of the visiting team. Some simple words can go a long way, but the visiting team is likely to depend on nursing staff and often, other families to help with conversations about indications, risks and alternatives to surgery.

8. *Economic burden*: Understand that many families travel a long distance to access surgical care and the decision to seek care is often an important economic decision for a family. Between forgone income, travel costs and upkeep while in the hospital, many families face a high toll and risk for impoverishing expenditure for surgical care (Meara, 2015). In many low-income countries, there is no insurance system for the poor, and although public facilities may be 'free' in name, the patients and families may be responsible for procuring the essential medications and supplies for an operation (fluids, sutures, dressings, etc.). Inpatient wards may be full with long backlogs for surgery, but many families may choose to stay to ensure they get care and because they have already invested in the transport.

9. *Basic resuscitation*: There may be a much more limited availability of emergency staff and critical care; therefore, one must be familiar with basic resuscitation skills (fluids, intravenous [IV] access, administration of oxygen and bagging and hemorrhage control, if necessary). Knowledge of Advanced Cardiac Life Support (ATLS) and ACLS can be critical.

10. *Doses of key medications for common conditions and pediatric doses*: Commonly available analgesics (i.e. Tylenol) and antibiotics (i.e. ceftriaxone/Flagyl). These can be kept on a handheld device or notebook for easy reference.

Case Selection

Many trainees take an elective to join a short-term surgical mission. Case selection is possibly the most critical aspect of a short-term surgical mission. Trainees may play a key role in the evaluation of patients for surgery, assisting in surgery and with postoperative care. Even if not on a surgical mission and working within the regular routine of care, OR time may be limited and triage for surgery a routine consideration. Below are a number of key elements to keep in mind:

1. You may work with the local team to prescreen the patients before you arrive, and complicated patients may also have been reviewed prior to the trip, especially for surgical sub-specialties.
2. Screening may continue every day as the community learns about the availability of increased surgical services. Nightly screening may be required, and a plan in place for managing patients who cannot be treated during the trip should be discussed.
3. The team should not take on cases outside their home scope of practice or above their skill level or without proper local licensure requirements. See the section 'Ethical Considerations'.
4. As mentioned above, advanced presentations of certain diseases are to be expected, and you and your team should be prepared for context-appropriate surgical strategies, given local pathology. Some operations that may occur, for example, in one stage may need to be staged in a resource-poor area; or cases that might require a longer, more risky operation in a high-income setting may need to be approached differently, given the absence of postoperative critical care support. Numerous resources and aids are available to prepare for critical care in resource-poor areas, especially for acute patients who require resuscitation (WHO, 2011). If going as part of a general surgery elective, you may also be exposed to other sub-specialty pathologies requiring obstetric, orthopedic, neurosurgical or urologic interventions. You should acquaint yourself with common procedures in these specialties and not perform them unless you are comfortable performing them or you are precepted by someone who is.
5. The team may start with straightforward cases (e.g. inguinal or umbilical hernia) to test workflow and anesthesia equipment and troubleshoot other OR equipment such as electro-cautery. Some teams also prefer to perform complex cases early in the first few days of the trip, to be present if there are early postoperative complications that need to be addressed.
6. Considerations for more complex cases:
   a. What are the chances that critical care will be required (i.e. ventilator or central line)? Most environments will not have critical care resources for their patients. It is not uncommon for a slightly more complex case where for example, a patient requires bagging of the airway, for the family to be responsible for this in recovery or on the ward.
   b. Are blood products required and are they available? For cases with a significant risk of blood loss, this may preclude the operation being done. Similarly, will parenteral nutrition be required? Again, this is likely not available in most settings and may impact case selection.
   c. Diagnostic imaging: Consider what imaging is absolutely essential for patient safety to determine operative candidacy. As many investigations are costly, anticipate the need to fund some of these investigations locally if needed or work with the host team to waive fees if possible.
   d. Equipment: That is, casting, supplies and dilators. Ostomy appliances are not to be expected, and most families will use rags to wrap around the ostomy to collect stool. Specialized equipment for necessary surgical sub-specialities may need to be brought by the outside team (i.e. casting, dilators, retractors). Other supplies you may be used to relying on such as urimeters and ostomy appliances are not to be expected, and most families will use rags to

wrap around the stony to collect stool. Familiarizing yourself with the available resources and local customs in peri-operative care in low-resource settings can be invaluable.

  e. Follow-up is critical, and a close working relationship with the host team can help to have a mutual agreement about who will care for patient once you leave if a complication occurs or for routine postoperative care or if further interventions such as staged procedures are necessary.

  f. Number of cases selected every day may depend on available resources, specifically anesthesia and equipment/supply availability. Major cases (especially those done simultaneously) may need to be limited. Smaller cases may need to be performed in a fashion that preserves the number of sterile drapes, gowns and instruments if sterilizing process is a rate-limiting step. Likewise, there may not be 'extra gowns' for students to scrub as this may deprive another patient of an operation.

  g. Be prepared to make difficult ethical decisions and choices, such as a higher-risk operation with a low chance of success but certain risk of morbidity or mortality if not attempted, versus smaller cases with a higher chance of success. These decisions are best made as a group and should involve the family in a culturally appropriate manner as necessary.

  h. Providers must weigh the service delivery/education balance as per the agreement and emphasis areas with the host team. An over emphasis purely on case volume may detract from teaching/training and sustainable change and capacity-building.

Preoperative Care

1. Hydrate patients (some may have travelled for days and have been made NPO).
2. Bowel preps may need to be done in the OR.
3. Make sure the equipment works.
4. Review consent and mark site.
5. Take a careful history about respiratory and GI symptoms. Chronic illness such as undernutrition, malaria with anemia and respiratory illnesses are common and can compromise surgical outcomes. Families may not fully disclose comorbidities to not 'miss the chance' for surgery, however, safety should not be compromised.

Intraoperative Care

1. Take a timeout: Familiarize yourself with the WHO Safe Surgery Checklist (WHO, 2016).
2. Anticipate instrument and consumable need for every case and minimize resource utilization to the greatest possible degree. This may include, for example, minimal use of gauze sponges and laparotomy pads and use of instrument ties rather than hand ties to absolutely conserve maximum suture. It is common for gowns and drapes to be recycled; be cognizant of how to economize on the use of drapes without compromising safety. In some places, even gloves may be recycled; therefore, bringing your own surgical gloves can be beneficial.
3. Basic suturing and knot-tying skills should be learned.
4. Be prepared to assist in anesthesia such as obtaining IV access – these skills are invaluable.
5. Trainees may be responsible for completing the postoperative note – often it is handwritten. It is critical to leave as much detail as needed. Leave your team's contact information on the op-note, if findings are unusual or if there has been a complication.

6. As a trainee, be cognizant always of the learning priorities of the host team, especially in the OR, and never take away a hands-on learning experience from a host trainee. This is best discussed before scrubbing on the case.

7. Many hospitals do not have a well-developed surgical assistant cadre, and trainees may be tasked with handling instruments during cases. Familiarize yourself with available instruments at your site. This experience exposes the trainee to a higher risk of needle-sticks and other injuries; therefore, the importance of this task should not be minimized, and careful attention should be paid at all times to the handling of the instruments.

Anesthesia Aspects

1. Machines may be old and medications dated. In rural areas of many LMICs, Epstein, Macintosh, Oxford (EMO) vaporizers are still common, as is ether anesthesia, due its cost (Enright, 2013).

2. Especially in smaller regional or general hospitals, most theaters may not be equipped for longer cases and time is often of the essence to finish operations as quickly as possible.

3. Pulse oximeters are likely the most critical instrument and if you can bring one along, it pays tremendous dividends.

4. Recovery rooms are not commonplace and perioperative care is lacking – extra effort as a trainee in the postoperative period to check on patients can make a big difference.

5. Analgesics – local Tylenol, at a minimum, can be helpful; pain medications are often in very short supply.

Ethical Considerations

There are numerous ethical considerations when on a surgical elective in a resource-poor area (Butler et al., 2014; Ahmed et al., 2016) and ample resources to prepare (Kingham et al., 2009; Ramsey, 2008).

1. *Several of the 'seven sins of humanitarian medicine' are worth emphasis, such as 'leaving a mess behind'*: This can overburden local providers and even undermine the confidence of the local community in the healthcare system. After all, the first principle of medicine is to 'do no harm' (Welling et al., 2010; Nthumba, 2010). This can be avoided through some of the key steps above and guidelines for responsible voluntarism and avoidance of 'itinerant surgery' or 'medical tourism'. Complications are inherent to surgery but must be anticipated when possible, and when unexpected, should be discussed with the local team and the patient/family.

2. *'Going where not wanted or needed, or being poor guests'*: Well-established organizations make a continuous assessment of needs and fit interventions to meet those needs. Above all, remember you are an ambassador for your organization and while there may be substantial challenges, there is never any excuse for being critical or frustrated with the local team.

3. *Being there for the wrong reasons*: There are substantial educational benefits to trainees from high-income countries that participate in these electives, such as seeing unique pathology. However, partnerships and programs should be established with mutual benefits in mind.

4. *Inappropriate donations and technology*: Many collaborations send medical equipment and supplies to LMICs. Much of it, unfortunately, may be obsolete and unable to be maintained locally, sometimes adding to the 'equipment graveyards' already present in these locations. The WHO guidelines for appropriate donations are a valuable resource, as are the presence of biomedical technicians and engineers, an overlooked part of the surgical team at home, but a critical part abroad (Howie et al., 2008).

5. *Creating a culture of dependency on foreign groups to provide care*: This of course also holds for other areas of healthcare and underscores the importance of knowing the overall goals of the group that you are working with. If the goal is at least partially to assist in capacity building, there must be clear opportunities for skills transfer, both through didactic courses and in the OR. These goals are important to know as a trainee, as it can better define your role and areas where you can make a contribution.

6. *Operating without adequate supervision*: Trainees may be asked to independently perform procedures for which they may not be prepared since this may be the norm in the local environment, and the host teams may lack familiarity with the seniority and skill set of a student or resident. This is especially true for trainees who are not part of a specific program and those who are either not traveling with a surgeon from their own institution or who do not know the skill level of the local provider they will be working with.

7. *Informed consent*: International regulations require voluntary informed consent for research and procedures (CIOMS, 2002; UNESCO, 2008); however, in practice, especially in rural areas there are many challenges experienced by doctors obtaining consent. These include differing cultural ethos, language barriers, poverty, education and power asymmetry. Attention should be paid towards these issues in an effort to remedy deficiencies in obtaining consent with special consideration and explanation of the trainee's role in the procedure and medical care (Chima, 2013; Khoury et al., 2012).

Conclusion

Recent years have seen a surge of interest in surgical electives in resource-poor areas from trainees in high-income countries. In addition, recent work has emphasized the prominent role of surgery in global public health. Getting involved in an elective as a trainee is a critical first experience for many providers who may go on to dedicate part of their career to surgical care for vulnerable populations globally. There are many factors to consider for surgical electives and resources to help the trainee prepare. Unfamiliar and advanced disease conditions, resource limitations and ethical challenges all must be navigated on these electives. While electives are by definition self-limited, relationships developed through these opportunities can be long-lasting and can allow for more sustainable capacity building activities.

References

Ahmed F, Wong KY, Citron I, Lavy C. Global surgery and the role of trainees. *Br J Hosp Med.* 2016; 77(4): 202–03. doi:10.12968/hmed.2016.77.4.202.

Ameh E, Bickler S, Lakhoo K, Nwomeh B, Poenaru D., (eds.). *Pediatric Surgery: A Comprehensive Textbook for Africa.* Seattle, WA: Global HELP, 2011.

Ameh E, Abantanga F. Surgical complications of typhoid fever. In *Pediatric Surgery: A Comprehensive Textbook for Africa*, (eds. Ameh E, Bickler S, Lakhoo K, Nwomeh B, Poenaru D.). Seattle, WA: Global HELP, 2011.

Butler MW, Ozgediz D, Poenaru D, Ameh E, Andrawes S, Azzie G, Borgstein E, Deugarte DA, Elhalaby E, Ganey ME, Gerstle JT, Hansen EN, Hesse A, Lakhoo K, Krishnaswami S, Langer M, Levitt M, Meier D, Minocha A, Nwomeh BC, Abdur-Rahman LO, Rothstein D, and Sekabira J. The global paediatric surgery network: A model of subspecialty collaboration within global surgery. *World J Surg.* 2014; 39(2): 335–42. doi:10.1007/s00268-014-2843-1.

Calland JF, Petroze RT, Abelson J, Kraus E. Engaging academic surgery in global health: Challenges and opportunities in the development of an academic track in global surgery. *Surgery.* 2012; 153(3): 316–20.

Carter LL. Principles of Plastic Surgery in Africa: Pan African Academy of Christian Surgeons. 2003. https://cmda.org/library/doclib/PAACS-Bulletin-106-Mar-2013.pdf

Charles AG, Samuel JC, Riviello R, Sion MK, Tarpley MK, Tarpley JL, Olutoye OO, Marcus JR. Integrating global health into surgery residency in the United States. *J Surg Educ.* 2015; 72(4): e88–93.

Chima SC. Evaluating the quality of informed consent and contemporary clinical practices by medical doctors in South Africa: An empirical study. *BMC Med Ethics.* 2013; 14(Suppl 1): S3. doi:10.1186/1472-6939-14-s1-s3.

Chu K. Open letter to young surgeons interested in humanitarian surgery. *Arch Surg.* 2010; 145(2): 123–4.

Chu K, Rosseel P, Gielis P, Ford N. Surgical task shifting in sub-Saharan Africa. *PLOS Medicine.* 2009; 6(5): e1000078.

Council for International Organizations of Medical Sciences (CIOMS). *International Ethical Guidelines for Biomedical Research Involving Human Subjects.* Geneva, Switzerland: CIOMS. 2002.

Cunningham CM. Pursuing a career in humanitarian and rural surgery: When is the best time to start? *Bull Am Coll Surg.* 2013; 98(2): 18–21.

Enright A. Review article: Safety aspects of anesthesia in under-resourced locations. *Can J Anaesth.* 2013; 60(2): 152–8.

Gosselin R, Spiegel D, Foltz M. *Global Orthopedics.* New York, NY: Springer, 2014.

Giannou C, Baldan M. *War Surgery: Working with Limited Resources in Armed Conflict and Other Situations of Violence.* Geneva, Switzerland: ICRC, 2009.

Henry JA, Groen RS, Price RR, Nwomeh BC, Kingham TP, Hardy MA, Kushner AL. The benefits of international rotations to resource-limited settings for U.S. surgery residents. *Surgery.* 2013; 153(4): 445–54.

Howie SR, Hill SE, Peel D, Sanneh M, Njie M, Hill PC, Mulholland K, Adegbola RA. Beyond good intentions: Lessons on equipment donation from an African hospital. *Bull World Health Organ.* 2008; 86(1): 52–6.

Khoury, A, Mendoza A, Charles A. Cultural competence: Why surgeons should care. *Bull Am Coll Surg.* 2012; 97(3): 13–8.

King M, Bewes P, Cairns J, Thornton J. *Primary Surgery: Non-Trauma Volume 1.* Oxford, UK: Oxford University Press, 1990.

Kingham TP, Muyco A, Kushner A. Surgical elective in a developing country: Ethics and utility. *J Surg Educ.* 2009; 66(2): 59–62.

Leow JJ, Groen RS, Kingham TP, Casey KM, Hardy MA, Kushner AL. A preparation guide for surgical resident and student rotations to underserved regions. *Surgery.* 2012; 151(6): 770–8.

Lorich, D. Open letter to community published in article by Jones, V. Trauma surgeon flees chaos of Haiti: Needed protection of Jamaican soldiers with M-16s to escape alive. *Better Health Network.* January, 2010. http://getbetterhealth.com/trauma-surgeon-flees-chaos-of-haiti-needed-protection-of-jamaican-soldiers-with-m-16s-to-escape-alive/2010.01.24

Meara JG, Leather AJ, Hagander L, Alkire BC, Alonso N, Ameh EA, Bickler SW, Conteh L, Dare AJ, Davies J, Mérisier ED, El-Halabi S, Farmer PE, Gawande A, Gillies R, Greenberg SL, Grimes CE, Gruen RL, Ismail EA, Kamara TB, Lavy C, Lundeg G, Mkandawire NC, Raykar NP, Riesel JN, Rodas E, Ro2 Roy N, Shrime MG, Sullivan R, Verguet S, Watters D, Weiser TG, Wilson IH, Yamey G, Yip W. Global surgery 2030: Evidence and solutions for achieving health, welfare, and economic development. *Surgery.* 2015; 158(1):3–6.

Mitchell KB, Tarpley MJ, Tarpley JL, Casey KM. Elective global surgery rotations for residents: A call for cooperation and consortium. *World J Surg.* 2011; 35(12): 2617–24.

Mock CN, Donkor P, Gawande A, Jamison D, Kruk M, Debas H. Essential surgery: Key messages from disease control priorities, 3rd edition. *Lancet.* 2015; 385(9983): 2209–19.

Nthumba PM. Blitz surgery: Redefining surgical needs, training, and practice in sub-Saharan Africa. *World J Surg.* 2010; 34(3): 433–7.

Ozgediz D, Wang J, Jayaraman S, Ayzengart A, Jamshidi R, Lipnick M, Mabweijano J, Kaggwa S, Knudson M, Schecter W, Farmer D. Surgical training and global health: Initial results of a 5-year partnership with a surgical training program in a low-income country. *Arch Surg.* 2008; 143(9): 860–5.

Operation Giving Back. 2016. http://www.operationgivingback.facs.org/

Philpott J. Training for a global state of mind. *Virtual Mentor.* 2010; 12(3): 231–6.

Ramsey KM. International surgical electives: Reflections in ethics. *Arch Surg.* 2008; 143(1): 10–1.

Semer N. *Practical Plastic Surgery for Nonsurgeons.* New York, Lincoln, and Shanghai: Authors Choice Press, 2007.

Swaroop M, Krishnaswami S. *Academic Global Surgery.* Cham, Switzerland: Springer, 2015.

Tarpley J, Tarpley M, Meier D, Meier P. Operating in the global theater. *Surg Rounds.* 2007; 11: 509–17.

UNESCO. International Bioethics Committee (IBC) Report of the International Bioethics Committee of UNESCO on Consent. Social and Human Sciences Sector, Division of Ethics of Science and Technology, Bioethics Section. SHS/EST/CIB08-09/2008/1, 2008.

Welling DR, Ryan JM, Burris DG, Rich NM. Seven sins of humanitarian medicine. *World J Surg.* 2010; 34(3): 466–70.

World Health Organization (WHO). Surgical Care at the District Hospital. http://www.who.int/surgery (accessed August 29 2016).

WHO. *IMAI District Clinician Manual.* Geneva, Switzerland: World Health Organization, 2011.

WHO. Patient Safety. 2016. http://www.who.int/patientsafety/safesurgery/en/ (accessed April 1 2016).

WHO. 2003. Surgical Care at the District Hospital. http://www.who.int/surgery/publications/en/SCDH.pdf

WHO. Strengthening Emergency and Essential Surgical Care and Anaesthesia as a Component of Universal Health Coverage. http://apps.who.int/gb/ebwha/pdf_files/EB135/B135_3-en.pdf

Chapter 21

Dentistry and Oral Health

Brittany Seymour, Hawazin Elani and Jane Barrow

Contents

Introduction to Global Oral Health

For the first time in global history, we have access to global burden of oral disease data that we can compare across decades and nations; we can analyse demographic, epidemiologic and nutritional trends in order to develop evidence-based interventions and measure long-term program impact on oral health. In response to evolving trends affecting health and human development, this chapter discusses a series of guiding principles for dental volunteering to achieve continued oral health improvement globally and more sustainable development in the long term.

Notably, 2011 was the first time that the burden of oral diseases was recognized in a United Nations resolution as a major problem (Benzian et al., 2012). Oral conditions, most of them largely preventable, negatively affect 3.9 billion people worldwide. Of the 291 diseases and conditions assessed in the 2010 Global Burden of Disease Study, caries was the most prevalent disease. Edentulism ranked 36 of all 291 conditions (Marcenes et al., 2013). Higher disease burden combined with less access to care is consistently reported among disadvantaged and marginalized populations, especially in developing countries (Elani et al., 2012). The combination of increasing exposure to common risk factors for many diseases (such as unhealthy diet high in sugars or tobacco use), a lack of population-wide preventive programs and an insufficient oral health workforce results in a generally increasing burden of oral diseases globally (Donoff, McDonough, and Riedy, 2014; Varenne, 2015). Although more people are keeping their teeth longer, due to a growing, aging population with rising non-communicable disease rates, they are experiencing more complicated health needs, both oral and general, across their lifespan (Glick et al., 2012). All of this is further compounded by a low political prioritization of oral health, leading to a spiral of neglect and increasing challenges (Varenne, 2015). These circumstances leave the dental profession with a heavy burden and a unique global responsibility. Further details about oral disease burden, current and recommended oral health practices and geographic comparisons across the global can be found in the Fédération dentaire internationale (FDI) World Dental Federation Oral Health Atlas: The Challenge of Oral Disease (FDI World Dental Federation, 2015). On average, the world is seeing rising oral disease rates, specifically dental caries, in middle-income countries in particular; these regions of the world are experiencing wider availability of foods and beverages high in sugar and low in nutritional value but at the same time suffering from a lag in available oral healthcare services to address increasing disease rates (FDI World Dental Federation, 2015).

Volunteering Globally

Dental volunteering in the global setting can take several forms. Service projects provide urgent care to local communities; though valuable in the short term, they have been criticized for their lack of sustainability and for their absence of continuity of care. Training and education projects are designed to empower local providers and include promoting oral health education and training local health providers with practical dental skills. The most sustainable volunteer models, and often the longest term, focus on capacity building through collaborative work with local partners to address community-driven priorities and oral health needs (Hardwick, 2009). This chapter provides a modern lens for global oral health electives within the context of the emerging 'sustainability era'. It is up to you, today's students, to fully bridge the gap between traditional models of dental volunteering (still largely short term and established well before we had access to the kind of global data we have today), and the necessary sustainable efforts needed to adequately address and reduce oral diseases and inequities across the world.

Before You Go

Appropriate preparation is discussed in another chapter and applies to dental volunteering; thus, this section considers a few 'red flags' to watch out for when selecting your elective.

The following are red flags for global oral health electives (Hartman, 2015):

■ They promise big changes in a short amount of time. Measureable community oral health improvement cannot be achieved through the brief experience of a volunteer. You should never be encouraged to celebrate high-volume treatments in short periods of time.

■ They don't pass the '90-second rule'. If they promise you will perform dental screenings, exams, or treatments on children before they've requested information about your training or background, they don't pass.

■ They glorify the volunteers and their contributions to the community through images and text on their website and/or printed materials. These actions devalue community partnership and local leadership.

■ Meaningful stories about long-term impact and outcomes are absent. If an organization is unable to demonstrate improvement in the oral health status of their community members in the long term, their activities are likely geared much more towards satisfying your expectations and less towards the community's goals and interests.

■ They imply dental experience and/or interesting clinical experiences as a strategy for moving you forward in your career. Without adequate understanding of how you will engage with the country's dental licensure status, local rules and regulations, the assurance of providing dental care should never be promised to you, or any volunteer, up front.

If you encounter any of these basic points in your global oral health elective plan, you likely need to reconsider the appropriateness of your selected experience and evaluate alternative options.

While You're There

The provision of clinical care thus remains the most common model for dental global health electives. Even if students are focusing on activities other than provision of dental care during their elective, it is very common for communities to request treatment by dental volunteers, because resources and access to oral health services are often scarce and need is high.

Clinical Considerations for Global Oral Health Electives

Standards for providing dental care are too often lowered in resource-challenged settings. Dental volunteers may opt out of rules and regulations where they are volunteering, that would otherwise guide the safe ethical treatment of patients in the United States, because adhering to these rules isn't always possible in global settings. The provision of high-standard voluntary dental care during short-term global health electives is challenging and often unrealistic. Intimate familiarity with the standards described below can allow for atypical procedural set-ups that still align with standard guidelines. If dental care cannot be delivered in a low-income global community under the same standards as in the United States, then alternative volunteer activities should be selected and clinical care should be paused in the interim. Reliance on outsiders who cannot perform their clinical responsibilities optimally is not considered an acceptable form of global oral health electives. Instead of clinical care, elective activities could include assisting communities in developing dental supply chains, strengthening their own regulatory processes, or other related supportive activities.

1. Licensure
   It is important to consider licensure policies and regulations for visiting and volunteer dentists. Many countries have regulations in place, and students participating in clinical activities under the supervision of a volunteer dentist should be aware of and respect any national policies for temporary licensure to provide dental care. The process can be as simple as providing U.S. dental education and licensure status and paying a nominal fee.
2. World Health Organization Basic Package of Oral Care (BPOC) (WHO, 2002)
   BPOC is an evidence-based clinical approach to care designed for ethical use in resource poor and underserved settings.
   - Oral Urgent Treatment (OUT). Emergency care and acute pain alleviation and management.
   - Affordable Fluoridated Toothpastes (AFT). Creating access to affordable and available fluoride sources.

  – Atraumatic Restorative Treatment (ART). Although evidence of the effectiveness of ART is favourable, this method is most appropriate in areas where a patient will eventually be able to access more permanent treatment.

3. Dental Assisting

   Dental students who do not provide direct dental care to patients during their global oral health electives may instead provide dental assisting services. Many states have dental assistant licensure requirements (Commonwealth of Massachusetts, 2014) including 'on-the-job' training requirements. The Dental Assisting National Board defines a formal Code of Professional Conduct (Dental Assisting National Board, Inc., 2007) such as respecting patients' legal rights and performing services only when qualified and properly trained. Dental students should be familiar with their state requirements and perform dental assisting duties responsibly in the global community, just as they would at home.

4. Preventive Care

   This would include fluoride gels or foams delivered in trays, dental sealants and fluoride tablets. However, fluoride varnish is probably the most common and convenient method of administration in a low-resource setting, requiring less time, follow-up and supervision and is often applied after restorative procedures by dentists, given a lack of hygienists in a short-term volunteer setting. As Class II Medical Devices approved by the Food and Drug Administration (FDA), fluoride varnishes must be administered by a licensed healthcare provider in most states. They are considered 'off-label' use for prevention of dental caries. If dentists use fluoride varnish for prevention purposes, they have the responsibility to be well informed about the product and its scientific basis for use. Evidence suggests that for optimal effectiveness, fluoride varnish must be applied at least twice biannually for at least 2 years (Association of State and Territorial Dental Directors, 2007).

5. Additional Considerations for Standard of Safe Care

   a. Occupational Safety and Health Administration (OSHA): Dental students who intend to participate in clinical global health electives should be familiar with how OSHA's standards can be adapted for blood-borne pathogens, including for exposures, personal protective equipment, regulated waste including biohazard and medical waste and training (United States Department website of Labor as of September 1, 2016, https://www.osha.gov/SLTC/dentistry/).

   b. Centers for Disease Control and Prevention (CDC) *Guidelines for Disinfection and Sterilization in Healthcare Facilities*: Detailed sections outline many different options and products for achieving adequate sterilization. The guidelines include a section specifically for dental instruments that can help dental teams determine what supplies and equipment need to be sterilized and how (CDC, 2008) even in atypical treatment settings.

   c. Alternative Dental Operations: Some states have protocols in place for obtaining permits for portable or alternative dental operations, defined as any non-facility where the practice of dentistry is performed on a temporary basis (Commonwealth of Massachusetts, 2011). Many global volunteer settings where dentistry is performed meet this definition. Some states mandate minimum emergency equipment and drugs be available, such as ammonia inhalants and defibrillators.

6. Collaborating with experienced dentists who are familiar with the above standards and primed to practice under resource-strained circumstance in global settings should be mandatory for any dental student participating in a clinical global oral health elective.

When You Return

Reflection, introspection and development of a framework for a long-term relationship with the community are important steps once you return from your global health elective. These processes are discussed in another chapter and can help you in your career decision-making pathways and participation in future global health electives.

Conclusion

Oral diseases, their risk factors and solutions require careful collaboration and planning across boundaries, cultures and disciplines. Determinants of oral health are multidimensional, and include biological, structural, behavioural, environmental and social factors. The dental profession has a unique and tremendous responsibility to our global population. Oral disease burdens are high, while adequately trained workforce and funded dental delivery infrastructures are low. Instinctively, it may appear that the clinical skills of trained dental volunteers are needed now more than ever. But deeper understanding of the principles of global health theory and practice demands a paradigm shift in global oral health electives for dental students (Seymour, Benzian, and Kalenderian, 2013). Clinical care is now just one option on the broader global oral health agenda, especially when it cannot be performed up to the highest of standards. Whether in low-income neighbourhoods in the United States or low-income countries around the world, global oral health electives for students must focus on key themes and principles for optimal long-term impact reiterated throughout this book.

The following are examples of strong global oral health electives for students:

1. *University of California San Francisco (USCF) Global Oral Health Community Partnership: Research*

   This University of California San Francisco School of Dentistry program strives to add a rigorous evaluation or investigation component to an existing program, moving students away from one-off dental volunteering and more towards research-oriented work. Projects are selected after competitive review and require ethics board approval. Ultimately, these programs aim for sustainable oral health improvements by researching the structural causes of poor oral health around the world and in their own neighbourhoods.

2. *University of Colorado (CU) School of Dental Medicine's Global Health Program: Clinical Care*

   The University of Colorado School of Dental Medicine and the Center for Global Health (CGH) at the Colorado School of Public Health have partnered with Agro-America, a private family-owned Guatemalan banana and palm oil agro-business, in an innovative private sector/university partnership. This interdisciplinary clinic provides primary medical care, prenatal and maternal health services, comprehensive dental care to both children and adults and laboratory services. Student volunteers are always supervised by CU dental faculty who maintain active temporary licenses issued by the Guatemalan Dental Board. The program, entrenched in the local culture, implements U.S. regulatory standards of care regarding charting, sterilization, X-ray and clinical protocols.

3. *University of California (UC) Berkeley Children's Oral Health and Nutrition Program: Prevention*

   The Children's Oral Health and Nutrition Program, based at UC Berkeley School of Public Health, is a multidisciplinary global public health program that aims to improve the health of young children by promoting early childhood nutrition and oral health, and preventing dental caries and malnutrition in several countries around the world. Students are required to participate in a series of team meetings to prepare for the onsite work and volunteer under the direct mentorship of both U.S.-based and local health professionals.

In summary, this chapter aims to improve upon long-standing dental volunteer models in light of new data and evolving opportunities that employ students' valuable skills and knowledge well beyond the dental chair. With appropriate support, mentorship and proper selection of global oral health electives, dental students who engage in these programs can serve as global citizens proficient in global health diplomacy and sustainable professional practice.

References

Association of State and Territorial Dental Directors, Fluorides Committee Research Brief. September 2007. *Fluoride Varnish: An Evidence-Based Approach.*

Benzian H, Bergman M, Cohen L, Hobdell M, Mackay J. 2012. The UN high-level meeting on prevention and control of non-communicable diseases and its significance for oral health worldwide. J Pub Health Dent.;72(2):91–3.

Centers for Disease Control and Prevention (CDC). 2008. *Guidelines for Disinfection and Sterilization in Healthcare Facilities, 2008.* http://www.cdc.gov/hicpac/pdf/guidelines/Disinfection_Nov_2008.pdf (Accessed September 1, 2016).

Commonwealth of Massachusetts Division of Health Professions Licensure Board of Registration in Dentistry. 2014. *Initial Dental Assistant Licensure Application Instructions.* http://www.mass.gov/eohhs/docs/dph /quality/boards/dentist/dental-asst-appl.pdf (Accessed September 1, 2016).

Commonwealth of Massachusetts Division of Health Professions Licensure Board of Registration in Dentistry. 2011. *Portable Dental Operation (PDO) – Permit M – Dentist Application information and Instructions.* http://www.mass.gov/eohhs/docs/dph/quality/boards/dentist/dentist-permit-m-pdo.pdf (Accessed September 1, 2016).

Dental Assisting National Board, Inc. Adopted August 2007, revised April 2015. DANB's Professional Code of Conduct. http://www.danb.org/The-Dental-Community/Professional-Standards.aspx (Accessed July 10, 2016).

Donoff B, McDonough J Riedy C. 2014. Integrating oral and general health care. *N Engl J Med*;371(24):2247–49.

Elani HW, Harper S, Allison PJ, Bedos C, Kaufman JS. 2012. Socio-economic inequalities and oral health in Canada and the United States. *J Dent Res*;91(9):865–70.

FDI World Dental Federation. 2015. *The Challenge of Oral Disease – A Call for Global Action. The Oral Health Atlas.* 2nd ed. Brighton, United Kingdom: Myriad Editions.

Glick M, Monteiro da Silva O, Seeberger GK, Xu T, Pucca G, Williams DM, Kess S, Eiselé JL, Séverin T. Dec. 2012. FDI Vision 2020: Shaping the future of oral health. *Int Dent J*;62(6):278–91.

Hardwick KS. 2009. Volunteering for the long-term good. *Compend Contin Educ Dent*;30(3):126, 128.

Hartman E. 2015. *7 Red Flags When Considering an International Volunteer Program. Matador Network.* http://matadornetwork.com/pulse/7-red-flags-considering-international-volunteer-program/(Accessed September 1, 2016).

Marcenes W1, Kassebaum NJ, Bernabé E, Flaxman A, Naghavi M, Lopez A, Murray CJ. 2013. Global burden of oral conditions in 1990-2010: A systematic analysis. *J Dent Res*;92(7):592–97.

Seymour B, Benzian H, Kalenderian E. October 2013. Voluntourism and global health – an evolving dental curriculum to prepare students. *J Dent Educ*;77(10):1252–57.

Varenne B. 2015. Integrating oral health with non-communicable diseases as an essential component of general health. WHO's strategic orientation for the African Region. *J Dent Educ*;79(5 Suppl):S32–7.

World Health Organization Collaborating Center for Oral Health Care Planning and Future Scenarios. 2002. *Basic Package of Oral Care (BPOC).* Nijmegen, the Netherlands: WHOCC.

Chapter 22

Eye Care

Dan Hayhoe

Contents

Introduction

After completing a 2-year residency, I went to Nigeria in 1976 to help establish the first sub-Saharan optometry school (outside South Africa). Over the last 40 years, I have also worked in Ghana and Malawi, liaising with Malawian colleagues to forge an ongoing partnership between the University of Waterloo and Lions Sight First Eye Hospital. I draw on such experiences to provide you with a theoretical and practical basis for your rotation in the Global South.

Following an overview of eye health and health systems, we discuss challenges inherent to working in the Global South, concluding with an examination of the importance of community partnership and appreciation of indigenous knowledge and skill. This structure follows my own progression of orienting myself within wholly different and sometimes confusing healthcare systems in the early years, to the challenges of dealing with local obstacles in the decades that followed, to finally coming to observe, learn from and work within local communities in the Global South.

My greatest regret is my hubris at the outset, and my most profound satisfaction is in what I have learned from my colleagues, students and patients in Africa. My hope is that you will begin where I left off.

What Should I Know before I Go?

As a prospective participant in an eye care elective in the Global South, it is essential for you to appreciate challenges and opportunities for learning inherent in a short-term rotation. You must research host demographics, the status of healthcare delivery systems and your place within that framework, local language, history and culture, ethics, mores and (often spiritual) worldviews. In addition, it is important for you to appreciate the availability and possible limitations of equipment, pharmaceuticals and levels of tertiary care as well as the barriers to timely access and ongoing patient compliance. This chapter focuses on a broad spectrum of issues, both clinical and cultural, with an emphasis on Africa but with applicability across other demographics in the Global South.

The Global Burden of Eye Disease with a Focus on the Global South

About 285 million people are estimated to be visually impaired worldwide (39 million blind and 246 million with low vision). This latter category comprises moderate to severe visual impairment defined as best corrected visual acuity from 6/18 to 6/60 in the better eye. Approximately 90% of the world's visually impaired live in low-income countries. Globally, uncorrected refractive errors are the main cause of moderate and severe visual impairment, while cataracts remain the leading cause of blindness in low- and middle-income countries (LMICs) (WHO Fact Sheet 282, 2014). There are less than five ophthalmologists per million population in LMICs as opposed to 80 per million in high-income countries. Analysis shows that it will take 97 years at the projected population and educational trajectories to achieve parity (Resnikoff, 2012). In Africa, 200–400 cataract operations are performed per million compared to 4000–6000 in industrialized countries (Lewallen and Courtright, 2001).

Of those living with blindness, 82% are aged 50 and above. An estimated 19 million children below the age of 15 are visually impaired, of whom 12 million (62%) have uncorrected refractive errors which are easily diagnosed and corrected. In studies of self-presenters in South Africa, Nigeria and Uganda, refractive error (mostly presbyopia) was found to be the single most frequent diagnosis (Lewallen and Courtright, 2001). Overall, 80% of all visual impairment can be prevented or cured (WHO Fact Sheet 282, 2014) with cataract and uncorrected refractive error accounting for 33% and 42%, respectively (Pascolini and Mariotti, 2011).

Over the past 20 years, diseases affecting the eye have been reduced by prevention and cure, including infections such as onchocerciasis and trachoma by improvement in sanitation and living standards, measles by immunization, trichiasis by surgery, antibiotics, facial cleanliness and environmental improvements and nutritional issues such as vitamin A by supplementation. Countries such as Brazil, Morocco, China and India have made investments in public healthcare for the poor or specific initiatives to treat glaucoma or cataracts (WHO Fact Sheet 282, 2014).

Understanding Health Systems

There are three levels of care in a number of areas of the Global South. Primary Care Facilities may include rural outposts for outreach including human immunodeficiency virus/acquired immune deficiency syndrome (HIV/AIDS) awareness and counselling; ante- and postnatal care; under-five immunizations; vitamin A distribution and eye camps for screening, medical treatment and referral. Secondary Care Facilities are located at the District Hospitals and may include all of the above plus X-ray capabilities, ambulances and an operating theatre. Tertiary Care Facilities are located in the urban centres and, in addition to the above, may provide specialist services as well as laboratory and sometimes imaging capabilities (Malawi National Health Plan 1999–2004, Volume 2: National Health Facilities).

In all three tiers, the shortage of supplies, medical personnel and delivery systems frequently impact healthcare. In Malawi, for example, there are fewer than 300 medical doctors in the entire nation, representing 1/50,000 population (WHO Malawi Country Fact Sheet, 2014).

Under colonial rule healthcare was frequently undertaken by mission organizations (Ngalande-Banda and Simukonda, 1993), with national governments assuming more responsibility post-independence. Consequently, two independent healthcare systems often exist today.

The cadres of health workers may typically include health surveillance assistants, who have minimal training but are utilized effectively in rural outreach programs (community-based health education services, immunizations, mosquito net distribution and vision screening), medical assistants, nurse midwife technicians, clinical officers, registered nurse midwives and medical doctors.

A two-tiered health system is utilized throughout the Global South, with those who can afford to pay for optical services and spectacles doing so. For the rural poor in particular, a model of a consortium of care providers, international service clubs, locally operating NGOs and government or mission hospitals collaborating with trained local screeners, followed by eye camps and appropriate referrals to the tertiary care hospital is effective. The cost to the patient, including transportation and spectacles, is virtually zero.

Barriers to Eye Care Delivery and Utilization

Global inequality in eye health may be measured using disability-adjusted life years (DALYs). For non-communicable eye diseases, the major contributor is refractive errors, regardless of economic status. 'Creating new eye health services for refractive errors and reducing the unacceptable eye health disparity in refractive errors should be the highest priorities for international public health services in eye care' (Ono et al., 2010). Barriers to eye care delivery and utilization include cost, accessibility, awareness, trust in the outcome and cultural/social impediments (Sherwin et al., 2008).

Refractive errors have not received much attention because many definitions of blindness have been based on best-corrected distance acuity (Dandona and Dandona, 2001). 'If the presenting near visual acuity was taken into consideration, the imbalance of refractive errors would be greater for females since they are less likely to be able to afford spectacles for presbyopia' (Ono et al., 2010). A perception of a lesser need for eye care, particularly for women, may profoundly reduce economic opportunities in the form of Income Generating Activities (IGAs) such as tailoring, which requires good near vision.

Cost is a mitigating factor in the Global South where, in a country such as Malawi, close to 75% live below the poverty level of $1.25 per day. 'Children from the poorest households are more likely to be exposed to health risks, be malnourished, experience reduced access to preventive and curative healthcare services, and consequently, die in childhood' (Ustrup et al., 2014). Although advances have been made in indicators like the infant and under-five mortality rates, the poorest children have benefitted the least. Consequently, inequities in health and access to healthcare disfavouring the poor have persisted and widened (Ustrup et al., 2014).

A shortage of medical staff is ubiquitous due to poor working conditions, low wages and the migration of skilled personnel to developed countries (Ustrup et al., 2014), and accessibility is a significant problem in rural areas which are typically underserved by health facilities, exacerbated by a lack of transport and poor road conditions. Travel time becomes costly in terms of lost opportunity to obtain income and ensure basic food security, especially in demographics dependent on subsistence agriculture.

Social and cultural barriers are real considerations, particularly in rural areas where there is a lack of education and awareness of potential benefits, and a fear of harm associated with medical and surgical intervention. In one initiative, of 12 candidates selected for cataract surgery, 9 refused to attend due to fear of Western biomedical treatment. Those who did attend only did so because they were told they would undergo a routine eye wash. Once the three candidates returned with restored vision, others were convinced to participate. Likewise, while simple spectacle correction of presbyopia is accepted in the Global North, in the rural Global South, acceptance of uncorrected vision is the norm.

Access to Instrumentation and Pharmaceuticals

We take for granted full-scope diagnostic capabilities (including Optical Coherence Tomography, digital retinal imaging, automated visual fields and even the basic spectrum of tonometry, gonioscopy, pachymetry, fundus biomicroscopy and binocular indirect ophthalmoscopy) unavailable in many clinical settings in the Global South. Diagnostic pharmaceutical agents such as tropicamide and cyclopentolate may also be unavailable. In many countries, chloramphenicol is widely used, whereas fourth-generation fluoroquinolones and many topical steroids are unavailable. Topical drugs for glaucoma therapy are often rare and glaucoma is frequently left untreated. A trabeculectomy as a 'one time' surgical intervention for primary open-angle glaucoma (POAG) may be the most viable option (Sherwin et al., 2008).

There may be very few pharmacies in rural areas stocking eye medicines, but when they do exist, they carry the added advantage that the shopkeeper is one of the local villagers integrated into the social network providing transparency and legitimacy (Bisika et al., 2009).

Indigenous Belief Systems and Challenges

Your mindset as a visiting team member must be one of respectful collaboration and learning. The local Global South team leader will possess an intimate knowledge of indigenous beliefs, traditional medical practitioners/healers (TMPs), traditional eye medicines (TEMs), spiritual worldviews and the pitfalls of assuming an understanding and acceptance of 'modern medicine' by the local population.

Healthcare practiced in the Global South is frequently characterized by medical pluralism. The biomedical model is present alongside non-Western ethnomedical systems that often do not make the distinction between mind and body (Locke and Scheper-Hugues, 1996), systems which are not mutually exclusive. Unlike the Global North, 'lay' practice is the core of medical knowledge to which specialists only add (Bisika et al., 2009).

Cultural and religious practices also come into play. A patient may present with classic symptoms of dry eye syndrome. The usual regimen of clinical tests may be less important than the observation on gross inspection of a significant application of home-made kohl (a dark composition of lead and admixture of other elements) on the lid margins. In addition to the mechanical blockage of the Meibomian gland orifices, this substance may have a significant negative impact on ocular health. The resolution of the issue must be undertaken with a very real sensitivity to the patient's cultural background and reasons for use of the kohl. Your local partners could tell you that its use ranges from cosmesis in adults to warding off 'the evil eye' in infants.

An 'African Perspective on Visual Impairments' presented to UNESCO states 'societies in most underdeveloped nations such as those in Africa look at disabilities as curses or punishment inflicted upon them for their sins . . . this not only demoralize(s) disabled people but also denies them the opportunity to participate in socio-economic activities such as education and the job market' (Belay, 2005, 1). Their access to education, employment and social interaction is limited, leading to pervasive marginalization, increasing poverty and vulnerability to a plethora of health problems.

The Role of TMPs and TEMs in Africa

Rural communities have strong faith in traditional healers who provide the first line of medical attention, where modern medical services are inaccessible (Ebeigbe, 2013). Traditional medicine remains the most widely accessible form of healthcare in Africa (Chan, 2008). An estimated, 135 interactions occur between traditional healers for each interaction between biomedical eye care personnel and village personnel. Cataract accounted for 61.4% of visits to the traditional healer, conjunctivitis 31% and trachoma 6.8% (Courtright, 1995).

In Nigeria, traditional beliefs differ from one ethnic group to another, but belief in the influence of ancestral spirits is prevalent. TMPs claim to heal utilizing plants through consultation with ancestral spirits (Ebeigbe, 2013). A survey of 68 TMPs in Benin City, Nigeria, revealed that 100% treated conjunctivitis (all redness was treated as conjunctivitis), itching and poor or cloudy vision, followed by cataract (76%), chalazion (68%), corneal ulcer (53%), entropion (35%) and glaucoma (12%). Recommended treatments may include sugar solutions, urine, local gin, saliva, water and breast milk (Bisika et al., 2009; Nwosu, 2005). Couching for cataracts was performed by 38% of the TMPs using a needle or thorn to pierce the cornea or globe and push the crystalline lens back and down into the posterior chamber (Ebeigbe, 2013).

The most commonly used TEMs are plant extracts, herbs and roots which may be toxic, cause corneal ulceration, opacification and perforation, even leading to endophthalmitis (Nwosu, 2005). Of the TMPs surveyed, 51% reported they never referred a case to a hospital or clinic. If the practitioner believes the ancestors have given him/her the power to cure all conditions, a case would never be referred to a biomedical practitioner (Ebeigbe, 2013).

There is limited success in expanding referrals, unless the concept is presented as a collaborative activity with the healer as a vital link in the process. TMPs are plentiful and culturally accepted throughout much of the Global South, and programs encouraging cooperation show that they have the potential to bring a positive contribution to community-based blindness prevention (Courtright, 1995; Courtright et al., 2000).

Self-Treatment

Self-treatment for ophthalmic disease was chosen by 22% of rural Malawians (Bisika et al., 2009). A contributing factor is that herbal medicine (found locally) is common knowledge and considered a continuum of acceptable ways of managing ocular disease (Bisika et al., 2009). Traditional eye medicines are expected to require more time before a 'cure' is achieved, partially explaining why there are long delays in seeking biomedical care (Courtright et al., 1996). Medical specialists, whether biomedical or traditional, are consulted only in special situations. In a study in rural Malawi, self-treatment increased significantly with decreasing socio-economic status (Bisika et al., 2009). Among the population reporting self-treatment, 72% reported using TEMs. Of this 72%, 55.4% used plants growing near their house (Bisika et al., 2009).

The Importance of Integration with Local Professionals

Community Ophthalmology is a broad based and multidisciplinary approach utilizing personnel drawn from local communities to conduct needs assessments, educational outreaches and to plan and implement strategies and interventions (Lewallen and Courtright, 2001). This has major implications for the effective delivery of eye care in the Global South. The resultant local 'buy in' through trust and communication is unattainable if outside personnel act alone.

While training and expectations may differ, the observation of your local counterpart skillfully assessing, diagnosing and treating ocular disease without sophisticated diagnostic tools, advanced technology or pharmaceutical agents engenders respect and insight into challenges and solutions.

The University of Waterloo School of Optometry interns travel to Malawi annually to complete a Primary Care externship as part of the local team with a Malawian community ophthalmologist acting as preceptor who formally evaluates the visiting team members from the Global North. The rotation includes observation in the operating theatre, field work and eye camps with the Malawian staff as well as participation in the trachoma eradication program. Partnership with Lions International and other local NGOs to facilitate delivery systems is extremely effective. In rural areas, externs observe local screeners – with no instrumentation – identify 'white eyes', the appearance of a mature cataract in the pupil. Phacoemulsification is not utilized for cataract extraction, but intraocular lenses are readily available. The lack of pre- and postoperative refraction yields less than optimal visual acuity by the standards of a more resource-rich country, but the results are life changing.

The benefits of partnering with local mentors in the Global South are numerous. You will observe the diagnosis and treatment of ocular pathologies rarely seen at home, and certainly not seen in such advanced stages of presentation. In addition, you will experience the privilege of working alongside colleagues who practice effectively with limited resources. In some regions of the Global South, it is not uncommon to watch a clinical officer in a brightly lit ward diagnose acute anterior uveitis by observing cells in the anterior chamber with nothing more than a direct ophthalmoscope. Ultimately, you will appreciate the life-altering experience of seeing patients who may well have already self-treated, consulted a TMP or utilized TEMs.

The Role of Preceptors

Preceptors and team leaders should be drawn from the local cadre of service providers. These preceptors can be essential in increasing your cultural competency. What, for example, would you have assumed to be the presenting symptoms of a child in southeastern Nigeria

(Biafra) whose mother brought him in during the late 1960s reporting he had Harold Wilson Syndrome? The answer is layered with geopolitical nuances impossible for you as an 'outsider' to understand. In fact, the diagnosis would have been Kwashiorkor, bitterly labelled as Harold Wilson Syndrome, in reference to the British Prime Minister at the time largely blamed by the Igbo people during the civil war for implementing the blockade of the region that lead to massive starvation.

You must constantly communicate with your local preceptors to identify the meaning behind indigenous use of the language. In one instance, for example, a local staff member commented 'these people have tubular vision, they're fish eaters'. The reference to visual field loss due to a high incidence of glaucoma was linked to an ethnic group who had been fishermen for generations; however, the moniker 'fish eaters' was used as an identifier of the group, not a causative agent. At first, you may have been tempted to interpret her comments as a locally observed correlation, but in fact the staff member was making a joke, not a diagnosis.

Reflection

It is the province of knowledge to speak and it is the privilege of wisdom to listen.

Oliver Wendell Holmes

Knowledge may mean that you have a grasp of facts and statistics as they apply to a particular demographic. Wisdom, however, entails the application of that knowledge with humility and understanding, in collaboration with your colleagues who know more than you ever will about the culture, worldview, beliefs, customs and challenges of those with whom you work in the Global South (Box 22.1).

BOX 22.1   PRE-DEPARTURE CHECKLIST

1. Do I understand the status of eye care in the host country? What are the potential barriers and opportunities for symbiosis and shared learning? As a visitor you must be proactive in eliminating silos of information.
2. Do I have a knowledge of the host team including their training, roles and responsibilities? Do I know my role place on the team?
3. Do I have an overview of the prevalence of ocular pathologies and their presentation in more advanced stages due to delay in seeking treatment?
4. Have I role played a basic case history and examination cross linguistically?
   Non-verbal body language and gestures are vital but easily misinterpreted. A skilled translator may well report that the patient has a family history of 'water on the eye'. This is an example of the need to apply the nuances and multiple meanings of your own language. A cataract is also a waterfall, rapids or whitewater in English (as in the six cataracts of the Nile). The term is used as such in the vernacular of other languages to signify the visual consequences of a lenticular cataract as though one were looking from behind a waterfall.

5. Have I completed a hands-on session in alternative instrumentation? For example, in many situations, it will be necessary to rely on direct ophthalmoscopy rather than slit lamp, fundus biomicroscopy and binocular indirect ophthalmoscopy.

6. Have I discussed the enhanced role of the extended family in patient care? This may include interpretation, transportation, obtaining medications and ultimately providing food and some degree of care during a hospital stay.

7. Have I investigated cultural sensitivities and attitudes towards Western medicine, philosophies of life, spiritual beliefs and worldviews as they pertain to my intended destination? These concepts might include: Ubuntu (Southern Africa), Yoruba spiritual beliefs and medicine (West Africa), Juju (West Africa), Sangomas (Africa), Karma (Asia and beyond), Yin and Yang (China and beyond).

8. Have I discussed mental health issues, culture shock and medication-related complications (e.g. mefloquine) in team dynamics?

9. Do I have an overview of possible challenges upon return? One possible challenge might be the 'refrigerator phenomenon' in which 5 minutes into your impassioned and eloquent recounting of your experiences, your listener, with glazed eyes, interjects 'my mother just got a new refrigerator'.

10. Have I met with previous participants in the elective? A database of information should be an ongoing process with updates on current challenges, status of facilities, cultural sensitivities and pitfalls to avoid.

References

Belay TE. 2005. African Perspective on Visual Impairments. *A paper presented to UNESCO at the World Summit on the Information Society Workshop on ICT and persons with disabilities*, Tunis, Tunisia, November 16.

Bisika T, Courtright P, Geneau R, Kasote A, Chimombo L, and Chirambo M. Self treatment of eye disease in Malawi. *Afr J Tradit Complement Altern Med.* 2009; 6(1): 23–29. Pb online 2008 Oct 25 www.ncbi.nlm.nih.gov/pmc/articles/PMC 2816523/

Chan M. (2008). Address to the WHO *Congress on Traditional Medicine* WHO 2008, 66 Beijing, People's Republic of China, Nov 7,2008.

Courtright P. Eye care knowledge and practices among Malawian traditional healers and the development of collaborative blindness prevention programs. *Soc Sc Med.* 1995; 41: 1559–1575.

Courtright P, Lewallen S, Chirambo M, Chana H, and Kanjaloti S. *Collaboration with African Traditional Healers for the Prevention of Blindness.* 2000. Singapore: World Scientific Publishing. ISBN 978-981-02-4377-7.

Courtright P, Lewallen S., and Kanjaloti S. Changing Patterns of Corneal Disease and associated vision loss at a rural African hospital following a training programme for traditional healers. *Br Journal Ophthalmol* 1996:80:694–697.

Dandona R and Dandona L. Refractive error blindness. *Bull World Health Organ.* 2001; 79(3): 237–243.

Ebeigbe JA. Traditional eye medicine practice in Benin-City, Nigeria. *African Vision and Eye Health; South African Optometrist.* 2013; 72(4): 167–172.

Lewallen S and Courtright P. Blindness in Africa: Present situation and future needs. *Br J Ophthalmol.* 2001; 85: 897–903. doi:10.1136/bjo.85.8.897

Locke M and Scheper-Hugues A. A critical-interpretive approach in medical anthropology;rituals and routines in discipline and dissent. In Sargent and Johnson (Eds) *Medical Anthropology: Contemporary Theory and Method.* Westport: Praeger, pp. 41–70, 1996.

Malawi National Health Plan 1999-2004, Vol 2: National Health Facilities. http://www.chikupirafoundation.co.uk/single.htm ipg=5973

Ngalande-Banda EE and Simukonda HPM. The public/private mix in the health care system in Malawi. *Health Policy Plann*. 1993; 9(1): 63–71.

Nwosu SN. Destructive ophthalmic surgical procedures in Onitsha, Nigeria. *Niger Postgrad Med J*. 2005; 12: 53–56.

Ono K, Hiratsuka Y, and Murakami A. Global inequality in eye health: Country-level analysis from the Global Burden of Disease Study. *Am J Public Health*. 2010 September; 100(9): 1784–1788.

Pascolini D, Mariotti SP. Global estimates of visual impairment: 2010. *Br J Ophthalmol*. 2012; 96(5): 614–618.

Resnikoff S. The Global Burden of Eye Disease: Can Ophthalmology Meet the Public Need? *International Council of Ophthalmology 9th World Roundtable* November 10, 2012.

Sherwin JC, Dean WH, and Metcalfe NH. Causes of blindness at Nkhoma Eye Hospital, Malawi *Euro J Ophthalmol*. 2008; 18(6): 1002–1006.

Ustrup M, Ngwira B, Stockman LJ, Deming M, Nyasulu P, Bowie C, Msyamboza K, Meyrowitsch K, Cunliffe NA, Bresee J, and Fischer TK. Potential barriers to healthcare in Malawi for under-five children with cough and fever: A national household survey. *J Health Popul Nutr*. 2014 March; 32(1): 68–78.

World Health Organization. 2014. WHO Media Centre Fact Sheet 282. Visual impairment and blindness, August 2014. Available at: www.who.int/mediacentre/factsheets/fs282/en/

World Health Organization. 2014. WHO Country Cooperation Strategy at a glance, May 2014 Malawi. Available at: http://who.int/iris/handle/10665/136935

Chapter 23

Global Public Health: Preparation and Training

Michelle M. Amri

Contents

Background

Global health refers to any health issue that concerns many countries or is affected by transnational determinants, such as climate change or urbanization, or solutions, such as polio eradication (Koplan et al., 2009). The topic of global public health is similarly vast and expansive, and as a practitioner you will need to know about a range of topics. This includes specific subject areas, such as understanding, managing and preventing communicable or infectious diseases; and understanding macro-level topics, such as long-term societal trends of chronic non-communicable diseases, the importance of creating policy across government sectors and collaborating across different levels of government and non-government sectors (multisectoral collaboration, for example, in applying the Health in All Policies approach). The connections between social determinants of health, trade, economics, community development and globalization are also crucial areas to understand as a foundation for global public health training and practice.

This chapter is meant to provide practical information regarding the preparation for your placement. It also seeks to provide global health trainees, such as yourself, with information on fundamental training areas for global public health. Additionally, it provides assistance in guiding the development of training programs in upcoming years, as gaps will be easily identified and provide guidance to students in areas they may seek to divert further effort in. Ultimately, it may help accompany practical education, such as graduate training, to better prepare you for a meaningful career in public health.

Preparing for Your Placement

In your global public health placement, you may be doing one or more of many tasks. One student may work more strictly on epidemiology, studying a specific disease and mapping using statistical data. Another student may be meeting with various stakeholders, such as government and non-governmental organizations (NGOs) and trying to ignite action on a particular issue. A third may be conducting an evaluation of a project by designing and distributing a survey, conducting interviews and analysing results. Because these placements can vary drastically, it is difficult for any school to provide all necessary training to students. However, many public health schools give little attention to any training required for endeavours abroad, which can have impacts on a student's work if impressions greatly differ from realities. There are some areas in particular that you should be aware of, as discussed in this section.

Knowing the levels of government and understanding the responsibilities of ministries and arms-length organizations is critical. For example, in the Philippines, the municipal level breaks down even further to the Barangay level. Understanding whether health promotion falls under the jurisdiction of a ministry of health or an external agency solely dedicated to health promotion provides insights into bureaucracy in a nation and whether or not health promotion is a government priority. Having a stronger understanding of this climate in which public health operates will allow you to gain an understanding of government priority areas. This may potentially help in framing decisions to gain buy-in and understanding which of the options are unlikely.

You should also make yourself knowledgeable of the politics not just within your office, but within and between different levels of government and beyond, such as at a global or national level. This will help ensure what you are working on or proposing will materialize. This knowledge of politics extends to the roles of international organizations. It is important you know who is funding the project and understand the roles of various development partners. For example, when working with different partners, whether NGOs, government or the United Nations, it is important to know which organization is meant to lead, and what relevant information you might have that they lack.

Working in any new culture requires skills in cultural competency, and understanding how to communicate effectively and politely with people of different backgrounds; for example, understanding the beliefs of a nation, which may trickle down into the clothing, where in some cultures a more revealing dress may be seen as disrespectful. In Lao People's Democratic Republic, the majority of women wear traditional skirts (sinhs) that end below the knee, and while shorter dresses may be seen around town, it is unusual to see a shorter length in a professional setting. In Tanzania, failure to recognize appropriate dress proved a barrier for public health students doing grassroots work in the community. Because many students were used to cooler climates, they wore minimal clothing in the field, which made them less relatable to locals, ultimately impacting their work.

Cultural clashes can also present themselves in other ways. In some cultures, direct communications and contentious topics are avoided, whereas in others, they are not. It is equally important to understand hierarchy and whom you should report to, and to ensure respect of authority figures. For example, formalities involved in creating partnerships with a Ministry of Health may require a letter to be sent straight to the cabinet with carbon copy inclusion to relevant department heads, rather than sending it solely to the relevant departments. It is important you practice patience, understanding there may be language barriers when working with those of different cultures. In order to enhance your understanding of cultural complexities, reach out to your global health department for advice and resources on cultural competency and travel safety and health. In addition, you must conduct your own research on the country and city, prior to departure.

Many individuals on a global health placement in the Global South are from the Global North. As a result, there may be a power imbalance, and the individuals you may be working with may perceive you as an authority. In this scenario, you must clearly explain your intended role and limited experience. Ensure all local voices are heard and respected, since these individuals have knowledge of the local context, laws and previous activities; and it is they who will lead the change once you leave. Instead of working to simply provide health education to the community, work to build capacity; developing training for a cadre of specially selected community health workers who understand their privileged role in the community for educating and training future staff has proven more effective in ensuring sustainability of programs in India.

Consider the unintended consequences of measures to deal with diseases such as malaria or to provide water and sanitation. Without adequate consideration and preparation, your mosquito nets for malaria prevention may be used instead as fishing nets. Building wells without consulting communities, you may find them unused, as women prefer social time going to fetch water in the local river. Projects bringing students to build latrines, while useful to students, may be wasted on the community if you do not realize that homes already have latrines, students' work needs to be revised by local tradespeople or that local cultural norms where it is unacceptable to regularly remove waste manually are not considered. Always begin by conducting a 'needs assessment', humbly asking simple but critical questions of your local partners. Providing education through the distribution of leaflets in the local language along with your mosquito nets may be useful.

In other instances, locals may not have adequate resources to apply interventions suggested by global health students. In trying to curb guinea worm in Papua New Guinea, a couple of projects proved unsuccessful. First, when advised to boil the water, locals found this ineffective, as they lacked funds to purchase firewood or time to boil. And second, the cotton cloth distributed for straining larvae from drinking water was used for clothing or decorations. To combat these ineffective measures, pipe filters were later distributed – requiring no additional cost or time for the one drinking the water.

Global Health Careers Landscape

As a global public health student, you may be wondering what employment opportunities lie ahead. Recent debate suggests that the abundance of global health students graduating from Global North schools may exceed demand (Eichbaum, Evert, and Hall, 2016) and I beg to differ. Resources will need to be continually and unpredictably devoted to emerging areas. Recent examples would be the emergence of zika and ebola or managing antimicrobial resistance. As a result, new opportunities are available in these areas. However, choices for masters graduates will be restricted by two key variables:

1. **The student's interest**
   If you have a particular interest in a specific topic, you may look for roles in those fields, such as interest in the following:
   - A specific mental health issue: You may choose to work for a NGO which provides programming to populations that require services.
   - Physical activity: You may work for a research centre that publishes guidelines and resource books.
   - Healthcare policy analysis: You may choose to work for a provincial/territorial or federal government.

■ A specific disease or chronic condition such as human immunodeficiency virus (HIV)/ acquired immune deficiency syndrome (AIDS): You may apply epidemiology skills and work for a local health authority to analyse disease trends within a city.

Because the opportunities for graduates are vast, this list is not exhaustive. However, it demonstrates the types of roles that you may want to consider. Certainly, there may be an analogous role in a field that is of particular interest to you. Alternatively, as a recent graduate, you may apply to organizations over specific topic area.

2. **Opportunities available**

For those alumni applying to organizations, depending on the organization and role an individual is seeking to fill, the training required can vary substantially. Below are some simple examples that will give prospective students, hopefully, a sense of the unique training and skill sets required. For example, some potential opportunities and associated skill sets required include the following:

■ Program and policy roles at the World Health Organization require skills in research, program evaluation and report writing.
■ Service delivery roles at a grassroots organization require skills in survey and qualitative research, stakeholder relations and marketing.
■ Epidemiology roles include skills in data collection, analysis, statistical software and critical thinking.
■ Health education roles include skills in public speaking, developing presentations, stakeholder relations and technical knowledge.
■ Research roles include skills in qualitative and quantitative statistical methods and potentially, report writing.

Because some of these skills overlap, you may want to focus on developing these skill sets over learning technical content knowledge of a specific health issue.

Current Training Programs

Global health placements can provide many benefits, to either students or host institutions or potentially both. A study evaluated students who engaged in global health placements and found students value the opportunity to make cross-country comparisons, experience the role of international organizations and to learn concrete skills in project design, questionnaire formulation, qualitative and quantitative analysis and write-up (Cole, Plugge, and Jackson, 2013).

However, some students leave their training feeling unprepared in skill sets required in the field, due in part to the current structure of masters-level training in global health. In many high-income countries, you can choose from two 'global health' options: (1) training in a Master of Public Health (MPH), where the focus is on a specific field, such as epidemiology or health promotion, with the option to enrol in global health elective credits or (2) a Master of Science in Global Health (MScGH), where the focus is typically on global issues in low- and middle-income countries with a research thesis component. These formal education options may not satisfy your desires for a well-rounded education, and you may very well need to seek skills and competencies not formally taught in order to better prepare for a career in global health.

The exact balance of masters-level training is difficult to design to ensure it meets the needs of all students. For example, students with moderate prior experience in global health reported greater satisfaction with a global health concentration of their MPH at one university, whereas students with lower prior experience wanted more courses and support with practicums (Jackson and Cole, 2013).

1. **Master of Public Health (MPH)**
   This program is typically offered as a 1–2-year degree with graduates beginning employment with both non-government and government entities. Some MPH programs require work experience prior to acceptance; however, this is not a standard requirement.

   Mandatory classes, such as biostatistics, research methods, theory courses and occasionally health policy provide a basic level of public health understanding but may not address macro-level issues, though electives in global health or healthy public policy are possible. Practicums, either from a list of the school's opportunities or arranged by students with approval of faculty, may include global health practicums. One might have opportunities to conduct research with a host university, apply public health training to conduct fieldwork with a community organization or create policy with an international organization.

   The Association of Schools and Programs of Public Health (ASPPH)'s Education Committee has identified a MPH Core Competency Model, which highlights five core competencies which graduates should be competent in before degree completion. These core competencies are biostatistics, environmental science, epidemiology, health policy and management and social and behavioural science. In addition, ASPPH has identified seven interdisciplinary/cross-cutting competencies: communication and informatics, diversity and culture, leadership, public health biology, professionalism, program planning and systems thinking. All 12 domains are considered to be the foundation of graduate public health studies (ASPPH, 2006).

2. **Master of Science in Global Health (MScGH)**
   The 'newer' MScGH is most often a 1-year degree and includes a choice between traditional coursework and a practice-based placement or a research thesis. While similar to an MPH with core courses in research methods and health policy, remaining core courses such as globalization and evaluation methods are at best elective options in MPH programs.

   Similar to the core competencies outlined for MPH training, the ASPPH has developed a global health competency model. This model identifies five core competencies for students studying global health, which graduates should be competent in before degree completion. These are in addition to training in other fields, such as public health, and are capacity strengthening, collaborating and partnering, ethical reasoning and professional practice, health equity and social justice and program management (ASPPH, 2011).

Connecting Skills-Training to Key Competencies

While you may seek to further your content knowledge and expertise on a specific health issue, it is also wise to focus your training on developing crucial and transferrable skills, such as epidemiology, research and health promotion. You may now be wondering what other key competencies exist.

These key competencies include understanding how broader policy decisions have profound impacts on health outcomes – as health does not operate in a vacuum. You should strive to understand not only policies that target and impact the social determinants of health, such as those focusing on income or education, but also attempt to understand policy areas that are not typically directly linked to health. These indirect policy areas can directly affect health outcomes, as well. For example, transportation policies can create a more 'liveable' built environment, with aesthetic appeal and bike lanes, which can actually increase active transport and potentially physical activity levels. Or there are areas that lie under the broad topic of health but action needs to be taken in other areas. For example, applying the 'One Health' approach, an understanding that the health of people is connected to the health of animals and the environment, warrants targeting the agriculture and livestock sectors to overcome overuse of antibiotics in animals, which results in antibiotic resistance. Hence, you should appreciate that health considerations need to be given to all policy areas, known as 'Health in All Policies', and appreciate why there needs to be multi-sectoral collaboration.

If you are able to enhance these competencies, you will inevitably increase your chances of adapting to and positively participating in global health work abroad. Therefore, you may find it valuable to enrol in public policy courses or self-study, to better understand legislative systems, how laws and bills are passed, jurisdictions of different levels of government, the policy cycle, policy tools (such as moral suasion, legislation and regulation) and how policies can be framed. You may also find utility in following news channels, focusing on not only local news but also international.

Schools of public health can look to utilize a framework, such as one put forward by the World Health Organization, to gauge progress in promoting health systems that possess a balance between relevance, quality, cost-effectiveness and equity, ultimately to understand impact on social accountability (World Health Organization, 1995). While the framework mentioned has been proposed for those in medicine and the validity needs to be ensured, schools of public health can look to expand a similar framework for trainees.

Conclusion

Global health is an attractive area for many students. There are many opportunities that cover various interest areas and require different skill sets. In order to best prepare for a role in global health, it is important you focus on developing not only technical or subject matter knowledge, but also key competencies. While many key competencies are not offered in masters-level programs, you should look to develop these skills through alternative avenues. You may even consider advocating for inclusion of these competencies for all masters-level students at your institution. Administrators should seek to promote developing these competencies through pre-existing required courses or consider developing a competency course in addition to theory and methods courses.

Using the knowledge from this chapter, such as awareness of previous mishaps in the global health field and striving to develop key competencies and learning from others mistakes, you will well equip yourself for a career in global public health. I wish you the best of luck and good health on your journey; the world is your oyster.

References

Association of Schools and Programs of Public Health. (2011, October 31). Global Health Competency Model. Final Version 1.1. Retrieved from: http://www.aspph.org/educate/models/masters-global-health/

Association of Schools and Programs of Public Health Education Committee. (2006, August). Master's Degree in Public Health Core Competency Development Project. Version 2.3. Retrieved from: http://www.aspph.org/app/uploads/2014/04/Version2.31_FINAL.pdf

Cole, D.C., Plugge, E., and Jackson. S. (2013, June). Placements in global health masters' programmes: What is the student experience? *Journal of Public Health*, 35(2): 329–337. doi:10.1093/pubmed/fds086.

Eichbaum, Q., Evert, J., and Hall, T. (2016, October). Will there be enough jobs for trained global health professionals? *Lancet*, 4: e692–693.

Jackson, S. and Cole, D. C. (2013, May). Graduate global public health education: Activities and outcomes in relation to student prior experience. *Journal of Global Health Sciences*, 5(3): 54–63. doi:10.5539/gjhs.v5n3p54.

Koplan, J. P., Bond, T. C., Merson, M. H., Reddy, K. S., Rodriguez, M. H., Sewankambo, N. K., and Wasserheit, J. N. (2009, June 6). Towards a common definition of global health. *The Lancet*, 373: 1993–1995. Retrieved from: https://www.globalbrigades.org/media/Global_Health_Towards_a_Common_Definitition.pdf

World Health Organization. (1995). Defining and Measuring the Social Accountability of Medical Schools. Retrieved from: http://apps.who.int/iris/bitstream/10665/59441/1/WHO_HRH_95.7.pdf

Global Health Research: Practical Guidelines

Mary T. White, Jason T. Blackard and Caley A. Satterfield

Contents

An increasing number of undergraduates, medical, nursing and allied health students, medical residents and students of other disciplines are interested in conducting research during the course of short-term global health electives, either as their primary focus or in addition to other service or educational activities. Ideally, trainees performing global health research will have prior experience in global health, epidemiology, social and behavioural determinants of health and research methods. As formal instruction in these areas is frequently unavailable in standard undergraduate or pre-professional curricula (Wallace and Webb, 2014; Eley and Wilkinson, 2015; Cluver et al., 2014), this chapter reviews what is typically involved in global health research conducted by trainees on short-term experiences in global health (STEGHs). While the structure of such experiences can vary – whether sponsored by home institutions with established overseas partnerships, offered by independent non-governmental organizations (NGOs) or initiated by individual trainees – the essential elements of successful global health research apply equally to all elective settings. This chapter is structured as a step-by-step roadmap of the research process, each step accompanied by discussion of the essential knowledge, attitudes and skills necessary for its successful completion.

Research has been defined as 'a systematic investigation, including research development, testing and evaluation, designed to develop or contribute to generalizable knowledge' (U.S. CFR, Title 45, Part 46). For an activity to be considered as research, data must be systematically gathered to address a specific question, ideally of relevance to a recognizable need, with generalizable implications. When findings are not generalizable, as in some program evaluation or quality improvement studies, they may nonetheless be of great value even if not viewed as formal research. A goal of this article is to ensure that trainees aspiring to conduct research will have a clear understanding of what constitutes research and what the research process involves.

Like the concept of research, global health may also be understood in a variety of ways, often emphasizing international medicine, tropical disease or international public health. One broadly accepted definition is that of Koplan et al. (2009): *Global health emphasizes transnational health issues, determinants and solutions; involves many disciplines within and beyond the health sciences and promotes interdisciplinary collaboration; and is a synthesis of population-based prevention with individual-level clinical care.* Given the broad scope of global health, there is an infinite number of possible research questions. At one author's university, research in which trainees have participated includes studies of cardiovascular disease and human immunodeficiency virus (HIV) in Kenya, malnutrition in Peru, water sanitation in the Dominican Republic and literature reviews. Through another author's university partnership in Botswana, trainees have conducted laboratory-based research focused on viruses of public health importance. As in public health, much global health research is population-based, exploring questions related to disease prevention, social, behavioural and environmental determinants of health, advocacy for vulnerable populations and population-based policies and interventions (Fried et al., 2010). Relevant research modalities include epidemiology, biomedical and clinical research, quality improvement, health policy analysis and interdisciplinary studies.

For trainees with limited experience and time, it is often easiest to join a pre-existing study, if such is available, at their elective site. This can provide valuable research experience but bypass the intellectual work of developing a research question and protocol. Alternatively, pending host-site support, a variety of non-interventional studies may be feasible and useful to the site. These include outcomes and quality improvement studies using previously collected, anonymized data. As long as the studies are retrospective and findings will not be disseminated beyond the host site, the studies may be exempt from ethical oversight or receive expedited review. However, some study modalities, including prospective studies comparing different clinical approaches, merit ethical oversight as research (Bellin and Dubler, 2001). Other observational or descriptive studies may also be possible and worthwhile, perhaps those on barriers to access, resource utilization or the epidemiological characteristics of a particular disease. For students lacking a research mentor or host-site support, feasible options include literature reviews, case studies, health policy analysis or global health education research.

In any field, challenges for researchers include developing a research question and method, the logistics of study implementation and data analysis. In global health research, when these activities will be done in an unfamiliar setting, with limited infrastructure and funding, often in an unknown language and culture, with variable mentorship and local support, these challenges are compounded. Given the complexity and challenges of global health research, emerging literature on global health research conducted by trainees indicates that strong mentorship, ideally from both the home institution and the elective setting, is invaluable (Shah et al., 2011). Experienced mentors can provide numerous forms of support. They may connect trainees with pre-existing studies, guide the development of research questions, identify potential research partners, help navigate ethics and human subjects protection approval, help secure funding, expand the trainees' professional networks, and support the development of abstracts, papers and presentations. Mentors from the host site can ensure the research question is relevant, feasible, and culturally and politically acceptable and, if necessary, help to recruit participants. In these and other ways, having multiple mentors to provide guidance and oversight can greatly improve the likelihood that research will be successful (see also Chapter 5).

Regardless of the topic area or method, research is a carefully defined process that can be divided into several discrete steps. At the most basic level, these include the following five steps:

1. Developing the research question
2. Identifying appropriate research methods; developing a protocol
3. Implementing the protocol
4. Data collection and analysis
5. Dissemination of findings

Developing the Research Question

The first of these steps – developing the research question – is frequently the most challenging for researchers. A prerequisite for global health research is a basic grasp of the primary sources of morbidity and mortality around the world, including the diverse socioeconomic, environmental and behavioural contributors to health; communication skills that reflect awareness of and respect for cultural diversity; and commitment to professionalism, ethical accountability, respect for human rights and social responsibility (Jogerst et al., 2015; Provenzano et al., 2010). In addition to this general background, researchers need a working knowledge of the country, region and specific location where they plan to visit and work. This includes the basic health demographics of the area, the healthcare system and local healthcare infrastructure and elementary language skills. Without a broad understanding of the country and the specific research setting in which they will be working, trainees can have difficulty managing daily social, cultural, logistical and professional challenges. While the sending and host institution can assist in preparing trainees for their international experience, ultimately it is each individual's responsibility to ensure that s/he is prepared. Those trying to participate in global health electives or conduct research *without* this basic knowledge are likely to find the experience disorienting and frustrating, lacking the context necessary to develop a meaningful research question and work effectively.

Trainee-researchers should make every effort to choose a country and research topic of interest to them, ideally in a setting in which there is support for research. When research is to be conducted in a foreign setting, a central ethical principle is that research must respond to needs and priorities identified by the host community (CIOMS, 2002, Guideline 10). For this reason, researchers should make every effort to work with host-site preceptors to develop their research question. Host colleagues can ensure that a study question is meaningful and that a proposed study design is logistically and socioculturally feasible. Feasible research opportunities will vary with the size, activities and resources of a site, whether research is an established activity at the site and whether faculty mentors from the home institution or host site will be available during the elective. If host-site support is not available, research options will be limited to projects that researchers can do independently.

Aspiring researchers should keep in mind that they are visitors, dependent on their hosts for their opportunities. What may not be evident to them is the degree to which the resource disparities between them and their host communities impact their hosts' behaviours and choices. Where resources and opportunities are severely limited, negotiations are not conducted on a level playing field. Hosts may agree to support research projects that are in fact burdensome to their clinical staff or surrounding communities. Aspiring researchers, eager to collect data and publish for their own interests, may be unaware of their impact on host clinical settings and communities. Researchers should be aware that when they request permission to conduct research, that permission, even if granted, may be based on very different expectations than their own. Clear articulation of the expectations by the mentee, the host institution and the mentor prior to initiation of the research project may partially alleviate this concern.

With or without input from the host site, the next step in developing a research question is to explore topic areas of interest using the published literature. Given the paucity of literature on healthcare in many less-developed countries, studies that are several decades old or conducted in different geographic regions may be all that is available. It is always easier to develop a research question when substantial literature already exists. Biomedical or clinical research must always be situated within what is already known about a given topic, typically requiring an extensive literature review. A broad literature review enables the identification of gaps in what is known, which provides the starting point for a research question. There are many methods for conducting literature reviews, but a general comprehensive literature review should be sufficient for this step. An excellent resource describing how to conduct a literature review is available at http://www.istl .org/09-spring/experts1.html.

Questions to consider include the following:

- How many articles related to the research topic can be found in the published literature? (Relevant databases include PubMed, Medline, PsycInfo, CINAHL, Google Scholar.)
- How many articles related to the research topic are specific to the country or region in which you plan to work?
- Are there any relevant review articles available?
- Do any studies appear to be the close in scope and methodology to the one you are considering?
- What factors distinguish your study from previously published studies? Can you clearly describe the innovation and uniqueness of your study question and/or study design?

Note: A more rigorous type of literature review is a *systematic* review – a review of a clearly formulated question that uses explicit, systematic methods to identify, select and critically appraise relevant research and to collect and analyse data from the studies that are included in the review (see http://www.cochrane.org). These reviews differ substantially from narrative-based reviews or synthesis articles. Statistical methods (meta-analysis) may or may not be used to analyse and summarize the results of the included studies.

The extensive research involved in developing a research question can seem long or perhaps even unnecessary to students who are eager to gather and analyse data. However, a thorough literature review is absolutely essential for substantive research – findings are meaningless devoid of context. Discussions with expert researchers, presentations to students, and work-in-progress group discussions can also help sharpen the focus of a research project and are highly recommended. Good research questions are narrowly focused, answerable given the time and resources available and expected to yield meaningful findings.

This first step in the research process – developing the research question – requires commitment to the process, a passion for the project, respect for one's mentors at home and abroad and open-mindedness to feedback. The ability to synthesize the literature and situate a focused research question within this larger context calls for disciplined intellectual and analytical skills. Because the knowledge, attitudes and skills required in research are at their most demanding in this step, the ability to develop an informed, focused, relevant and feasible research question may be indicative of an individual's readiness for the challenges of global health.

Selecting a Method and Developing a Protocol

Once a research question has been identified, a feasible method must be developed and articulated in a protocol. Developing a method is largely a skill based on research experience, awareness of the resources and constraints of a particular setting; here, mentoring guidance on study design can be particularly helpful. The most straightforward methods are those for literature reviews or observational studies that involve no interventions or participants other than the researchers. Experimental studies, including those that require human participants, typically involve materials, technology and support staff, necessitating funding, logistical and ethical considerations.

It is very difficult to anticipate the specific logistics required to implement a research protocol in an unfamiliar setting. Background research can help, as can informal discussions with mentors familiar with the partner country or institution. If face-to-face conversations are not possible, e-mail or Skype calls may substitute and should be included as an integral part of the protocol development process. Regardless of the approach, the need for substantive contact between the researcher, the host institution, and mentor prior to initiation of research is paramount. It is most important to submit the draft protocol for review by content experts, country experts (rarely the same as the former) and host preceptors, all of whom may raise important concerns. Trainees should recognize that the more that informed individuals review their protocols constructively, the greater the likelihood that their final protocols will be conceptually sound and logistically feasible.

Researchers must also be familiar with ethical requirements at both their home institution and in the country where they plan to conduct their study (U.S. CFR Title 45, Part 46; OHRP, 2016). Training in research methods can be obtained through didactic coursework, online training or from mentors and Institutional Review Board (IRB) personnel. Studies involving identifiable humans or human data will require prior approval from an IRB at the researcher's home institutions and often from a comparable committee in the host country. The U.S. Department of Health and Human Services publishes a list of research regulations, by country, that is updated annually (OHRP, 2016). While capacities for research review and oversight are rapidly expanding globally, the quality and time required for review vary considerably from place to place. Visiting researchers should not assume that because a host site has approved their protocol as ethical, that it will be perceived or experienced as such by the host community. Visitors need to do their own due diligence to ensure their proposals are ethically acceptable both at home and abroad. Even studies for which the data are de-identified must petition both home and host ethics review committees for study exemption. Because this takes considerable advance planning, most novice researchers on short-term electives will not find it possible to develop and implement an original protocol using human participants.

Study Implementation

When visitors from high-income countries visit low-income countries, they are often surprised by the lack of infrastructure and resources that are part of daily life at home. When they require support for their research activities, they can draw host personnel away from their other duties, disrupting routines. This disruption is significant and should not be dismissed or overlooked. When designing a study, visiting researchers should anticipate the likely impact of the research activity on the host site and personnel and make every effort to minimize it and compensate for it (Crump et al., 2010; Provenzano et al., 2010). This may involve regular evaluation of the research activities, with input from host personnel, in terms of the time and the financial resources required, as these may change over time.

The challenges of protocol implementation are as varied as the protocols. Table 24.1 illustrates a range of study types and methodologies for a single disease (hepatitis B virus) in a single country. If human participants or identifiable medical data are necessary for the study, informed consent is required. Informed consent refers to the act of telling the potential participant what the study is about, the risks, benefits and alternatives of participation, the right to withdraw without penalty and assurances of confidentiality. This information sharing is followed by asking the participant

Table 24.1 Example Global Health Research Projects

Project Description	Type of Research	Research Methods
Prevalence of HBV in Botswana	Clinical – Observational	• IRB approval • Patient enrolment • Sample collection and processing • Laboratory testing of markers of HBV infection • Statistical analysis
Optimal treatment strategies for HBV in Botswana	Clinical – Interventional	• IRB approval • Patient enrolment • Sample collection and processing • Laboratory testing of markers of HBV infection • Safety monitoring for adverse events • Statistical analysis
Occurrence of hepatocellular carcinoma in Botswana	Clinical – Chart review	• IRB approval (expedited review) • Patient data collection • Clinical laboratory testing of serologic markers of HBV infection[a] • Statistical analysis
Occurrence of hepatocellular carcinoma in HBsAg-negative individuals in Botswana	Clinical – Case series	• IRB approval (expedited review) • Patient data collection • Laboratory testing of markers of HBV infection[a] • Statistical analysis (if necessary)
Occult HBV in a previously vaccinated injection drug user	Clinical – Case report	• IRB approval (expedited review) • Patient data collection • Laboratory testing of markers of HBV infection[a]
Detection of HBV drug resistance mutations in HIV-positive persons in Botswana	Laboratory – *In vivo* and *in vitro*	• IRB approval (expedited review) • Patient data collection • Laboratory testing of markers of HBV infection[a] • Laboratory testing: PCR, cloning, sequencing • Bioinformatics analysis • Statistical analysis (if necessary)

(Continued)

Table 24.1 (*Continued*)   Example Global Health Research Projects

Project Description	Type of Research	Research Methods
Functional analysis of HBV drug resistance mutations in Botswana	Laboratory – *in vitro*	• IRB approval (not likely to be necessary) • Patient data collection (in aggregate, de-identified form) • Laboratory testing of markers of HBV infection[a] • Laboratory testing: PCR, cloning, sequencing • Bioinformatics analysis • Statistical analysis (if necessary)
Increasing awareness of HBV in at-risk individuals	Educational	• IRB approval • Patient enrolment • Survey and focus group data collection • Statistical analysis
Cost-effectiveness of HBV screening in Botswana	Outcomes	• IRB approval (not likely to be necessary) • Patient data collection (in aggregate, de-identified form) • Economic modelling • Statistical analysis

HBV, hepatitis B virus; HBsAg, hepatitis B virus surface antigen; IRB, institutional review board; PCR, polymerase chain reaction.

[a] Previously completed as part of routine clinical care.

to sign a form stating that they understand what they have heard and are willing to participate in the study. Notably, in order to be approved by a U.S. IRB, consent forms and spoken scripts must be translated into the local languages and back again into English.

While the informed consent process is familiar in North America, it can be difficult to implement in low-income countries if the researcher does not speak the local language, the potential participant is illiterate, or has reasons (sometimes due to recent political history) to avoid signing or marking a consent form. Importantly, there are many cultures worldwide in which individual autonomy and rights are not a moral, legal or political priority, where the norm may be for a community leader to represent a group, a male head of the house to represent his spouse, and where social inequality across racial and ethnic lines is the norm. Local staff may not understand the need for autonomous decision making and may try to persuade prospective participants to enrol. Inducements and incentives, even small ones such as a bag of rice in return for participation, may sway decisions. These and many other local variants can make Western ethical norms difficult to uphold. Such cultural and educational differences may call for some modification of study protocols, but modifications, if made, must be reviewed and approved by ethics committees at the home institution and the host country equivalent. As the right to informed consent is the founding principle of Western research ethics, ensuring that it is upheld is one of the central responsibilities of IRB review. Where this principle is not a priority, finding ways to respect local norms while upholding Western ethical standards is nonetheless essential. When abuses occur, they jeopardize the reputations of individual researchers, their institutions and the research enterprise as a whole.

Other logistical challenges in global health research may involve patient recruitment, needs for laboratory equipment and diagnostic technologies, quality control procedures, and literacy barriers and cultural resistance to surveys and focus groups. International research ethics guidelines also call for equitable distribution of benefits and burdens in selecting candidates for research participation, special protections for minors, women of childbearing capability, prisoners and the mentally ill (and by implication, refugees) and for host communities to have access to products of research (CIOMS, 2002). While much medical research conducted during short-term electives may not involve these concerns, particularly non-interventional observational research or literature reviews, researchers should be aware of the general ethical requirements governing international research and uphold them to the greatest extent possible.

Data Management

The logistics of data collection, data management and data analysis should be planned well in advance of arriving at the field site location. Failure to do so frequently leads to insufficient quantity or quality of data for analysis and/or other issues that may lead to project failure. In developing the protocol, if data are to be gathered, researchers should do the following:

- Generate a list of all study-related variables that will be collected.
- Create a data entry form for those variables.
- Discuss the anticipated data and means of recording these data with a local statistician to ensure accurate data collection and entry (including how to code individual variables).
- Discuss the protocol in general terms with the statistician to confirm study design and consider sample size and power calculations.
- Discuss who will do the analysis – the researcher or a statistician collaborator.

In addition to personnel support, effective data management requires reliable technology and infrastructure. The local power supply necessary for reliable computer use should be ascertained, as well as needs for adaptors for local voltage. Related considerations include confirming Internet connectivity, methods to secure data integrity, and plans for regularly backing-up data to a secure site. When travelling with computers and other technology necessary for work, it may be advisable to investigate any regulations at the home institution regarding international travel with university-owned equipment (laptop computers or tablets), relevant home country export control laws, encrypted computers, and software.

A note of caution: In these days of social media, blogging, and so forth, while researchers may be tempted to report on their activities while abroad, it is risky, unprofessional and unethical to do so. Misunderstanding, breach of confidentiality and premature sharing of findings are all possible. Researchers share ownership of data with their host collaborators. Any unauthorized sharing of data risks violating professional commitments and suggests an exploitive attitude of researchers towards their hosts.

Dissemination of Findings

For their own professional development, trainees should seek as many opportunities to present their research as possible. The more presentations they give, the more individuals they will reach and the more constructive input they will receive related to their research project. A presentation of the research protocol before their elective begins can be a valuable chance to receive feedback. At the completion of the elective, at least one presentation should be given prior to the trainee's return home to ensure that personnel representing the host institution have the opportunity to review the student's findings and that the on-site supervisor and other institutional leaders and stakeholders are acknowledged for their contributions. Once back at their home institution, students can present the research findings in a variety of formats including abstracts, posters, presentations and papers, in venues that include the following:

- Lab presentations
- Research seminars (which can be student-focused, works-in-progress or more formal departmental seminar series)
- Grand rounds
- An individual lecture in a related course
- Presentations to student groups interested in global health or studying in the same discipline as the research project
- Poster presentations (for PhD programs, medical student research, summer research or an organized research week or global health symposium)
- Poster or paper presentations at local, regional and national conferences

Importantly, in final publications and presentations, any members of the host community that contributed to the study design, data analysis and/or writing up the study should approve the work before it is publicly presented and be included as authors per usual standards of publication. If the study is to be presented at a national conference, every effort should be made to have collaborators from the host site be present. If the study is to be published in a peer-reviewed journal, the journal should be available to the host site free of charge.

Capacity Strengthening

While not strictly a step in the research process, a global health competency of relevance to research is that of capacity strengthening (Jogerst et al., 2015). Every year, as thousands of North American students travel to villages in low-income countries, they learn and serve in a variety of ways, often at their hosts' expense. Their hosts often accept this in hopes that over the long term some benefit may be gained from long-term relationships with individual visitors or their sending institutions. Indeed, sometimes this hope materializes. Electives may blossom into academic partnerships that may lead to research collaboration and bilateral exchanges. Students, on the other hand, argue that they want to see the world and try to help people who are less fortunate than they are themselves. While the activities in which they engage may seem modest, their goal – and the goal of the global health movement – is ultimately to promote the health of humans and the environment around the world. While students may feel their electives are too short to make much of a difference, they are never too short to make a friend, discover a future colleague, leave a happy memory or make a bad impression. Positive connections are the currency of the elective experience, one important measure of its success. If maintained, these relationships may lead to a return trip from the trainee or fund-raising efforts on behalf of the community, development of an NGO or a stronger institutional partnership. What makes lasting connections possible is the visitor's attitude. Ideally, this will be one of respect, humility and willingness to learn; resilience in the face of discomfort, frustration and exposure to suffering; and most of all, genuine interest in the lives of the people encountered. These qualities are both innate and can be developed. If trainees achieve at least this much in their international electives, they will have provided some benefit and perhaps laid the groundwork for future, more substantive engagement.

Conclusion

This brief discussion has outlined the basic steps involved in global health research in view of the central challenges involved – the unfamiliar setting, language and people; resource and infrastructure limitations; social, cultural, linguistic and political considerations, and unforeseeable logistical complications. The challenges are substantial, yet countless young researchers are eager to contribute to the task. The next steps involve the development and cultivation of global health research competencies for trainees and strengthening the research capacities of universities and healthcare institutions around the world. With these competencies in place, it is reasonable to expect that trainees from diverse disciplines may serve as a vital global health research workforce around the world.

References

Bellin E and Dubler NN. 2001. The quality improvement–research divide and the need for external oversight. *Am J Public Health* 91(9): 1512–17.

Cluver JS, Book SW, Brady KT, Thornley N, Back SE. 2014. Engaging medical students in research: Reaching out to the next generation of physician scientists. *Acad Psychiatry* 38(3): 345–49.

Council for the International Organizations of Medical Science (CIOMS). 2002. *International Ethical Guidelines for Biomedical Research Involving Human Subjects* (1993, 2002) http://www.recerca.uab.es /ceeah/docs/CIOMS.pdf

Crump JA, Sugarman J, Working Group on Ethics Guidelines for Global Health Training (WEIGHT). 2010. Ethics and best practice guidelines for training experiences in global health. *Am J Trop Med Hyg* 83(6): 1178–82.

Eley DS and Wilkinson D. 2015. Building a teaching-research nexus in a research intensive university: Rejuvenating the recruitment and training of the clinician scientist. *Med Teach* 37(2): 174–80.

Fried LP, Bentley ME, Buekens P, Burke DS, Frenk J, Klag MJ, Spencer HC. 2010. Global health is public health. *Lancet* 375: 535–37.

Jogerst K, Callender B, Adams V, Evert J, Fields E, Hall T, Olsen J, Rowthorne V, Rudy S, Shen J, Simon L, Torres H. 2015. Identifying interprofessional global health competencies for 21st century health professionals. *Ann Glob Health* 81(2): 239–47.

Koplan JP, Bond TC, Merson MH, Reddy KS, Rodriguez MH, Sewankambo NK, Wasserheit JN. 2009. Towards a common definition of global health. *Lancet* 373: 1993–97.

Office for Human Research Protections, U.S. Department of Health and Human Services. 2016. *International Compilation of Human Research Standards*, 2016 Edition. Available at http://www.hhs .gov/ohrp/international/index.html. Accessed February 29, 2016.

Provenzano AM, Graber LK, Elansary M, Khoshnood K, Rastegar A, Barry M. 2010. Short-term global health research projects by U.S. medical students: Ethical challenges for partnerships. *Am J Trop Med Hyg* 83(2): 211–14.

Shah SK, Nodell B, Montano SM, Behrens C, Zunt JR. 2011. Clinical research and global health: Mentoring the next generation of health care students. *Glob Public Health* 6(3): 234–46.

U.S. Code of Federal Regulations. 2009. Title 45, Part 46, Federal Policy for the Protection of Human Subjects. http://www.hhs.gov/ohrp/humansubjects/commonrule/

Wallace LJ and Webb A. 2014. Pre-departure training and the social accountability of international medical electives. *Educ Health* 27(2): 143–47.

MOVING ON

Chapter 25

Returning Home: Debriefing and Managing Reverse Culture Shock

Kevin Chan

Contents

The global health experience doesn't finish when your project is complete. There are important elements that include debriefing and managing reverse culture shock that are as important as the project itself, and if managed correctly enhance the global health experience.

Debriefing is the 'Skilled facilitation of an in-depth conversation' and 'is an important dimension of education in the health professions' (Bender and Walker, 2013). The purpose of debriefing, in general, is to help facilitate a structured conversation about one's experience with an expert facilitator to help guide learning to help stimulate future practice. Nauzley Abedini, in 'Shades Off', highlights that reflection on one's practice in a global health experience, both during the experience and afterwards, presents an opportunity to become more immersed in the global health experience and provides an opportunity to learn lessons going forwards, both in global health and in one's career (Abedini, 2016).

Debriefing after a global health experience is as important as preparing to go abroad. For first-time global health participants, re-entry back home is underappreciated as a stressful part of the project. Global health debriefing requires two core components: (1) debriefing with host participants and (2) debriefing upon return home.

Over the past decade, debriefing has been increasingly used by programs and projects to ensure feedback is provided to host organizations and to provide information for future participants in international projects. Debriefing is also used to ensure participants adjust and reintegrate back home, while minimizing reverse culture shock. Debriefing should provide support and counselling if the experience was negative, but should also excite, challenge and provide an opportunity to learn, if the experience was positive. Although there is a paucity of literature on debriefing in global health, the few articles looking at debriefing see it as a beneficial and essential component of a global health experience, if formalized (Evans et al., 2013; Purkey and Hollar, 2016), but it may result in long-term emotional challenges if not done well (Balmer, 2016).

Bender and Walker highlight one conceptual model of debriefing, in which there are components of a welcome, check-in, debrief and check-out (Bender and Walker, 2013). Purkey and Hollar highlighted that there were five key components: evaluation of elective, experience, knowledge translation, review of health and safety, and reintegration (Purkey and Hollar, 2016).

Debriefing Starts in Your Host Country

One of the most important things to do at the end of a global health project or experience is to provide feedback to your global health hosts, especially before you go home. Often, we forget that we're a guest abroad. Spending time thanking hosts and providing appropriate, culturally sensitive feedback may help improve long-term relationships and improve projects abroad.

At the start of the project, you should make it clear to the hosts that you'd like time to be set aside during the project and at the end of project to provide mutual feedback in order to discuss what worked well in the project and what elements could be improved. Taking your hosts out to dinner and providing small gifts especially from home often go a long way in cementing friendships and partnerships (Table 25.1).

Table 25.1 Potential Topics to Discuss in Debriefing on a Project with Host Partners

• Orientation in-country to the project
• Expectations on both sides – what were achieved and what gaps were not met

• Accommodations and lodging
  • Housing
  • Food, cooking facilities
  • Recreational opportunities

• Travelling within country
• Financial considerations
• Cross-cultural experiences   • If applicable, experience with translators

• Personnel and staff
  • Interpersonal interactions
  • Strengths and weaknesses

• Specifics about the project   • Things that could be improved
• Elements (equipment, personnel, restructuring of relationships) that would strengthen the project

Debriefing Back Home

Prior to going abroad, make an appointment with your advisor to discuss your global health experience upon your return home. Preferably, this is someone with global health experience who can help you sort through your emotional, cultural and spiritual experience. You might also begin this process while in-country to process such experiences with weekly e-mails to a preceptor or alumnus of your program (Table 25.2).

Table 25.2 Potential Topics to Discuss in Debriefing with Your Advisor

• Pre-departure orientation
  • What were its strengths and weakness to help prepare you for the project?
  • What suggestions would you make to make the experience better?
  • Did you have enough training with regard to personal safety, health, language, cultural competences and ethics? Was this training sufficient?

• Logistics
  • Travel to the country
  • Travel within country
  • Housing/accommodations
  • Packing checklist – correct?

• Was in-country orientation sufficient and appropriate?
• Why did you want to go on the elective? Have the reasons changed after having gone there?
• What cross-cultural experiences did you have? Were your belief systems challenged? How has this changed your view on equity and justice issues and evidence-based medicine? Was it what you were expecting? What things were unexpected and novel? Did it scare you or excite you? What memory stands out for you?
• How would you evaluate the location? Was it safe? Did it have appropriate facilities for a global health experience?
• What type of partnerships did you build personally and professionally? With whom did you have the strongest connections? Were you able to share with others to make this a two-way exchange?
• How was your interaction with the hosts? Were there any problems with staff? Colleagues? Fellow travellers? Did you feel that you were part of the community?
• Did you have enough funds to do what you wanted to do at the host site?
• How do you feel about your impact on those with whom you worked? How did you ensure that you were not a drain on the system? Did you feel that you were impeding the training of local medical students and health professionals?

• What were the strengths and weaknesses of the global health experience?
  • If clinical, did you get the clinical exposure that you hoped to get? Did you have appropriate supervision?
  • If research, did you have the appropriate support structures in place to get the research done?
  • If public health/community oriented, did you have appropriate access to the community leaders and to voices of interest?

• What advice would you provide for future groups interested in going to this site?

Reducing Reverse Culture Shock

As discussed in Chapter 10, 'Culture shock is a sense of confusion and uncertainty sometimes with feelings of anxiety that may affect people exposed to an alien culture or environment without adequate preparation'. Reverse culture shock takes place when we return to our culture of origin after growing accustomed to a new culture – the issues of re-entry back into your home environment sometimes are as big a problem (Balmer et al., 2015; Uehara, 1986; Westwood et al., 1986).

It's important to spend time preparing to go home. It's common to want to spend more time abroad and to not want to go home. One of my first global health experiences was in rural Africa. When I returned home, there were many elements I wasn't used to, from the speed of the cars travelling by, looking the wrong way for traffic (they drive on the left side of the road in English Africa), to issues that I wanted to talk about and my friends really didn't really want to hear.

It's also not unusual to have a 'hero' syndrome – where you feel that you can 'fix' things in a locale abroad and why isn't everyone interested in helping your cause? It's easy for us to get frustrated when returning to a high-resource context to see waste and materialism in our home communities and workplaces. When you get little or no response, it isn't unusual to get frustrated with people back home.

As the Uehara (1986) study noted, the change in values often prompts reverse culture shock. However, at the same time, these transformative processes in the global health experience may be the impetus that allows us to affect change. Finding people with similar experiences or who are willing to listen can reduce the reverse culture shock experience. Taking the time to explore one's feeling and perspectives may go a long way to enhancing your own global health experience, the experience of others and your relationships with your hosts aboard (Table 25.3).

Time for Reflection

Throughout your global health experience and upon returning home, a useful thing to do is to set aside time to reflect. This can be done as a self-reflective exercise, reflection with an advisor, friend or colleague and/or in group format. It is important to look at things that you learnt while you spent time abroad. Included in these lessons are both the 'good' experiences and the 'bad' experiences (see the section 'About the "Bad" Experience') (Table 25.4).

Table 25.3   Elements to Help Reduce Reverse Culture Shock

• Spend some time in the country enjoying activities/culture/fun things before going home. Just like you should give yourself some time to adjust to a new country during orientation, you should give yourself some time to adjust to going home.
• Give yourself time prior to return to normal activities. Don't fly home and return to school or to work the next day. Provide an appropriate adjustment period.
• Reflection (see the section 'Time for Reflection') is an essential element to reducing culture shock. Being aware of how the experience has affected you both positively and negatively can help reduce culture shock.
• Take a token of the culture home. It may be a sculpture, music, literature or some other aspect of culture.
• Teaching and disseminating the experience is a great way to help reduce culture shock.
• Do something you enjoy when you return home!

Table 25.4 Potential Topics for Reflection

• If you're with a group, it's very useful to get together to discuss the good and bad parts of a project together, over dinner or coffee.
• Writing down your thoughts in a notebook or in a journal is often extremely therapeutic.
• Identify any ethical challenges, your reactions (both good and bad) to certain situations, and how you dealt with these challenges.
• Looking at what the 'ideal' experience is and how that could be constructively achieved is often very helpful.
• Look at your personal reactions to situations while abroad and upon return to home. In particular, many global health participants may find themselves 'in-between' cultures, and find that they see increasing problems with their own home culture.
• Be cognizant of how the experience changes you as a person.
• If the experience was conducted individually, it's useful to be able to talk to someone (can be an advisor, a friend or a colleague with global health experience).
• How will you keep this global health experience alive? What subjects would you like to learn more about and explore?

Some of my most experienced global health colleagues will phone me up after a mission to talk about their issues while abroad. Sometimes, they need that ability to express their frustrations or challenges while having someone be supportive and non-judgmental.

About the 'Bad' Experience

In global health, things change constantly. Sometimes, the global health experience doesn't follow expectations – logistics don't work out, the project plans don't come through or a supervisor gets sick or they're not available. Or worse, something catastrophic may happen – you get sick or are in a car accident and it aborts your elective.

One of my most frustrating experiences was as a resident. I went to a country to teach pediatrics to find the main university/teaching hospital on strike for 8 of the 9 weeks I was there. Instead, we did pediatric clinics around the country. But there were days when I did next to nothing.

Every global health experience, including the 'bad experience', is an opportunity to learn and grow from. You may learn the value of politics and socio-economic status and other social determinants of health and how big a role they play on healthcare itself. You may work on projects and other endeavours that were not part of your original medical objectives. Often, other opportunities arise that can fill your time.

If the truly catastrophic event occurs, it's the optimal time to re-evaluate if you really want to do global health. But at the same time, it's important to reflect on what went wrong, and if there was anything in advance that could have prepared you better to the challenges that you faced.

It's also important to feed that back to your global health advisor and/or programs.

The challenge is to be objective to try and find out what the issues are, and how these can be addressed. In particular, what is the problem? Logistics? Personnel? Safety issues? Language? Attitudinal? Something else? A self-reflective process would provide a lens to reflect on the issues and perhaps provide a solution.

One of the toughest elements after a 'bad' experience is to objectively evaluate if the project/program should continue or not. Major projects may be discontinued with a single 'bad' experience. It's important to have this discussion with your advisor and teams.

Disseminating Information to Future Groups

If the global health experience is to continue in future years, it's important to disseminate information to future individuals or groups that may be continuing with this global health experience. Dinners or after-school talks are very useful. Being part of the next participating individual's or group's orientation also provides a very helpful handover of information and acts as a way of disseminating and imparting knowledge (Table 25.5).

Conclusion

Debriefing is an important element of any global health project and opportunity. It's important to have the opportunity to express, verbalize and synthesize what has occurred after a global health experience. Debriefing begins with partners abroad and should be formalized with an advisor upon returning home.

Debriefing is an important component in reducing culture shock and requires time for reflection, especially after a bad experience (Table 25.6).

Finally, it's important to disseminate information to future groups on an on-going project.

Table 25.5 Disseminating Information to Future Groups

• Logistics
  • Travel to the country
  • Travel within country
  • Housing/accommodations

• Cross-cultural experiences
• Personal health

• Interactions with hosts
  • Key contacts and informants
  • Awareness of interactions

• If clinical
  • Support personnel
  • Key diseases/challenges
    • Preparation and/or information sources to understand key diseases/challenges

• If research
  • Key research equipment, support
  • Research knowledge required to go abroad

• If public health/community oriented
  • Key personnel/community leaders
  • Experiences/challenges/opportunities in community

• Anecdotal stories are important to provide about the challenges and opportunities that lie ahead for the next group

Table 25.6   Debriefing Write-Up (A Short-Form Feedback for the Global Health Experience)

A. General
Please provide a detailed description of the project/learning experience that you partook in, including the following sections (maximum 500 characters per section):
Project information:
Project title
Region (drop-down list: North America, Latin America and the Carribbean, Europe, Middle East and North Africa, sub-Saharan Africa, Asia, Asia-Pacific)
Country
Location city or rural
Type of opportunity (drop-down list: Pre-clinical, clinical, research, other. If other, please specify)
Participant Information:
First name
Last name
Approximate total cost of the elective
General breakdown in terms of transportation, accommodation, food, outings, etc.
Duration of experience (include start and end date)
Hours worked per week
Organization information
Name of organization hospital/clinic
Description of site: Address, postal/zip code, phone number, e-mail address, fax number, website
Medical superintendent and supervisor: Minimum time commitment, availability (time of year)
B. Project Evaluation
Please describe your experience, including the following sections (maximum of 350 words per section). Responses may be in point form, if easier.
1. Please evaluate the organization you worked with regarding their planning, reliability and the appropriateness of the tasks assigned to you. Why did you choose this organization?
What did you like about your elective experience? What did you not like?
Explain the level of professional support you received on your elective (a nurse, doctor, etc.).

(*Continued*)

Table 25.6 (*Continued*)   Debriefing Write-Up (A Short-Form Feedback for the Global Health Experience)

Did you perceive that you made any negative or positive impacts on the organization you worked with (e.g. resources used, exchange of information)? Would you go with the organization again and why?
1. Did you struggle with any issues while on elective, and what support would be desirable? Specifically, did you struggle with any cultural, language, safety, personal health or ethical issues? If yes, do you feel you would have benefited from further pre-departure training addressing these issues, and if so, what type of training?
Do you feel you would have benefited from having an 'on-call' faculty contact back home to liaise with in order to help resolve safety, ethical or medical issues that arose during your experience? Were things urgent? Would e-mail with 24-hour turnaround time be sufficient?
Would you be interested in attending a debriefing session in which students can get together, eat, chat and share their travel experiences?
C. Logistics
Please provide information on the logistics of your elective, including the following sections (maximum 1250 characters per section):
Main language spoken:
Other languages:
Was there translation facility available? If so, how much did it cost, and who absorbed the cost?
Travel arrangements
• How did you get there?
• What was the cost from airport, cost of local internal transportation?
• How often did you have to use local transportation?
Religion/gender
• Were there any differences from home in appropriate behaviour between genders (especially with respect to dress code)?
• Which religious groups were dominant in the country? Any issues between religious groups?
• How about sexual orientation?
Housing details
• What type of housing did you live in? What was the cost? How close was it to the hospital? Who managed your accommodation?

References

Abedini, Nauzley. 2016. Shades off. In *Reflection in Global Health: An Anthology*, eds. Thuy Bui et al. San Francisco, CA: Global Health Collaborations Press, pp. 4–6.

Balmer, Dorene F., Stephanie Marton, Susan L Gillespie et al. 2015. Reentry to pediatric residency after global health experiences. *Pediatrics.* 136: 680–686.

Bender, Amy and Pamela Walker. 2013. The obligation of debriefing in global health education. *Med Teach.* 35: 1027–1034, accessed October 9, 2016, 10.3109/0142159X.2012.733449.

Evans, Rachel, Catherine Dotchin and Richard Walker. 2013. Maximising the value from the elective experience: Post-elective workshops. *Clin Teach.* 10: 362–367, accessed October 9, 2016. 10.1111/tct.12033.

Purkey, Eva and Gwendolyn Hollar. 2016. Developing consensus for postgraduate global health electives: Definitions, pre-departure training, and post-return debriefing. *BMC Med Educ.* 16: 159, accessed October 9, 2016, 10.1186/s12909-016-0675-4.

Uehara, Asako. 1986. The nature of American student reentry adjustment and perception of the sojourn experience. *Int J Intercult Relat.* 10: 415–438.

Westwood, Marvin J, W. Scott Lawrence, and David Paul. 1986. Preparing for re-entry: A program for the sojourning student. *Int J Adv Couns.* 9: 221–230.

Chapter 26

Moving Forward

Neil Arya and Carolyn Beukeboom

Contents

Well now that you're back, you want to get 'more involved' in global health? Some of you just want to stay in touch, be informed, work with underserved populations at home or advocate for change, while others wish to pursue further education, consider going on short-term trips or do more long-term work.

Carolyn's Journey

There are different paths you might choose, each with various pauses and different endings. My passage is an example of a global health career journey, with different forks in the road I have taken, and is still unfinished. I hope that in following me back and forth through several phases in terms of experiences – hands-on, supervisory, development, health promotion, humanitarian assistance, research and education – and through further education in global health, tropical medicine, nurse practitioner (NP) and most recently a Master's of Science in Public Health, that you get a sense of the challenges and realities of life working overseas along with options combining international work with work at home.

Initiation of a Global Health Journey

For as long as I can remember, I have wanted to care for others in a developing country; I thus chose to become a nurse. During my third year of university, I applied for MedOutreach, a student-run organization for nursing and medical students to go to West Africa, and was thrilled when I was one of eight chosen for this experience. Two weeks into my first trip I remember feeling anxious and wondering how I ever thought that this could be a life vocation. We lived in a basic house with occasional electricity, minimal running water and poor sanitation. Out of fear of illness, I was reluctant to eat or drink anything apart from soda – luckily I had brought a large jar of peanut butter with me. The large spiders, the malaria-carrying mosquitoes, and the rats and mice were more than an irritation and became a constant fear. But, by the end of the 6 weeks, as I got to learn more about the local culture, make friends with locals and experience the basic healthcare system, I knew that I was interested in going beyond what this opportunity afforded me. Shortly after my return to Canada, my family went to a warehouse sale in Toronto – I remember feeling overwhelmed, almost suffocated by the consumerism and wealth. I could never be the same again.

Short- and Long-Term Work Experiences

After I completed my degree, I decided to work as a casual nurse in the hospital, so I had the opportunity to do a few 2–3 week missions to Central America. I also started to volunteer with an organization in my city that sponsors families and children in India. One day, the director of this organization approached me to offer an opportunity to help in various children's homes in India along with spending a couple of months working at Mother Teresa's homes, fulfilling a dream come true, as I had always admired Mother Teresa and longed to work with her.

Following other shorter-term missions, I chose an experience with a faith-based organization focused on development in the Andes, where I lived and worked for the next 3 years. I prepared through a 4-month program that involved workshops in cross-cultural skills, social justice issues, interfaith dialogue, theology, conflict management, adult education and self-awareness (communication skills, Myers Briggs test, stress management, etc.). I spent 5 months for Spanish language training living with a local family in a different South American country. For 2 years, I did not return to Canada. When I went back for my final year, I discovered that with better knowledge of the area, more connections and local friends, this would be my most productive and rewarding year.

These 3 years abroad taught me much about learning a new culture and language, conflict management and communication skills, as well as how to approach ethical dilemmas, for all of which I felt the benefits of the 4-month orientation program prior to departure.

Seeking New Skills

During my final year, having been frustrated at being the only medical provider in remote rural villages, I felt a need to expand my healthcare knowledge and skills and decided to return to school in Canada to become a NP. Though I had been to Liverpool for a 3-week Tropical Medicine course for nurses, this course was not as useful as I thought in the Andes. Only years later when I went to Africa did the benefits of that training become practical.

Balancing Work Opportunities at Home and Abroad

After receiving my NP certification, I decided to work at a community health center with patients who were new immigrants and refugees, had mental health issues, were impoverished or suffered from addiction. My prior overseas experiences, and in particular my Spanish language skills, helped me in this position. I could appreciate the new immigrants and refugees who come to this country with limited language skills and different cultural views, including sense of time, dress, privacy, food, and so on. Sometimes, I had even been to their countries and seen the devastating effects of poverty and war.

Through scoping out opportunities on the Internet, speaking to friends and acquaintances who had worked abroad, being attuned to e-mail invitations and attending evening educational sessions on working abroad through the university, I was presented with several unique opportunities. Flexible management and a collaborative colleague with whom I job-shared permitted me to be away for prolonged periods. I was able to take 3 weeks to go to Asia after an earthquake for disaster relief with direct hands-on care, working with healthcare professionals from all over the world. I worked in various capacities overseas: in a supervisory role with a well-known humanitarian assistance organization in the Horn of Africa for 9 months; hands-on care in a human immunodeficiency virus (HIV)/acquired immune deficiency syndrome (AIDS) clinic in South Africa for 5 months and short-term experiences in health promotion and education in South America.

This is not to say that each of these experiences was easy. There were challenges and stresses along the way. Especially having worked for long periods overseas, at one point, I lost a sense of where I belonged. My family and many of my friends had moved on in life, but I wanted these relationships with them to remain the same when I returned. Following some of my experiences abroad, witnessing poverty, suffering and sometimes hopelessness, I felt burnt out, lonely, depressed and demoralized. Family and friends could scarcely understand, and often wanted to hear only so much. The importance of seeking out others who had journeyed with me was very beneficial to debrief all that I had endured.

Moving on from Clinical Care – Need for New Skills in Research and Health Education

As my personal situation changed, more recently I sought out shorter-term opportunities. I now wanted to explore the bigger picture, to be involved in projects, research and educational ventures. I chose to do a Masters in Science in Public Health from the London School of Hygiene and Tropical Medicine – a program chosen for its reputation for international work. Since I had conducted a research project looking at the nutritional status of refugee children coming to Canada during my masters, I was offered an opportunity to evaluate a project implemented in West Africa through a reputable organization. With my knowledge of the region, I was asked to be part of a university-based development project teaching health promoters in the Andes. Opportunities have come through personal connections – those whom I know recommending me, relaying opportunities or mere chance meetings, through reading or via conferences. I now have a better understanding of the pros and cons of overseas work and the potential harms that could result, thus carefully choosing the organizations and people I work with.

Learning about the Broader Picture of Global Health

So how about you? Even if you would like minimal engagement in global health, you may still wish to read more on the culture, language, political situation or political economy and history of specific locations where you have been or wish to visit. Though your activities may be primarily medical or healthcare-related, reading more about poverty, bioethics, war and peace, social justice, public health and the environment, trying to understand aid, social entrepreneurship, international financial institutions, philanthropy and medical anthropology will only increase your appreciation of global health. This is what guided us. Such knowledge can be gained through non-fiction books, textbooks, websites, journals and conferences.

General Books

A few of our favourite non-fiction works:

Anthropology: *Infections and Inequalities*, Paul Farmer
Economics: *Dying for Growth*, Jim Kim (poverty debt); *Banker to the Poor*, Muhammad Yunus
Aid: *Dead Aid*, Dambisa Moyo; *End of Poverty*, Jeffrey Sachs; *When Helping Hurts*, Steve Corbett (religious perspective); *The Trouble with Africa – Why Foreign Aid Is Not Working*, Robert Calderissi
War: *War and Public Health*, Vic Sidel and Barry Levy; *Damned Nations*, Samantha Nutt
Humanitarian Assistance: *An Imperfect Offering*, James Orbinski
Societal Development: *Guns, Germs and Steel* and *Collapse*, Jared Diamond
Ecology: *Our Common Future*, http://www.un-documents.net/our-common-future.pdf; World Watch's annual *State of the World*, http://www.worldwatch.org/bookstore
Epidemiology: *The Wisdom of Whores: Bureaucrats, Brothels and the Business of AIDS*, Elizabeth Pisani

Global Health Texts

You might just want to understand global health better and just get a textbook rather than take a course. A few possibilities: Seear's *An Introduction to International Health Scholars*, Second Edition, reflects on issues related to foreign aid and development, including water and sanitation, primary care, developmental goals and human rights and understanding measurements such as disability-adjusted life years (DALYs); Lindstrand et al., *Global Health: An Introductory Textbook* (Professional Publishing, 2006), with Hans Rosling, famous for TED Talks, has illustrations related to Rosling's Gapminder; Skolnik's *Global Health 101*, Second Edition (Jones & Bartlett, 2012) is more structured and amenable as an introductory text; while Birn, Pillay and Holtz's *Textbook of International Health*, Third Edition (Oxford University Press, 2009) about to be published in 2017 as the *Textbook of Global Health*, Fourth Edition, includes historical, cultural, environmental, economic and political determinants of global health. For those interested in ecological issues, Brown et al., *Supporting Global Ecological Integrity in Public Health* (Earthscan, 2005), may be of special interest.

Websites

Some websites with interesting comparative stats:

Global Burden of Disease (*GBD*), http://www.healthdata.org/gbd, the largest and most comprehensive effort to measure epidemiological levels and trends worldwide, is headed by Chris Murray of the Institute for Health Metrics and Evaluation at the University of Washington, and funded by the Bill and Melinda Gates Foundation.

Gapminder, http://www.gapminder.org/, provides tools to analyze world statistics in easy graphics, founded by Hans Rosling of TED Talks fame, who is a Swedish medical doctor, statistician, and professor of International Health at Karolinska Institutet

Human Development Reports of UNDP, http://hdr.undp.org/en: The Human Development Index (HDI), co-founded by Indian economist Amartya Sen, is a composite statistic of life expectancy, education and per capita income, indicators which are used to rank countries into four tiers of human development. The United Nations Development Program issues annual and regional reports.

Global Goals for Sustainable Development SDGs, http://www.globalgoals.org/, follow on the Millennium Development Goals.

Journals

The Lancet and *Lancet Global Health* have many articles on global health issues. In addition, *BMJ*, *NEJM* and *JAMA* occasionally offer interesting articles in relation to global health. Although public health literature, especially *Global Public Health*, includes many more, *Social Science and Medicine* can have relevant articles related to humanities and the larger context. Don't forget development journals such as the *New Internationalist*; or political ones such as *Foreign Affairs* and *Foreign Policy*, the *Economist*; ones concentrating on conflict such as *Medicine, Conflict and Survival*, the online *Conflict and Health* or newspapers such as the *Guardian*.

Conferences

Conferences offer excellent places to not only expand your knowledge in the area of global health but also connect with people who have similar interests and (who knows?) may one day provide unique opportunities for you in the global health world.

The following organizations have annual conferences:

Global Health Council, http://globalhealth.org/; *Consortium of Universities for Global Health* (*CUGH*), http://www.cugh.org/ (related to educators); the *Canadian Society for International Health* (*CSIH*) (including policy, governmental and international organizations), http://www.csih.org/en/; *Unite for Sight*, http://www.uniteforsight.org/ (related to technology, entrepreneurship and students); *Mt. Sinai*, http://www.arnholdinstitute.org/ (focused on Global Health Offices and local/global linkages) and the Western Regional International Health Conference at the University of Washington (focused on students conducting research).

Discipline-specific organizations such as the the *World Organization of Family Doctors* (*WONCA*), http://www.globalfamilydoctor.com/; *American Public Health Association*, https://www.apha.org/; the *American Society of Tropical Medicine and Hygiene*, http://www.astmh.org/; the *International AIDS Conference*, http://www.iasociety.org/conferences each may have conferences where you can make wonderful contacts.

And let us put a plug in for our biennial PEGASUS Conference on PEace, Global health (local and international) And SUStainability, www.pegasusconference.ca, which brings together students, researchers, educators, practitioners, advocates and policymakers biennially to Toronto with a transdisciplinary approach to global challenges.

Considering a Career

Working abroad can be very rewarding, but also challenging, as you balance family and financial considerations, career development or maintaining a job in your own country with living abroad or getting time off work, and navigating between two (or more) countries and cultures. How will you engage family members and maintain friendships and relations in the process?

When pursuing a career in global health in your own country or abroad, you'll first need to consider what type of work interests you. This could be academic, advocacy, field work, research, consultation or evaluation; it could be in disaster relief, humanitarian aid or development; it might be short 2-week stints or more long term, up to several years; positions might be paid, stipended with expenses or volunteer.

Often various experiences abroad will be required to understand more fully the 'bigger' picture or to provide you the contacts required to expand your own interests. Having a mentor who has 'been there' or seeking out people who have taken similar paths will be beneficial. Networking, connecting with others in the field, may sometimes lead to opportunities when you least expect them.

Skills to Work

Perhaps you wish to gain more skills to return to a low- and middle-income country (LMIC) or to work domestically with those marginalized in high-income countries (HICs). So what are these skills, and how do you obtain them? In global health, your tasks might include developing, enabling, facilitating, managing, monitoring, researching or evaluating healthcare projects or programs to improve determinants of health, to strengthen systems or benefit local health systems. Whether you see yourself as an educator, outreach person or a volunteer in some capacity, each may require different skill sets. Some of you are thinking of humanitarian aid/emergency relief, where logisticians with specific skills to deal with crises are as important as professionals in healthcare, public health, nutrition or infectious disease. After the acute phase, development will involve public health, water, sanitation, agriculture, along with mechanical and civil engineering specialties. Whatever the task, before making the decision to go, reflect on what, with your current skill set, you really have to offer compared to the resources you may consume. You might also think a bit more about the value of other, less trained professionals with whom you have worked and what they can accomplish with a little training, should you decide to return.

What does a global health generalist need? Jogerst, working with the Consortium of Universities for Global Health, identified eight domains for a global citizen level (Jogerst et al., 2015). These included (1) global burden of disease, (2) globalization of health and healthcare, (3) social and environmental determinants of health, (4) collaboration, partnering and communication, (5) ethics, (6) professional practice, (7) health equity and social justice and (8) sociocultural and political awareness. Three other domains for the basic operational program-oriented level included capacity strengthening, program management and strategic analysis. These competencies were partly based on other work in public health (Ablah et al., 2014), medicine (Arthur et al., 2011) and nursing (Wilson et al., 2012).

Medical teachers or professional program leaders, particularly in academia, may be interested in two comprehensive books co-edited by Jessica Evert freely available on the web. The first on undergraduate health professional training *Developing Global Health Programming: A Guidebook for Medical Schools Developing Global Health Programming*, First Edition and *A Guidebook for Medical and Professional Schools Developing Global Health Programming*, Second Edition (Evert et al., 2014), has sections on the global health landscape, program structures and content, competencies, ethics, local global health, interdisciplinarity, advocacy, teamwork and networking. *Global Health Training in Graduate Medical Education: A Guidebook,* First Edition (Evert et al., 2008), and the Second Edition (Chase and Evert, 2011) includes profiles of existing programs for residency, fellowship and organizations for work later.

If you are doing community health work, the Hesperian series (http://hesperian.org/), which began with *Where There Is No Doctor,* may be appropriate. For those engaging in primary care, clinical care books such as Brett D. Nelson's *Essential Clinical Global Health* (Wiley, 2015) is more comprehensive, including specifics about pathology; or perhaps you might get a better understanding of infectious diseases through an *Oxford Handbook of Tropical Medicine* or Heymann's *Control of Communicable Diseases*. Remember that many countries are now going through a demographic transition and non-communicable diseases may play a larger role.

Education and Training

So maybe you need more training? What training is offered by universities, and what is sought by employers? Medical personnel may find clinical or research global health fellowships in emergency medicine, family medicine, internal medicine, pediatrics, women's health and surgery, involving domestic and international experiences and graduate-level coursework (Nelson et al., 2012).

Masters programs in epidemiology, public health, infectious diseases and global health offered by Harvard, Johns Hopkins and the London School of Hygiene & Tropical Medicine (LSHTM) are the most well known internationally oriented programs, but can be quite expensive. Depending on your current life situation, some offer programs at a distance, although these may not allow you the interactions and connections you would like. Shorter specific courses in Tropical Medicine for healthcare providers are taught in Liverpool and at LSHTM (usually 3-week or 3-month programs). Organizations such as the International Committee of the Red Cross (ICRC), World Health Organization (WHO) and Médecins Sans Frontières (MSF) offer their own training orientations to humanitarian aid work. SPHERE training is for those interested in humanitarian assistance and disaster relief response.

There may be opportunities for funding of mid-career post-doctoral fellowships or visiting scholar posts or work through governmental, international and private agencies focusing on global citizenship and scientific and cultural exchange, as well as development, civil society organizations, academic, private sector and professional associations.

Health professionals might even consider training beyond clinical provision and public health, to strengthening health systems, to disciplines in the social sciences such as developmental studies and human rights or law, business and administration, whose graduate degrees may be more useful for health systems work, disaster relief activities, policy reform, research and program management. Certificates in each of the aforementioned may also be possible.

Philanthropic organizations such as the *Bill and Melinda Gates Foundation,* http://www.gatesfoundation.org/, the largest private foundation in the world, funds healthcare with a goal to improve health through technology and reduce poverty; the *Rockefeller Foundation*, https://www .rockefellerfoundation.org/, funds projects in a variety of disciplines and the *Wellcome Trust*, https:// wellcome.ac.uk/, a biomedical research charity, will support research and delivery. *Grand Challenges in Global Health*, http://grandchallenges.org/; the *Population Council*, http://www.popcouncil.org/, and the U.S. Agency for International Development (USAID) may each fund evidence-informed ventures strengthening health education and delivery with public and private partnerships.

Several programs are modelled after the *Peace Corps Global Health Service Partnership*, https:// www.peacecorps.gov/volunteer/is-peace-corps-right-for-me/global-health-service-partnership/: fellowships from the Fogarty International Center of the U.S. National Institutes of Health (NIH) such as the *Global Health Program for Fellows and Scholars*, https://www.fic.nih.gov/Programs/ Pages/scholars-fellows-global-health.aspx, or *Global Health Corps*, http://ghcorps.org/. Fogarty also has a directory which lists non-NIH funding opportunities (award programs, open funding grants, travel awards and fellowships) for pre-doctoral/graduate students, post-doctoral students, faculty and health professionals. Such formative experiences and mentor networks can help transition to long-term employment opportunities. Internships might be available through organizations such as the WHO. You might consider volunteer service provision, education, technical assistance, and community development with NGOs such as *Voluntary Service Overseas*, https:// www.vsointernational.org/, or *CUSO*, http://www.cusointernational .org/.

Organizations to Consider for a Global Health Career

You may wish to explore research and academic institutions, international agencies, including non-governmental, multilateral and governmental agencies. Once again, whether or not you have a healthcare background, you might also think of work on service delivery, financing, governance, health workforce, health information systems and supply management systems. New organizations have sprung up dealing with climate change, vaccines and medicines, immigrant/refugee health, health professional education and the innovations of social entrepreneurship.

Governmental aid and research agencies include *AusAID*, http://dfat.gov.au/aid/pages/australias-aid-program.aspx; *Australian Research Council (ARC)*, http://www.arc.gov.au/; *Canadian Institutes of Health Research (CIHR)*, http://www.cihr-irsc.gc.ca/e/193.html; *Centers for Disease Control and Prevention (CDC)*, https://www.cdc.gov/; *Department for International Development (DFID)*, https:// www.gov.uk/government/organisations/department-for-international-development; *European Research Council (ERC)*, https://erc.europa.eu/; NIH, https://www.nih.gov/; and *USAID,* https://www.usaid. gov/, and many of these have postings on their organizational websites. The CDC website, for instance, allows you to explore jobs by topic area, including HIV/AIDS, measles, sanitation and hygiene, security, vaccination and water. CDC Global Health vacancies might fit epidemiologists, public health advisors, health scientists and medical officers.

You might consider the United Nations and subsidiary agencies of its UN Economic and Social Council, including the United Nations Children's Fund (UNICEF), United Nations Population Fund (UNFPA) and the United Nations Development Program (UNDP), United Nations Department of Humanitarian Affairs (including the World Food Programme [WFP]), UN High Commissioner for Refugees (UNHCR) and Food and Agricultural Organization (FAO), the World Health Organization and its member nations. The World Bank is a similar intergovernmental agency. Their respective websites should provide a search tool for current job openings and contacts for internships.

Bilateral agencies, non-governmental organizations, and faith-based organizations, including *World Vision and Catholic Relief Services, Oxfam, International Rescue Committee, CARE, Save the Children, Partners In Health*, www.pih.org/, PATH (Program for Appropriate Technology in Health), www.path.org/. may be worth exploring.

Books to Guide Your Career Search

One of our authors, Canadian pediatrician Kevin Chan, is an editor of Drain, Huffman, Pirtle and Chan, *Caring for the World: A Guidebook to Global Health Opportunities* (University of Toronto Press, 2009), which has practical resources for those seeking global health careers. Its pearls of wisdom about the global health landscape include websites and contact information for language courses, conferences, organizations and universities. Oxford's *Working in International Health* by Maïa Gedde, Susana Edjang and Kate Mandeville, part of the Successes in Medicine Series (2011 paperback), http://ukcatalogue.oup.com/product/9780199600717.do, may be of interest to professionals in international development, particularly in program management. 'How-to' texts on general international work include Jean-Marc Hachey's *The BIG* (1600 pages!) *Guide to Living and Working Overseas* (2004), which has Canadian and international resources, articles and stories, organizational profiles related to internships, volunteer work, study vacation, short-term diplomatic missions, private sector and non-health jobs, awards and education. Though the book has been around for two decades, Hachey, a political scientist and leading expert on global health careers, now has a website and is marketing to general undergraduate university students in Canada through *MyWorldAbroad*, http://myworldabroad.com/. Osborne and Ohmans' *Finding Work in Global Health: A Practical Guide* (Health Advocate's Press, 2005) is directed to job seekers. Edward O'Neill's *A Practical Guide to Global Health Service* (AMA, 2006), concentrates on health and safety but, other than a little discussion on the importance of culture, really doesn't address preparation. It does, however, include general reflections and profiles of 300 organizations. Mark Wilson's *The Medic's Guide to Work and Electives around the World*, Second Edition (CRC Press, 2009), http://www.medicstravel .co.uk/ Medics_Guide_To_Work_and_Electives_Around_The_World/The_Medics_Guide_to_Work_ and_Electives_Around_the_World.htm, is meant to be a 'Lonely Planet' for electives, in particular for British medical students, and includes information on different types of electives around the world in both the developed and developing worlds. While it includes small bits on preparation, personal safety, health prophylaxis, and so on, by focusing on specific countries (Global Health North and South), accommodation and contacts, this work may lack in aspects of general preparation. Funding opportunities mentioned seem more relevant to Europe.

Job Support and Specific Listings

University-based departments of global health support career development through job counselling, advice on building resumes, provide resources to develop interview skills and organize career fairs to link students with alumni. Web job postings in development, health, governance and legal reform, education, program administration, environmental, engineering and computer system support may be found at sites such as *GlobalHealthHub*, http://www .globalhealthhub.org/jobs-grants-listings/; *Akili Initiative*, http://www.mappinghealth.com/akili/; *Global Health Trials*, https://globalhealthtrials.tghn.org/research-careers/jobs/; PublicHealth.org; idealist.org; devex.org; globalhealthjobs.co.uk; *International Career Employment Weekly*, http:// www.internationaljobs.org/contents.html; the *Guardian,* jobs https://jobs.theguardian.com/; *Jobs4Development*, http://www.jobs4development.com/; *DevNetJobs*, http://www.devnetjobs.org/ and *SciDevNet*, http://www.scidev.net/global/content/jobs.htm.

Conclusion

Whatever the nature of level of engagement at this time or in the future, whatever your personal circumstances or profession, we wish you a successful journey and hope that this volume may be a resource, now and for years to come, to help you on this voyage.

References

Ablah E, Biberman DA, Weist EM, Buekens P, Bentley ME, Burke D, Finnegan JR, Flahault JA, Frenk J, Gotsch AR, Klag MJ, Rodriguez Lopez MH, Nasca P, Shortell S, Spencer HC. 2014. Improving global health education: Development of a global health competency model. *Am J Trop Med Hyg*, 90(3): 560–565. 10.4269/ajtmh.13-0537.

Arthur MA, Battat R, Brewer TF. 2011. Teaching the basics: Core competencies in global health. *Infect Dis Clin North Am*, 25: 347–358.

Chase J, Evert J, (Eds). 2011. *Global Health Training in Graduate Medical Education: A Guidebook*, 2nd Edition. San Francisco, CA: KGlobal Health Education Consortium.

Evert J, Drain P, Hall T. 2014. *Developing Global Health Programming: A Guidebook for Medical and Professional Schools,* 2nd Edition. San Francisco, CA: Global Health Education Collaborations Press. https://www.cfhi.org/sites/files/files/pages/developingglobalhealthprogramming_0.pdf.

Evert J, Stewart C, Chan K, Rosenberg M, Hall T. 2008. *Developing Residency Training in Global Health: A Guidebook*. San Francisco, CA: Global Health Education Consortium, 2008. https://www .mcgill .ca/globalhealth/files/globalhealth/GHECResidencyGuidebook.pdf.

Jogerst K, Callendar B, Adams V, Evert J, Fields E, Hall T, Olsen J, Rowthorn V, Rudy S, Shen J, Simon L, Torres H, Velji A, Wilson L. 2015. Identifying interprofessional global health competencies for 21st-century health professionals. *Ann Glob Health*, 81(2): 239–247. 10.1016/j.aogh.2015.03.006. http://www.sciencedirect.com/science/article/pii/S221499961501156X; https://www.cfhi.org/sites/files/files/pages/global_health_competencies_article.pdf.

Nelson BD, Kasper J, Hibberd PL, Thea DM, Herlihy JM. 2012. Developing a career in global health: Considerations for physicians-in-training and academic mentors. *J Grad Med Educ*, 4(3): 301–306. http://www.jgme.org/doi/full/10.4300/JGME-D-11-00299.

Wilson L, Harper DC, Tami-Maury I, Zarate R, Salas S, Farley J, Warren N, Mendes I, Ventura C. 2012. Global health competencies for nurses. *Am J Prof Nurs*, 28: 213–222. https://www.researchgate .net/publication/229434441_Global_Health_Competencies_for_Nurses_in_the_Americas.

Index